Disability and Rehabilitation

Disability and Rehabilitation

Shyam D Ganvir PhD PGDGC MBA
Principal and Professor
Department of Community Physiotherapy
DVVPF's College of Physiotherapy
Ahmednagar, Maharashtra, India

Forewords
GJ Ramteke
Umanjali Damke

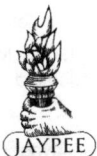

JAYPEE BROTHERS MEDICAL PUBLISHERS
The Health Sciences Publisher
New Delhi | London

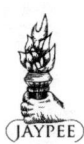 **Jaypee Brothers Medical Publishers (P) Ltd**

Headquarters

Jaypee Brothers Medical Publishers (P) Ltd
EMCA House, 23/23-B
Ansari Road, Daryaganj
New Delhi 110 002, India
Landline: +91-11-23272143, +91-11-23272703
+91-11-23282021, +91-11-23245672
Email: jaypee@jaypeebrothers.com

Corporate Office

Jaypee Brothers Medical Publishers (P) Ltd
4838/24, Ansari Road, Daryaganj
New Delhi 110 002, India
Phone: +91-11-43574357
Fax: +91-11-43574314
Email: jaypee@jaypeebrothers.com

Overseas Office

J.P. Medical Ltd
83 Victoria Street, London
SW1H 0HW (UK)
Phone: +44 20 3170 8910
Fax: +44 (0)20 3008 6180
Email: info@jpmedpub.com

Website: www.jaypeebrothers.com
Website: www.jaypeedigital.com

© 2023, Jaypee Brothers Medical Publishers

The views and opinions expressed in this book are solely those of the original contributor(s)/author(s) and do not necessarily represent those of editor(s) and publisher of the book.

All rights reserved. No part of this publication may be reproduced, stored or transmitted in any form or by any means, electronic, mechanical, photocopying, recording or otherwise, without the prior permission in writing of the publishers.

All brand names and product names used in this book are trade names, service marks, trademarks or registered trademarks of their respective owners. The publisher is not associated with any product or vendor mentioned in this book.

Medical knowledge and practice change constantly. This book is designed to provide accurate, authoritative information about the subject matter in question. However, readers are advised to check the most current information available on procedures included and check information from the manufacturer of each product to be administered, to verify the recommended dose, formula, method and duration of administration, adverse effects and contraindications. It is the responsibility of the practitioner to take all appropriate safety precautions. Neither the publisher nor the author(s)/editor(s) assume any liability for any injury and/or damage to persons or property arising from or related to use of material in this book.

This book is sold on the understanding that the publisher is not engaged in providing professional medical services. If such advice or services are required, the services of a competent medical professional should be sought.

Every effort has been made where necessary to contact holders of copyright to obtain permission to reproduce copyright material. If any have been inadvertently overlooked, the publisher will be pleased to make the necessary arrangements at the first opportunity.

Inquiries for bulk sales may be solicited at: jaypee@jaypeebrothers.com

Disability and Rehabilitation

First Edition: **2023**

ISBN: 978-93-5465-964-5

Printed at: Sterling Graphics Pvt. Ltd.

Contributors

Abhijit D Diwate
Professor
Department of Cardiovascular and Respiratory Physiotherapy
DVVPF's College of Physiotherapy
Ahmednagar, Maharashtra, India

Arijit Kumar Das
Professor
Department of Cardiovascular and Respiratory Physiotherapy
DVVPF's College of Physiotherapy
Ahmednagar, Maharashtra, India

Ashish Wasudeorao Bele
Professor
Department of Community Physiotherapy
Mahalaxmi Physiotherapy College and Rehabilitation Center
Satara, Maharashtra, India

Deepak B Anap
Professor
Department of Musculoskeletal Physiotherapy
DVVPF's College of Physiotherapy
Ahmednagar, Maharashtra, India

Deepali Nivrutti Hande
Professor and Head
Department of Community Physiotherapy
Dr APJ Abdul Kalam College of Physiotherapy (PIMS–DU)
Loni, Maharashtra, India

Deepti C Thokal
Associate Professor
Department of Community Physiotherapy
DVVPF's College of Physiotherapy
Ahmednagar, Maharashtra, India

Deepti Nandlal Wadhwan
Associate Professor
MVP's College of Physiotherapy
Nashik, Maharashtra, India

Maheshwari Harishchandre
Associate Professor
Department of Neurophysiotherapy
DVVPF's College of Physiotherapy
Ahmednagar, Maharashtra, India

Nitin Suhas Nikhade
Professor and Head
Department of Community Physiotherapy
MAEER's Physiotherapy College
Talegaon, Dabhade, Maharashtra, India

Pradnya Dumore
Assistant Professor
Department of Community Physiotherapy
DVVPF's College of Physiotherapy
Ahmednagar, Maharashtra, India

Pratima Sarwadikar
Assistant Professor
Department of Community Physiotherapy
Mahalaxmi College of Physiotherapy and Rehabilitation Center
Satara, Maharashtra, India

Sanjivani Kamble
Associate Professor
Dr DY Patil College of Physiotherapy
Dr DY Patil Vidyapeeth
Pimpre, Pune, Maharashtra, India

Saqib Syed
Associate Professor
Department of Musculoskeletal Physiotherapy
DVVPF's College of Physiotherapy
Ahmednagar, Maharashtra, India

Shrikant Bhimrao Darade
Associate Professor
Motiwala College of Physiotherapy
Nashik, Maharashtra, India

Shubhangi Patil
Professor
Ravi Nair Physiotherapy College
Sawangi (Meghe), Wardha, Maharashtra, India

Shwetanjali Bhagra
Assistant Professor
DVVPF's College of Physiotherapy
Ahmednagar, Maharashtra, India

Shyam D Ganvir
Principal and Professor
Department of Community Physiotherapy
DVVPF's College of Physiotherapy
Ahmednagar, Maharashtra, India

Sonyabapu Shewale
Assistant Professor
Department of Community Physiotherapy
DVVPF's College of Physiotherapy
Ahmednagar, Maharashtra, India

Suvarna S Ganvir
Professor
Department of Neurophysiotherapy
DVVPF's College of Physiotherapy
Ahmednagar, Maharashtra, India

Foreword

Physiotherapy is a "Novel" profession which includes all the novel therapeutic techniques and modalities for the betterment of patients. In the field of "community rehabilitation" physiotherapist plays an important role. For the development of good physiotherapy professional, the knowledge of specific area-centric approaches also important. This education also plays an important role in the development of physiotherapy education. I thankful to my best half, Dr Shyam D Ganvir, Principal, Dr Vithalrao Vikhe Patil Foundation's College of Physiotherapy, Ahmednagar, Maharashtra, India, who consistently educating the physiotherapy professional in view of "community development". He is being achieving numerous milestones in the field of physiotherapy and this book is the continuation of his hard work towards development of good physiotherapy professional.

I also thankful to my students, started their journey as my students and achieving milestones in the field of education as "Academician". Their participation in this book added the modern knowledge which is the integrated part of the modern physiotherapy.

I thankful to all contributing "authors" of this book for valuable contribution.

Last but not the least, I would like to recommend this "Novel" to all undergraduate and postgraduate students, especially final year physiotherapy students. This book will provide immense knowledge.

GJ Ramteke
Ex-Superintendent, School of Physiotherapy
Government Medical College and Hospital
Nagpur, Maharashtra, India
Ex-Principal, College of Physiotherapy
Datta Meghe Institute of Medical Sciences
Sawangi (Meghe), Wardha, Maharashtra, India

Foreword

Physiotherapy professionals consistently working for providing community health care. But to make better professional, it is important to provide concise knowledge to physiotherapy student during the education time.

In the field of making such physiotherapy professionals, I thankful to Dr Shyam D Ganvir, Principal, Dr Vithalrao Vikhe Patil Foundation's College of Physiotherapy, Ahmednagar, Maharashtra, India, who consistently working in the form of providing knowledge to students. This book is one of the contributing part of his effort.

I also thankful to all the contributing authors, not only playing important role in providing community health care but also adding up knowledge to their students as "Academician".

This book is highly recommended to all undergraduate and postgraduate students, especially final year physiotherapy students.

Umanjali Damke
Principal, School of Physiotherapy
Government Medical College and Hospital
Nagpur, Maharashtra, India

Preface

Physiotherapy or PT, is profession of the treatment and management after the clinical examination, assessment and diagnosis of the diseases for restoration of the neuromusculoskeletal and cardiopulmonary efficiencies, managing pain and certain integumentary disorders with the help of physical means like radiation, heat, cold, exercise, current, waves, manipulation, mobilization, etc.

The goal of this book has been to create a user-friendly textbook encompassing the breadth of the field of health, fitness, geriatrics, disability and community rehabilitation. Every health profession that provides care to elders has its own focus in the broader context of promoting successful aging and quality of life.

This book is designed to provide fundamental information about aging and strategies for supporting successful aging, maternal health and child health, physical fitness, and quality and legislation for disabled people. The language and style are simple, and attractive with emphasis on theory and intervention aspects which may be of utility not to undergraduates but even to postgraduates and teachers.

Also this book covers about physiotherapy in need of physiotherapy during pregnancy, fitness during pregnancy, exercise protocol during antenatal period, postnatal period, etc.

The book will be useful for students of physiotherapy to gain more knowledge about CBR, NGO's, Women's Health and Child Care, Healthcare System, Physiotherapy Management for all and detection and early identification of disability and polies for them.

Shyam D Ganvir

Contents

Section 1: Introduction to ICF, Disability Guidelines According to WHO

Chapter 1: International Classification of Functioning, Disability and Health   1
Shyam D Ganvir
- Aims *2*

Chapter 2: Disability, its Types, Guidelines for Permanent Physical Impairment and Disability Certification   5
Shyam D Ganvir, Saqib Syed
- Disability *5*
- Guidelines for Permanent Physical Impairment (PPI) *6*
- Disability Certification *7*

Chapter 3: Disability Models and Acts   9
Shyam D Ganvir
- Moral Models of Disability *9*
- Biomedical Model of Health *9*
- Medical Model of Disability *10*
- Rehabilitation Model *10*
- Social Model of Disability *10*
- Acts *11*

Chapter 4: Disability: Prevention, Management and Rehabilitation   17
Shyam D Ganvir, Deepti C Thokal
- Preventing Disability *17*
- Primary Prevention *17*
- Secondary Prevention *18*
- Tertiary Prevention *19*
- Management and Treatment of Disability *19*
- Rehabilitation of Disabled People *19*
- Sociovocational *21*
- Institution-based Rehabilitation *22*
- Community-based Rehabilitation *22*
- Home-based Rehabilitation Program *23*

Chapter 5: Home Exercise Programs for Various Classification of Disabilities   25
Shyam D Ganvir, Arijit Kumar Das
- Orthosis Use *34*
- Geriatric Homed-based Rehabilitation *35*
- Summary *38*
- Wheelchair Transfer Techniques *38*

Section 2: Community-based Rehabilitation

Chapter 6: Community Development 41
Shwetanjali Bhagra
- ❖ Definition of Community Development *42*
- ❖ The History of Community Development *42*
- ❖ Principles of Community Development *42*
- ❖ Values of Community Development *43*
- ❖ Characteristics of Community Development *43*
- ❖ Objectives of Community Development *43*
- ❖ Components of Community Development *44*
- ❖ The Method and Process of Community Development *44*
- ❖ Steps for Initiating Community Development *46*
- ❖ Types of Community *48*
- ❖ Types of Community Development Programs *48*
- ❖ Effective Approaches to Community Development *49*
- ❖ Importance of Community Development *49*
- ❖ Role of Community Development Worker/Community Developer *50*
- ❖ The Role of Physiotherapists in Community Development *51*

Chapter 7: The Link Between Institution-based Rehabilitation and Community-based Rehabilitation 53
Shwetanjali Bhagra
- ❖ Institutional Rehabilitative Strategies *53*
- ❖ Institutional Rehabilitation Programs *54*
- ❖ Links Between CBR and IBR *55*
- ❖ Gaps to be Filled by Local NGOs *56*

Chapter 8: Principles and Role of Community in Rehabilitation 58
Shubhangi Patil
- ❖ Definition of Rehabilitation *59*
- ❖ Goals of Rehabilitation *59*
- ❖ Objectives of Rehabilitation *60*
- ❖ Types of Rehabilitation *60*
- ❖ The Rehabilitation Team *62*
- ❖ Community-based Approach *65*
- ❖ Outreach Program for Rehabilitation *70*
- ❖ Principles of Rehabilitation *70*
- ❖ Role of Community in Rehabilitation *71*

Chapter 9: Evidence Based in Community Physiotherapy 74
Shrikant Bhimrao Darade
- ❖ Goals of EBP in Community Physiotherapy *76*
- ❖ Steps in Evidence-based Community Physiotherapy *76*
- ❖ Challenges to Implement EBP in Community Physiotherapy *79*
- ❖ Strategies for Effective Evidence-based Practice *79*
- ❖ Methodology for EBP in Community Physiotherapy *81*

Section 3: Basic Concepts of National and International Legislation for Persons with Disability

Chapter 10: Role of National Institutes, District Rehabilitation Center and Primary Health Center — 83
Deepali Nivrutti Hande
- Primary Healthcare Centers 84
- De-worming 86
- District Disability Rehabilitation Center 87

Chapter 11: Appropriate Technology, Assistive Devices Used for Disabled — 96
Shyam D Ganvir, Pratima Sarwadikar
- Appropriate Technology 96
- Assistive Technology 96
- Assistive Devices 97
- Home Automation 98
- Assistive Technology in Diabetic Foot 99

Chapter 12: Schemes and Legislations for Person with Disabilities — 100
Nitin Suhas Nikhade, Pradnya Dumore
- Provisions for Persons with Disabilities in Constitution of India 101
- National Policy for Persons with Disabilities 102
- International Legislations for People with Disability 119

Chapter 13: Accessibility for Persons with Disability — 123
Shyam D Ganvir, Deepak B Anap
- Handrails 131

Chapter 14: The UN Convention on the Rights of Person with Disabilities — 137
Shyam D Ganvir, Sonyabapu Shewale
- Article 1 137
- Article 2 137
- Article 3 138
- Article 4 138
- Article 5 139
- Article 6 140
- Article 7 140
- Article 8 140
- Article 9 141
- Article 10 141
- Article 11 141
- Article 12 142
- Article 13 142
- Article 14 142
- Article 15 143
- Article 16 143
- Article 17 143
- Article 18 144

- Article 19   144
- Article 20   144
- Article 21   145
- Article 22   145
- Article 23   145
- Article 24   146
- Article 25   147
- Article 26   148
- Article 27   148
- Article 28   149
- Article 29   149
- Article 30   150
- Article 31   151
- Article 32   151
- Article 33   151
- Article 34   152
- Article 35   153
- Article 36   153
- Article 37   154
- Article 38   154
- Article 39   154
- Article 40   155
- Article 41   155
- Article 42   155
- Article 43   155
- Article 44   155
- Article 45   156
- Article 46   156
- Article 47   156
- Article 48   157
- Article 49   157
- Article 50   157

Chapter 15: Early Identification and Intervention for Detection of Disability   158

Suvarna S Ganvir, Maheshwari Harishchandre
- Definition by WHO   158
- Locomotor Disability   159
- Evaluation of Disability   159
- Locomotor Disability   160
- Disability Evaluation of Spine   161
- Upper Limb Levels Percentage of Amputations   163
- Lower Limb Levels Percentage of Amputations   164
- Early Intervention Strategy   166
- Physiotherapist   170

Section 4: Elderly Individuals and their Services

Chapter 16: Health Care and Fitness — 171
Ashish Wasudeorao Bele
- National Healthcare Delivery System *171*
- Legal Rights and Benefits Related to Health *180*
- Principles of Fitness Training *189*
- Strategies of Health Fitness for Women and Geriatric *192*

Chapter 17: Geriatric Rehabilitation — 198
Shyam D Ganvir, Pratima Sarwadikar
- Rehabilitation for Specific Conditions *206*
- Arthritis and Related Musculoskeletal Problems *206*
- Stroke *207*
- Cardiac Disease *208*
- Hip Fracture *208*
- Amputation *208*
- Deconditioning, Sarcopenia, and Frailty *209*
- Falls *209*
- Pain *210*

Chapter 18: Elderly in India — 224
Shyam D Ganvir, Abhijit D Diwate
- Aging *224*
- Theories of Aging *225*
- Policy and Programs for the Welfare of Elderly in India *226*
- International Day for Older Persons and National Awards: Vayoshreshtha Samman *229*
- National Council for Older Persons/National Council of Senior Citizens *229*
- The National Policy on Older Persons *230*
- Benefits Extended by Other Central Ministries for the Welfare of Senior Citizens *230*
- Legislations *233*

Chapter 19: Wheelchair Management — 235
Shyam D Ganvir
- Wheelchair Users *235*
- Need for Wheelchairs *235*
- Rights to Wheelchairs *235*
- Benefit of Wheelchairs *236*
- Health and Quality of Life *236*
- Economy *237*
- Parts of Wheelchair *239*
- Wheelchair Services *239*
- Pressure Sore *245*
- Appropriate Wheelchair *247*
- Wheelchair Specifications *250*

- Cushion *252*
- Wheelchair Fitting *257*
- Transfers *262*
- Wheelchair to Bed *263*
- Wheelchair to Bed by Placing Legs on the Bed *263*
- Assisted Standing Transfer *264*
- Transfer Board *265*
- Emotional Health Problems *266*
- Energy and Emotions *266*
- General Health *268*

Chapter 20: Environment Modifications for People with Disabilities and Elderly Individuals — **270**
Deepti Nandlal Wadhwa
- Access to Building *270*
- Controls and Operating Mechanisms *275*

Chapter 21: Integrated Treatment Approach for Neuromuscular Dysfunction in Elderly — **279**
Sanjivani Kamble
- Ageing *279*
- Common Health Issues that Come with Ageing *279*
- The Brain's Aging *279*
- Key Elements of the Assessment of Neurologic Examination in Geriatric Population *280*
- Integrated Treatment Approach for Neuromuscular Dysfunction in Elderly *280*
- Health Advantages of Integrated Treatment Approach *283*
- What to Look for in a Long-term Care Setting for Integrated Therapy *283*

Appendices

- Appendix 1: Geriatric Assessment *285*
- Appendix 2: Orthosis Prescription Assessment *291*
- Appendix 3: Prosthesis Prescription Assessment *295*
- Appendix 4: Short Falls Efficacy Scale—International *302*

Index — **305**

Section 1 Introduction to ICF, Disability Guidelines According to WHO

CHAPTER

International Classification of Functioning, Disability and Health

Shyam D Ganvir

LEARNING OBJECTIVES

Through this chapter, the reader will be able to:
- Gain an introduction to ICF
- Describe the classification of ICF
- Use of ICF in clinical study and disability

■ INTRODUCTION

This volume contains the *International Classification of Functioning, Disability and Health,* known as ICF. ICF belongs to the "family" of international classifications developed by the World Health Organization (WHO) for application to various aspects of health. The WHO family of international classifications provides a framework to code a wide range of information about health (e.g., diagnosis, functioning and disability, reasons for contact with health services) and uses a standardized common language permitting communication about health and health care across the world in various disciplines and sciences.

ICF is WHO's Framework for Health and Disability

It is a universal classification of disability and health for use in health and health-related sectors. ICF therefore looks like a simple health classification, but it can be used for a number of purposes. The most important is as a planning and policy tool for decision-makers.

ICF is named as it is because of its stress on health and functioning, rather than on disability. Previously, disability began where health ended; once you were disabled, you were in a separate category.[1]

The Model of ICF

ICF follows the biopsychosocial model for disability, which integrates both the medical and social models. The reason for this integrated approach is that disability is undoubtedly a complex phenomenon, it is at the same time a problem at the level of a person's body, and a social phenomenon.

Disability represents the interaction of the features of a person and the features of the overall context in which the person lives and works, i.e., while some aspects of the disability are almost entirely internal to the person, others are entirely external.

In ICF, disability functioning are viewed as the outcomes of the interactions between health conditions (diseases, disorders, and injuries) and contextual factors.

The contextual factors include external environmental factors (e.g., social attitudes, architectural characteristics, legal and social structures, climate, terrain, etc.) and internal personal factors (e.g., gender, age, coping styles, social background, education, profession, past and current experience, overall behaviour patterns, character, etc.), which influence how disability is experienced by the individual.[2]

The **three levels of human functioning** classified by ICF are identified:
1. Functioning at the level of body or body part
2. The whole person
3. And the whole person in a social context

    Disability involves dysfunctioning at one or more of these three levels: impairments, activity, limitations, and participation restrictions.

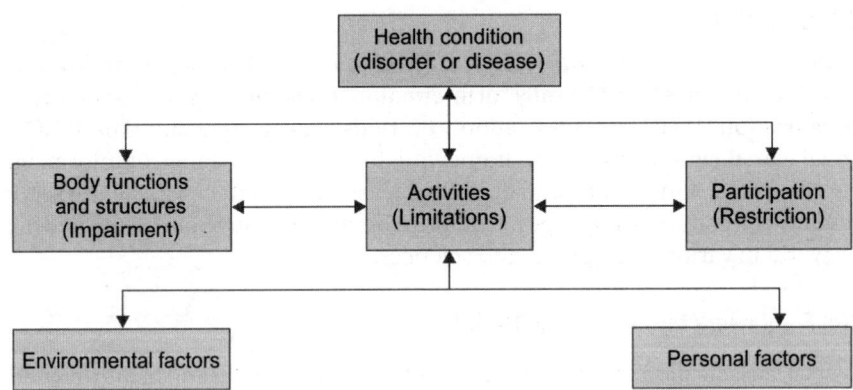

■AIMS

The aims of the ICF (WHO 2001) are to:
* Provide a scientific basis for understanding and studying health and health-related states, outcomes, determinants, and changes in health status and functioning;
* Establish a common language for describing health and health-related states in order to improve communication between different users, such as healthcare workers, researchers, policy-makers and the public, including people with disabilities;
* Permit comparison of data across countries, healthcare disciplines, services and time; and
* Provide a systematic coding scheme for health information systems.[2]

ICD-11 for Mortality and Morbidity Statistics (ICD-11 MMS)[3]

ICD-11 for Mortality and Morbidity Statistics

01 Certain infectious or parasitic diseases

02 Neoplasms

03 Diseases of the blood or blood-forming organs

04 Diseases of the immune system

05 Endocrine, nutritional or metabolic diseases

06 Mental, behavioural or neurodevelopmental disorders

07 Sleep-wake disorders

08 Diseases of the nervous system

09 Diseases of the visual system

10 Diseases of the ear or mastoid process

11 Diseases of the circulatory system

12 Diseases of the respiratory system

13 Diseases of the digestive system

14 Diseases of the skin

15 Diseases of the musculoskeletal system or connective tissue

16 Diseases of the genitourinary system

17 Conditions related to sexual health

18 Pregnancy, childbirth or the puerperium

19 Certain conditions originating in the perinatal period

20 Developmental anomalies

21 Symptoms, signs or clinical findings, not elsewhere classified

22 Injury, poisoning or certain other consequences of external causes

23 External causes of morbidity or mortality

24 Factors influencing health status or contact with health services

25 Codes for special purposes

26 Supplementary Chapter Traditional Medicine Conditions—Module I

V Supplementary section for functioning assessment

X Extension Codes

Disability, Impairment and Handicap

Impairment: Any loss or abnormality of psychological, physiological, or anatomical structure or function.

Disability: Any restriction or lack of ability to perform an activity in the manner or within the range considered normal for a human being.

Handicap: Disadvantage for a given individual, resulting from an impairment or a disability, that limits or prevents the fulfillment of a "survival role that is normal (depending on age, gender, and social, cultural factors) for that individual.

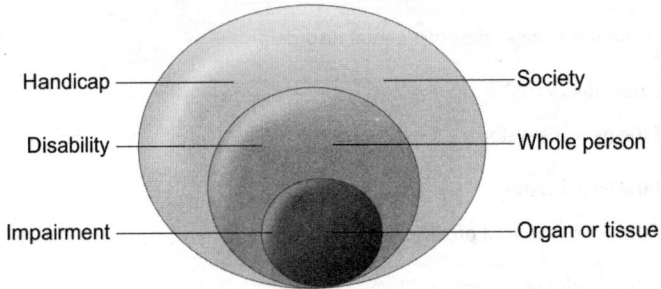

■REFERENCES

1. International Classification of Functioning, Disability and Health, Children and Youth Version, World Health Organization; 2007.
2. Towards a Common Language for Functioning, Disability and Health ICF, World Health Organization, Geneva, 2002.
3. Sunder S. Textbook of Rehabilitation, 3rd edition. Jaypee Brothers Medical Publishers (P) Ltd; 2010.

CHAPTER 2

Disability, its Types, Guidelines for Permanent Physical Impairment and Disability Certification

Shyam D Ganvir, Saqib Syed

LEARNING OBJECTIVES

Through this chapter, the reader will be able to:
- Gain knowledge about disability, it's types and grades.
- Understand guidelines for permanent physical impairment.
- Will have insight on guidelines for disability certification.

■ DISABILITY

According to World Health Organization "disability is any restriction or lack of ability to perform an activity in the manner or within the range considered normal for a human being."

Disabilities may be classified as mild, moderate, severe and profound. Categorization of disabilities is a difficult task.

Government of India has suggested certain norms. Disability Act of 1995 also specifies certain norms for classification based on severity to help certification for receipt of certain benefits under different schemes.

The government of India has put in place an Act for the disabled to make sure the disabled also form an important part of nation building.

The Persons with Disabilities (Equal Opportunities, Protection of Rights and Full Participation) Act, 1995 came into force on February 7, 1996. It is a significant step which ensures equal opportunities for the people with disabilities.

The Act provides for both the preventive and promotional aspects of rehabilitation like education, employment and vocational training, reservation, research and manpower development, creation of barrier-free environment, rehabilitation of persons with disability, unemployment allowance for the disabled, special insurance scheme for the disabled employees and establishment of homes for persons with severe disability, etc.[1]

Types of Disability

- Locomotor Disability
- Visual Impairment
- Hearing Impairment (Deaf and Hard of Hearing)
- Speech and Language Disability
- Intellectual Disability
- Mental Illness
- Disability caused due to Chronic Neurological Conditions
- Disability caused due to Blood Disorder
- Multiple Disabilities

Autism, learning disabilities, etc., emphysema, cancer, heart disease, multiple sclerosis, etc. are other types of disabilities. Disabilities may be classified as mild, moderate, severe and profound. Categorization of disabilities is a difficult task. Government of India has suggested certain norms. Disability Act of 1995 also specifies certain norms for classification based on severity to help certification for receipt of certain benefits under different schemes.[2]

Grades of Disability

- **Mild:** Less than 40%
- **Moderate:** 40% and above
- **Severe:** 75% and above
- **Profound:** 100%

For all concessions eligibility is only for those with 40% and above.[2]

■ GUIDELINES FOR PERMANENT PHYSICAL IMPAIRMENT (PPI)

- The estimation and measurement should be made when the clinical condition has reached the stage of maximum improvement from the medical treatment.
- Normally the time period is to be decided by the medical doctor who is evaluating the case for issuing the PPI certificate as per standard format of the certificate.
- The upper limb is divided into two components; the Arm Component and 'Hand Component'.
- Measurement of the loss of function of 'Arm Component' consists of measuring the loss of Motion, Muscle Strength and Co-ordinate Activities.
- Measurement of loss of function of Hand Component consists of determining the Pretension, Sensation and Strength.
- The impairment of the entire extremity depends on the combination of the functional impairments of both components.[3]

DISABILITY CERTIFICATION

Guidelines for Certification

Pursuant to the Rules on Persons with Disabilities (Equal Opportunity, Protection of Freedoms and Complete Participation), 1996 notified by the Central Government on 31 December 1995 in the exercise of the powers bestowed by Sections (1) and (2) of Section 73 of the Act on Persons with Disabilities, the person authorized to grant a disability certificate shall be a medical board; Consisting of at least three representatives, of which at least one is a professional in a particular area for the evaluation of locomotor/visual, including affected vision/hearing and speech impairment, intellectual retardation and leprosy, as the case may be, properly named by the federal and state governments.[2]

The specified tests, as indicated in the Guidelines, should be carried out by the Medical Board and recorded before the certificate I have issued. The certificate would be valid for a period of five years for persons whose disability I is temporary while it is valid for a lifetime in the case of permanent disability.[2,3]

The Director General of Health Services, Ministry of Health and Family Welfare will be the sole authority in the event of any dispute/doubt regarding the interpretation of definitions/classifications/assessments/tests, etc. In order to be eligible for any concession/benefit, the minimum level of impairment should be 40%. Various benefits, in accordance with and in accordance with the PWD Act, various benefits and allowances are to be given to affected persons.[3]

Guidelines for certification:
- The person authorized to grant a disability certificate shall be a medical board.
- Consisting of at least three representatives, of which at least one is a professional in a particular area for the evaluation of locomotor.
- The specified tests, as indicated in the guidelines, should be carried out by the Medical Board and recorded before the certificate I have issued.
- The certificate would be valid for a period of five years for persons whose disability is temporary while it is valid for a lifetime in the case of permanent disability.
- In order to be eligible for any concession/benefit, the minimum level of impairment should be 40%.[4]

Contents of Certificate

- **Type of disability:** Which are come under 21 types of disabilities.
- **Extent of disability:** Like in percent, verity of benefits from government associated with the degree of disability.
- **Permanence of disability:** It is mentioned that is it permanent or temporary.
- **Validity period:** It is according to Medical Association.[4]

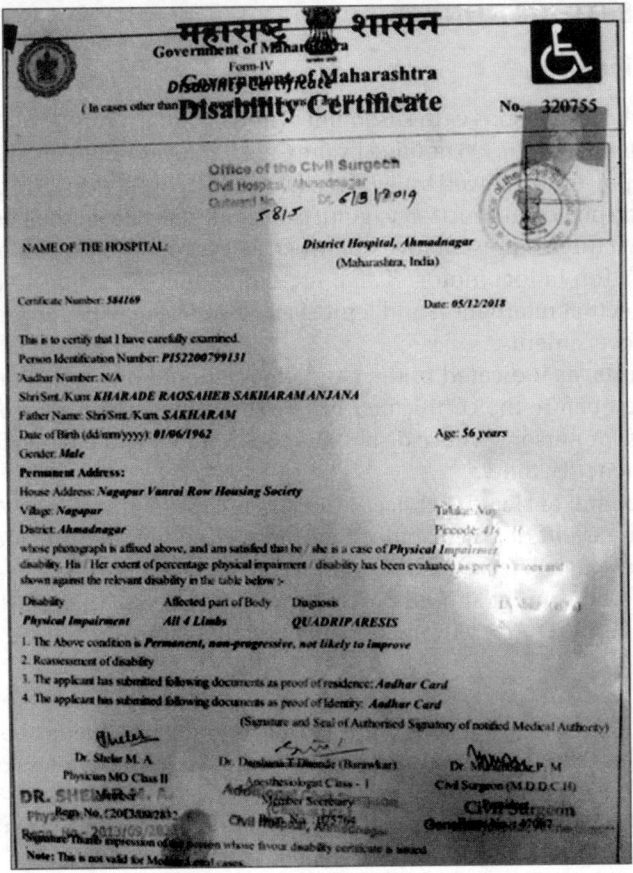

REFERENCES

1. https://www.disabilityaffairs.gov.in/content/page/guidelines.php
2. Disability Assessment and Certification: Based On Gazette Notification.
3. https://enabled.in/wp/guidelines-for-evaluation-of-permanent-physical-impairment-in-lower-limb/
4. https://www.vikaspedia.in/education/parents-corner/guidelines-for-parents-of-children-withdisabilities/disability-certificate

CHAPTER 3

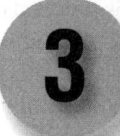

Disability Models and Acts

Shyam D Ganvir

LEARNING OBJECTIVES

Through this chapter, the reader will be able to:
- Understand in detail about models of disability.
- Gain knowledge about Acts and disability laws in India.

■ MORAL MODELS OF DISABILITY

It is the oldest practice, like other practices associated like wrongdoing and retribution, a feeling of remorse. This trend is associated with the shame of the entire nation. All this has affected the thinking and action of people with disabilities.[1]

The moral model is historically the oldest and least prevalent today. However, there are many cultures that associate disability with sin and shame, and disability is often associated with feelings of guilt, even if such feelings are not overtly based in religious doctrine. For the individual with a disability, this model is particularly burdensome.[1,2]

This model has been associated with shame on the entire family with a member with disability. Families have hidden away the disabled family member, keeping them out of school and excluded from any chance at having a meaningful role in society. Even in less extreme circumstances, this model has resulted in general social ostracism and self-hatred.

A good deal of history has viewed disability from a religious framework. Often disability has been seen as some kind of punishment for evil behaviour or as some kind of embodiment of evil itself. Those who gave birth to disabled people were tainted similarly. This influenced thinking and practices towards disabled people.[1,2]

■ BIOMEDICAL MODEL OF HEALTH

The biomedical model of health is the most popular in the western world and focuses mostly on wellbeing in terms of biological influences. The scientific concept of disease is used in the biological model of wellbeing. Similarly, it looks on illness mainly in terms of the treatment that the individual has. The biomedical model is usually contrasted with the biopsychosocial model.[1-3]

■ MEDICAL MODEL OF DISABILITY

The medical model of disability is provided by disability as an individual's problem, caused by illness, injury or other health condition, which therefore requires sustained medical assistance provided in the form of individual treatment by professionals. This approach is focused on the premise that disability-related problems will be met exclusively by people with disabilities.[1-3]

It views disability as a 'problem' that belongs to the disabled individual. It is not seen as an issue to concern anyone other than the individual affected. For example, if a wheelchair using student is unable to get into a building because of some steps, the medical model would suggest that this is because of the wheelchair, rather than the steps. Some examples of a medical model approach might:[1,2]

- ❖ A course leader who refuses to produce a hand-out in a larger font for a visually impaired student. The student cannot therefore participate in the class discussion;
- ❖ A member of staff who refuses to make available a copy of a PowerPoint presentation before a lecture. This creates a barrier to learning for the dyslexic students in the group who are likely to have a slower processing and writing speed and who will struggle to understand and record the key points.[1,2]
- ❖ A Students' Union society that organises an event that is not accessible to disabled members. This medical model approach is based on a belief that the difficulties associated with the disability should be borne wholly by the disabled person, and that the disabled person should make extra effort (perhaps in time and/or money) to ensure that they do not inconvenience anyone else.[5]

■ REHABILITATION MODEL

This is the same as the clinical paradigm utilized by people with disabilities to receive guidance, rehabilitation, medication or other services in recovery care.

It is similar to the medical model; it regards the person with a disability as in need of services from a rehabilitation professional who can provide training, therapy, counselling or other services to make up for the deficiency caused by the disability.[1,2]

Historically, it gained acceptance after World War II when many disabled veterans needed to be re-introduced into society. The current Vocational Rehabilitation system is designed according to this model. Persons with disabilities have been very critical of both the medical model and the rehabilitation model.[1,2]

While medical intervention can be required by the individual at times, it is naive and simplistic to regard the medical system as the appropriate locus for disability-related policy matters. Many disabilities and chronic medical conditions will never be cured. Persons with disabilities are quite capable of participating in society, and the practices of confinement and institutionalization that accompany the sick role are simply not acceptable.[2]

■ SOCIAL MODEL OF DISABILITY

The social model of disability places the challenge of disability as a societal problem and as a part of the full integration of individuals into society. Under this model, impairment is not a private characteristic, but rather a modest set of disabilities, all of which are created by the social environment. The management of the matter and document therefore involves government policy and the collective duty of society as a whole making the institutional improvements appropriate for the full inclusion of people with disabilities in all aspects of social life.[2]

It recognizes social discrimination as the most significant problem experienced by persons with disabilities and as the cause of many of the problems that are regarded as intrinsic to the disability under the other models.

This model draws on the idea that it is society that disables people, through designing everything to meet the needs of the majority of people[2] who are not disabled. There is a recognition within the social model that there is a great deal that society can do to reduce, and ultimately remove, some of these disabling barriers, and that this task is the responsibility of society, rather than the disabled person.[1,2]

The social model is more inclusive in approach. Pro-active thought is given to how disabled people can participate in activities on an equal footing with non-disabled people. Certain adjustments are made, even where this involves time or money, to ensure disabled people are not excluded. The onus is on the organiser of the event or activity to make sure that their activity is accessible. Examples might be:[2]

- A course leader who meets with a visually impaired member of the group before the beginning of a course to find out how hand-outs can be adapted so that the student can read them;
- A member of staff who makes PowerPoint presentations available on Blackboard to all members of the group before a lecture. This allows dyslexic students to look up unfamiliar terminology before the lecture, and gives them an idea of the structure that will be followed. This 'framing' helps students to understand and retain the information.[4]
- A Students' Union society that consults with disabled members before organizing an event in order to make sure that the venue is accessible.[1,2]

ACTS

- Persons with Disabilities Act, 1995
- Rights for Persons with Disability Act (2016).
- Mental Health Act, 2017
- RCI Act, 1992
- The National Trust for Welfare of Persons with Autism, Cerebral Palsy, Mental Retardation and Multiple Disabilities Act, 1999.

Persons with Disabilities Act, 1995

The Act provides for both the preventive and promotional aspects of rehabilitation like education, employment and vocational training, reservation.

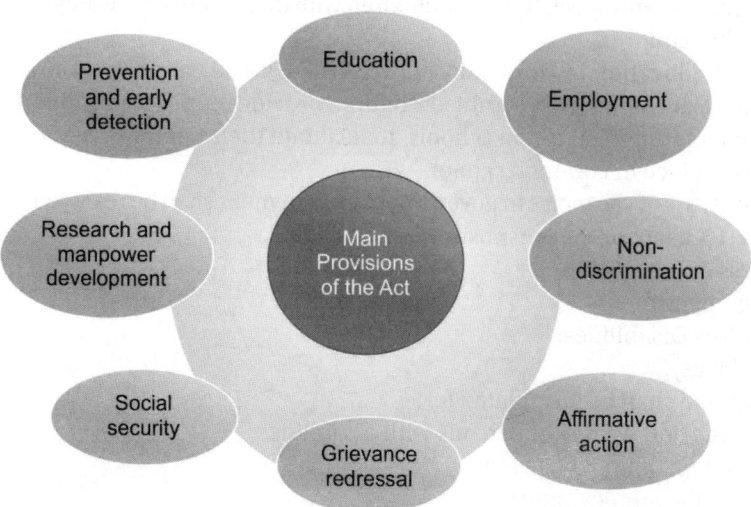

- ❖ Prevention and early detection of disabilities:
  - Surveys, investigations and research shall be conducted to ascertain the cause of occurrence of disabilities.
  - Various measures shall be taken to prevent disabilities. Staff at the Primary Health Centre shall be trained to assist in this work.
  - All the children shall be screened once in a year for identifying 'at-risk' cases.
  - Awareness campaigns shall be launched and sponsored to disseminate information. Measures shall be taken for prenatal, perinatal, and post-natal care of the mother and child.
- ❖ Education:
  - Every child with disability shall have the rights to free education till the age of 18 years in integrated schools or special schools.
  - Appropriate transportation, removal of architectural barriers and restructuring of modifications in the examination system shall be ensured for the benefit of children with disabilities.
  - Children with disabilities shall have the right to free books, scholarships, uniform and other learning material.
  - Special schools for children with disabilities shall be equipped with vocational training facilities. non-formal education shall be promoted for children with disabilities.
  - Teachers' training Institutions shall be established to develop requisite manpower.
  - Parents may move to an appropriate forum for the redressal of grievances regarding the placement of their children with disabilities.
  - Persons with Disabilities (PWD) Education Scenario in India:
  - The Bill provides for the access to inclusive education, vocational training and self-employment of disabled persons.
  - There should be equal opportunity in education for the persons with disabilities (WHO, 2015).
  - Kothari Commission (1964–66): The Kothari Commission officially first addressed issues of access and participation by all. It stressed a common school system open to all children irrespective of caste, creed, community, religion, economic condition and social status.
  - It was very first time in India Government of India took action for the Rights of Persons with disabilities and specially for the children with disabilities who wants to take education as like other children.
  - Integrated Education of Disabled Children (IEDC): The centrally sponsored scheme of Integrated Education of the Disabled Children provides educational opportunities for the disabled children in common schools, to facilitate their retention in the school system, and also to place in common school.
- ❖ **Employment:** 3% of vacancies in government employment shall be reserved for people with disabilities, 1% each for the persons suffering from:
  - Blindness or Low Vision.
  - Hearing Impairment.
  - Locomotors Disabilities.
  - Cerebral Palsy.

  Suitable scheme shall be formulated for:
  - The training and welfare of persons with disabilities
  - The relaxation of upper age limit
  - Regulating the employment

- Health and Safety measures, and creation of a non-handicapping, environment in places where persons with disabilities are employed.
- Government Educational Institutes and other Educational Institutes receiving grant from Government shall reserve at least 3% seats for people with disabilities.
- No employee can be sacked or demoted if they become disabled during service, although they can be moved to another post with the same pay and condition.
- No promotion can be denied because of impairment.

❖ Affirmative action:
Allotment of land shall be made at concessional rates to the people with disabilities for:
- House.
- Business.
- Special Recreational Centers.
- Special Schools.
- Research Schools.
- Factories by Entrepreneurs with Disability.

❖ Non-discrimination:
- Public building, rail compartments, buses, ships and aircrafts will be designed to give easy access to the disabled people.
- In all public places and in waiting rooms, the toilets shall be wheel chair accessible. Braille and sound symbols are also to be provided in all elevators (lifts).
- All the places of public utility shall be made barrier-free by providing the ramps.

❖ Research and Manpower Development:
Research in the following areas shall be sponsored and promoted.
- Prevention of Disability.
- Rehabilitation including community-based rehabilitation.
- Development of Assistive Devices.
- Job Identification.
- On site Modifications of Offices and Factories.
- Financial assistance shall be made available to the universities, other institutions of higher learning, professional bodies and non-government research-units or institutions, for undertaking research for special education, rehabilitation and manpower development.
- Financial assistance to non-government organizations for the rehabilitation of persons with disabilities.
- Insurance coverage for the benefit of the government employees with disabilities.
- Unemployment allowance to the people with disabilities who are registered with the special employment exchange for more than a year and could not find any gainful occupation.

❖ Social Security:
In case of violation of the rights as prescribed in this Act, people with disabilities may move an application to the:
- Chief Commissioner for Persons with Disabilities in the Centre; or
- Commissioner for Persons with Disabilities in the State.

Rights for Ppersons with Disability Act, 2016

❖ Respect for human rights, moral liberty, including the right to make one's own decisions, and the equality of persons.
❖ Non-discrimination in rights.
❖ Total and successful engagement and involvement in society

- ❖ Respect for the distinctions and recognition of people with disabilities as part of individual diversity and humanity
- ❖ Equal opportunities
- ❖ Accessibility of access
- ❖ Equality for men and women
- ❖ Respect for the evolving capacities of children with disabilities and respect for the right of children with disabilities to pre-serve their identities.[1-3]
  - Adopt legislation and other appropriate administrative measures where needed.
  - Modify or repeal laws, customs, or practices that discriminate directly or indirectly.
  - Include disability in all relevant policies and programmes.
  - Refrain from any act or practice inconsistent with the CRPD.
  - Take all appropriate measures to eliminate discrimination against persons with disabilities by any person, organization, or private enterprise.[1-3]

Mental Health Act, 2017

Mental impaired people are applicable to the following rights:

The right to be diagnosed and cared for in psychiatric hospitals or nursing homes founded or operated by the government or any other body for the treatment and care of mentally ill persons.

Mental ill people have the right to access from the State controlled, directed and organized mental health services. The Central Authority and the State Authorities established pursuant to the Act are responsible for such regulation and for issuing licenses for the establishment and maintenance of psychiatric hospitals and nursing homes.[1-3]

Treatment in the Government Hospitals and Nursing Homes mentioned above may be received either as a patient or on an outpatient basis. Mental patients may request voluntary admission to these hospitals or nursing homes, and minors may request admission through their guardians.

Mental ill people have the right to be released when they are cured and have the right to 'leave' a mental health institution in compliance with the rules of the Act.[3]

The Rehabilitation Council of India Act (RCI), 1992

This Act offers assurances to ensure the high nature of the facilities provided by the different recovery workers.

- ❖ To retain the privilege to be represented by skilled and certified health practitioners whose identities are kept in the Record held by the Council.
- ❖ To ensure the preservation of the minimum levels of education necessary for the acceptance of recovery qualifications
- ❖ To insure that the principles of ethical behaviour and integrity are upheld by recovery practitioners in order to defend from fines.
- ❖ To have the guarantee of the regulation of the profession of rehabilitation professionals by a statutory council under the control of the central government and within the limits laid down in the statute.[2,3]
  - **The National Trust for Welfare of Persons with Autism, Cerebral Palsy, Mental Retardation and Multiple Disabilties Act, 1999**
    - The Central Government is expected to create the National Trust for the Welfare of Persons with Autism, Cerebral Palsy, Mental Retardation and Multiple Disability in New Delhi, in compliance with this Act and for the benefit of the disabled.[2]

- The National Trust, formed by the Central Government, shall ensure that the items that have been defined as enshrined in the Act are located.
- This is the duty on the part of the Board of Trustees of the National Trust to provide for an appropriate quality of life for any recipient specified in any order this receives, and to offer financial support to designated entities for the execution of any authorized plan for the benefit of the impaired.[1,2]
- Affected people have the option to be put under the tutelage designated by the local level councils in compliance with the rules of the Act. The guardians so named shall be expected to be liable for the affected individual and their properties and to be accountable for the alternative.
- A person with a disability has the right to have his guardian removed under certain conditions. These include abuse or neglect of the disabled, or neglect or misappropriation of the property under the care of the disabled.[3]
- If the Board of Trustees is unwilling or persistently refuses to fulfil its functions, a recorded disabilities organization.
- The National Trust shall be bound by the provisions of this Act with regard to its accountability, financial supervision, accounts and audit.[1-3]

Disability Laws in India

The Preamble to the Constitution of India is dedicated to maintaining civil, economic and democratic fairness for all its people. The definition of justice is also focused on various conceptions of liberty, morals, health, pleasure, democracy and equality.[3]

Social justice requires the reduction of all sorts of inequality that result from disparities in wealth, employment, position, race, religion, etc.

To order to promote the goal of social justice, the Constitution sets out guidelines for the State and aim and eradicate disparities to wealth, services and resources, to reduce income differences, to guarantee equitable and humane working and maternity benefits; to avoid the abuse of children in jobs and industry; to include quality primary education for all; to promote educational and economic interests of the backward classes; to provide that the ownership and security of the material resources used for the community.[3]

Justice VR Krishna Iyer argued that the State is equally concerned with securing justice, equality and dignity, indirectly even to the mentally and physically deprived parts of the population, as is evident from the provisions of Articles 15(4) and 16(4) of the Constitution.

Article 15 of the Indian Constitution limits discrimination on grounds of faith, race, caste, sex or place of birth.

❖ Access to markets, public restaurants, hotels and palaces for public entertainment, and
❖ Use of wells, reservoirs, bathing, roads and public resorts; are funded entirely or partially from State funds or devoted to the benefit of the general public.[5]

Article 16 of the Constitution of India deals with the issue of equal rights in matters of public employment.

Health Law

Article 47 of the Constitution places on the State a primary duty to lift the diet and quality of life of its citizens and to increase public safety, in particular with a view to banning the ingestion of intoxicating beverages and substances that are hazardous to one's wellbeing, except for medicinal purposes.[3-5]

Indian health law includes a range of guidelines for the elderly. Any of the acts that provide for the welfare of people, including those with disabilities, can be found in the Mental Health Act, 1987.

Education Law

The right to education is at the hands of all people, including the elderly.

Article 29(2) of the Constitution provides that no person is to be refused admission to any educational institution established by the State or to receive State assistance on grounds of religion, race, caste or language.

Article 45 of the Constitution orders the State to provide free and compulsory education for all children (including the disabled) before they reach the age of 14. No child may be refused admission to any educational institution operated by the State or obtain State assistance on grounds of religion, ethnicity, caste or language.

Family Law

Different marriage laws passed by the State for various populations apply similarly to the elderly. The rights and obligations of the parties to marriage, as in the case of polygamy, people with disabilities or people without disabilities, are regulated by the particular rules and regulations of the various marriage Acts, such as the Hindu Marriage Act, 1955, the Christian Marriage Act, 1872.

The Child Marriage Restriction Act, 1929, as amended in 1978 to prohibit the formalization of child marriages, also extends to individuals with disabilities.[1]

Labour Law

The rights of the impaired are not so explicitly laid out in labour law, but the rules pertaining to the impaired in their partnership with the workplace are laid down in subordinate laws, such as legislation, regulations and standing orders.[1]

■ REFERENCES

1. Ganvir S, Gundecha AA. Disability, laws and models: An overview. Vims J Physical Th; 2020.
2. Sawhney N, Bansal S. Disability: prevention, management and rehabilitation. PsycEXTRA Dataset[Pristupljeno: 25.5. 2021.]. Dostupno na: https://doi. org/10.1037/E670282012-172. 2021.
3. Bhattacharyya R. Disability Laws in India: A Study. 2014:1(4).
4. International Classification of Functioning, Disability and Health, Children and Youth Version, World Health Organization; 2007.
5. Math SB, Gowda GS, Basavaraju V, Manjunatha N, Kumar CN, Philip S, et al. The Rights of Persons with Disability Act; 2016.

CHAPTER 4

Disability: Prevention, Management and Rehabilitation

Shyam D Ganvir, Deepti C Thokal

LEARNING OBJECTIVES

Through this chapter, the reader will be able to:
- Gain knowledge on steps of prevention
- Understand home-based rehabilitation
- Gain knowledge about exercises for rehabilitation (CP, amputation)
- Learn about orthosis used in rehabilitation programme

■ PREVENTING DISABILITY

Steps of Prevention

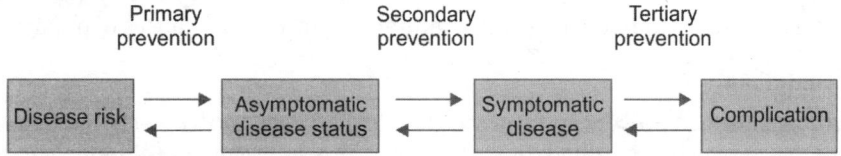

There are three levels of Prevention: Primary, Secondary and Tertiary.

■ PRIMARY PREVENTION

This involves the prevention of manifestation of disability. It may be universal for everyone or may be restricted to a selected population (high-risk group) or to an indicated population (individuals with an identified risk).

Primary prevention efforts should focus on the following (Batra, 2010):
❖ Care of pregnant and lactating mother.
❖ Immunization for pregnant mother and the newborn.
❖ Safety measures for the infant.

Care of Pregnant and Lactating Mother

Taking Care of the Surgical Scars

Especially in cases of cesarean section. Delivery and maintaining personal hygiene in normal vaginal deliveries. Unless taken care of properly complications such as fever, septicemia may arise.

- **Nutrition**: Iron supplementation, a proteinaceous diet, calcium supplementation is an essential part of postpartum care of the mother.
- **Avoidance of certain medications**: No medication should be taken by the mother in the lactation period unless advised by a physician, as these may enter the milk and affect the baby.
- **Emotional and psychological care**: Proper counselling should be done to avoid complications like baby and postpartum depression.

Immunization for Pregnant Mother and the Newborn

Immunization programs for the expectant mothers and the newborn child forms an important area of primary prevention. The immunization schedule which is followed by WHO and is also applicable in our country provides protection against diseases and subsequent disabilities.

Safety Measures for the Infant

The child is most vulnerable in the early years of life. In order to prevent disability, it is essential that:
- The child should not be left alone at doorsteps,
- Electrical appliances, medicines, pesticides and other hazardous materials should be kept in shelf away from the reach of the child.
- The child should not be left alone near stove or kitchen.
- The child should not be left alone near open drainages, main holes.

■ SECONDARY PREVENTION

Unlike primary prevention, which is provided to the general population, secondary prevention is aimed at particular groups of people who have "the highest likelihood of experiencing the target outcome (a high-risk group)" (Pianta, 1990, p. 307). These individuals have an increased vulnerability to certain biomedical or sociocultural/environmental causes of impairment.

Genetic Counselling

Genetic counselling can prevent some of the genetically-based birth defects. Some inheritable genetic conditions can be identified through medical procedures such as blood analysis. Some "high risk" groups have been subjected to mass screening to try to reduce the incidence of genetic conditions common within those segments of the population (Bennett, 1981).

Adolescent Pregnancy

Pregnant teenagers, especially very young ones, are another identified "at risk" group. Concern about teen pregnancy is increasing as there is some indication that the pregnancy rate among very young girls is rising (Leishman, 1980; Levy et al. 1992). Babies born to extremely young mothers are more at risk than those of older mothers.

Secondary Prevention of Disabilities in the Social Environment

A great deal of the secondary prevention effort is in the area of social environment. These efforts can be effective in preventing impairments at any stage of life, from the prenatal period to old age. Social prevention efforts include child protection to reduce the injury and neglect of children. These efforts may include the removal of youngsters from dangerous or negligent homes and placing them in foster care.

■ TERTIARY PREVENTION

Tertiary prevention includes all efforts designed to lessen the effects of an existing disability and improve a person's quality of life. This type of prevention is the most narrowly focused because the individual is actually affected. It may include medical intervention, social skills training, educational programming, or physical adaptations of the environment. Biomedical procedures classified as tertiary preventions can be extremely effective. Examples are: Phenylketonuria (PKU) and hypothyroidism. Both of these conditions can be diagnosed at birth, and both are highly treatable. PKU, an enzyme defect which can result in severe mental retardation, is treated by placing the child on a special diet. This diet completely prevents the disability (Coleman & Olson, 1987). The effects of hypothyroidism are prevented by giving the child thyroid hormone therapy (Fotheringham et al., 1983). Tertiary prevention in the education field has two goals: first, to teach a person to cope with a disability; and second, to help the person achieve the highest possible level of education, in spite of a disability. Figure below shows the normal route taken by families to reach the Early Intervention Centers.

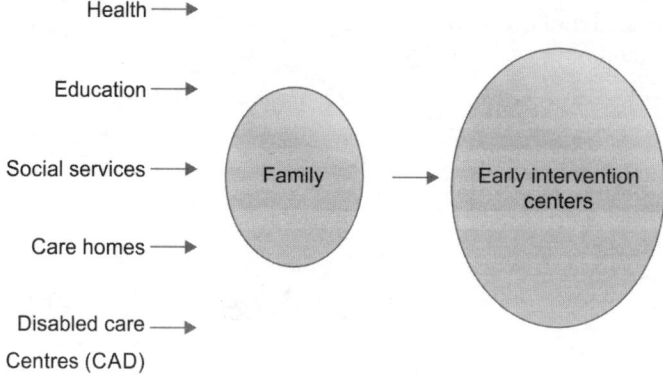

■ MANAGEMENT AND TREATMENT OF DISABILITY

Ministry of Social Justice and Empowerment (MSJE), Government of India, is the key line ministry with responsibility for disability, though there are several other ministries and government departments that are directly engaged with addressing the problem of disability in India, and many have earmarked funds to develop activities concerning disabled people.

■ REHABILITATION OF DISABLED PEOPLE

"**Rehabilitation**" means the establishment or the restoration of a disabled person to self-sufficiency at his highest attainable level provide such goods and services as he may consider necessary for the rehabilitation of any disabled person upon such terms and conditions as he may consider fit, and without limiting the generality of the foregoing, may provide or assist disabled persons by way of grant, loan or otherwise.

Rehabilitation programs for children and youth with disabilities are typically based on three assumptions:

❖ Services must be provided through **formal** organizational structures;
❖ Services must be provided by formally **trained and experienced** professionals; and

❖ Programs need to be **multifaceted, comprehensive**, and include a variety of specialists, materials, equipment and strategies in order to meet the complex rehabilitation and rehabilitation needs of persons with impairments (Helander 1993).

In 1979, the World Health Organization published its first version of the manual Training the Disabled in the Community (Helander, Nelson, and Goerdt, 1983).

Rehabilitation Team

The members of the team are classified according to their areas of specialization and function as Medical and Sociovocational teams.

Medical

There is hardly any area of medical specialization that has no bearing on the course of rehabilitation. The specialists interact with the rehabilitation team on a case-to-case basis. The neurologist, for example, would prescribe drugs for epilepsy, the plastic surgeon would treat the pressure sores and the rheumatologist would assess the patient with ankylosing spondylitis. The medical team members are:

❖ Physiatrist—the leader of the team
❖ Orthopedic surgeon
❖ Neurologist
❖ Neurosurgeon
❖ Plastic surgeon
❖ Psychiatrist
❖ Pediatrician
❖ Obstetrician
❖ Geneticist
❖ Neonatologist
❖ Rheumatologist
❖ Cardiologist
❖ Cardiac surgeon
❖ General surgeon
❖ Oncologist
❖ Urologist
❖ Ophthalmologist
❖ Otorhinolaryngologist
❖ General physician
❖ Family physician

Paramedical

❖ Physiotherapist
❖ Occupational therapist
❖ Creative movement therapist
❖ Recreation therapist
❖ Prosthetist-orthotist
❖ Rehabilitation nurse
❖ Speech pathologist
❖ Psychologist
❖ Biomedical engineer
❖ Horticultural therapist

Play and Drama Therapist
* Music therapist

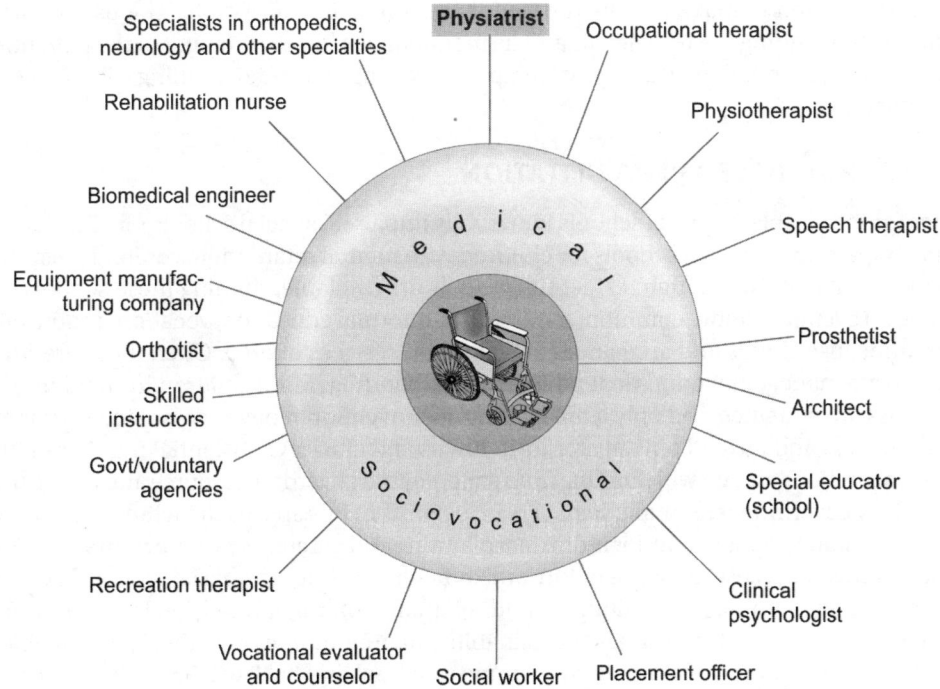

■ SOCIOVOCATIONAL
* Social worker
* Vocational counselor
* Vocational evaluator
* Skilled instructors
* Placement officers
* Child development specialist
* Special educator
* Employment agencies
* Industries
* Banks and funding agencies
* Nongovernmental organizations
* Community
* Family members

Role of Physical Therapist
The physical therapist assists the patient in movement restoration. He is a very important member of the rehabilitation team. He has to perform a thorough muscle strength evaluation and quantification, spasticity assessment, and measurement of joint range. On the therapeutic side he would have to perform exercises to maintain and increase joint range of motion, train sitting and standing balance, or increase strength, endurance, and coordination for specific muscle

groups or the entire body. During the course of therapy he would have to use various therapy modalities, such as heat and cold, as well as hydrotherapy techniques, electrical stimulation, traction and massage for pain relief. For those confined to home he would visit them and aid in home evaluation to make the environment barrier free and accessible. The use of various mobility aids including the wheelchair and its maintenance has to be taught to the patient. For those who are not ambulant, the physiotherapist does progressive gait training with or without ambulatory aids.

■ INSTITUTION-BASED REHABILITATION

Homes for the disabled, special schools for visually impaired, special schools for children with hearing impairment, special schools for children with mental retardation, cerebral palsy, have been the usual pattern. Though residential schools are available, running these schools from morning till evening is more common. Assessment, informal education, vocational counselling and training, use of aids and appliances are common services offered. Often these are run by NGO/private management and depend on external funding, more children from middle and upper class are benefited and only a meager number of children have access since number of schools are less and located only nearer to/in towns and cities. A substantial number of these kinds of institutions are run with funding from state/central government source and has been the approach by government for many years. Positive points in this approach include—more focus for special children, opportunity for individual planning and parents have time to attend to work. On the negative side, cost-intensive nature and difficulty to establish special schools in villages, towns and cities—number of institutions and rehabilitation manpower needed is enormous, parental involvement will be less and sustainability of programmes becomes questionable on long term, transportation of children from home to school and back will be a critical area.

■ COMMUNITY-BASED REHABILITATION

Community-based rehabilitation was mooted as part of primary health care approach at Alma Ata in 1979. While it is still in the stage of evolution in many developing countries, there is a need for auguring this process increasing the scale of operations. At this juncture it is worthwhile considering certain definitions, principles and approaches of community-based rehabilitation. ILO, WHO and UNESCO define community-based rehabilitation as—"Within Community Development ....the utilization (in an integrated programme) of approaches and techniques which relay on local communities as units of action and which attempt to combine outside assistance with organized local self-determination and effort and which correspondingly seek to simulate local initiative and leadership as the primary instrument of change".

Community-based rehabilitation focuses on the needs of disabled individuals as well as the involvement and responsibilities of the family and of the community in which the persons with disabilities are living.

The goals of community-based rehabilitation can be expressed as:
❖ To enable persons with disabilities to participate as fully as he or she chooses in family life and in other social activities.
❖ It provides opportunities for persons with disabilities to learn and to develop their abilities and skills to be able to participate and integrate fully in the society.
❖ To raise awareness in the community/society to achieve a barrier free environment, to enable the persons with disabilities to participate in all activities without discrimination.

Basic Principles of Community-based Rehabilitation

Though there is a debate on what precisely constitutes community-based rehabilitation, it is generally accepted that the following should be included in a programme that aims at integration and rehabilitation of persons with disabilities in the community.

- Shifting services from the institution to the homes of disabled people: It focuses on persons with disability living with their family, integrating them in the activities of the community, be it a village or in an urban area.
- Community-based rehabilitation enables people with disability to live independently, through training in activities of daily living skills (ADLS), education, skills development, employment opportunities, accessibility and social interaction with other members of the family and community.
- Interaction with other members of the community, without being neglected or discriminated.
- Shifting the services from professionals to trained community or family members: The purpose is to demystify that training and care for persons with disabilities can be done only by professionals. Members of the family and others have to be trained in giving these services, as often the professionals are unwilling to work in rural or other places where rehabilitation services are not available.
- Ensure that persons with disability have a say in planning and managing the programme: It should be ensured that disabled people are regarded both as recipients of services as well as contributors to managing the programme. To enable this to happen, disabled persons should be involved in taking decisions for the programme. They have to be trained to be able to play this role.
- Community-based rehabilitation programme should be flexible so that they can operate at the local level, using the locally available resource. A flexible, locally relevant programme will ensure community involvement, as they will have the capacity to manage it on their own. Agencies extending specialized services can play a supplementary role in service provision, which is not available locally.

■ HOME-BASED REHABILITATION PROGRAM

The disabled people are usually prescribed with home exercise program (HEP) by the treating physiotherapist with the objective of enhancing the functional potential of the disabled person considering their long-term disease condition. This HEP should be prescribed similar to that of a medicine drug dosage for an effective disability rehabilitation ensuring the importance of HEP in every disabled condition.

Home Exercise Program is a subcategory of physical exercise which is planned, structured, repetitive, and purposive which can be performed at home settings with or without supervision leading to improvement or maintenance of bodily functions.

The Home Exercise Programs (HEPs) for any disabled condition are very important resource that contributes to significant functional improvements.[1] Usually these HEPs are individualized based on the patient's condition, disability level, types, and family goals.[2,3] The success of disability rehabilitation depends on various factors among which the HEP and adherence to HEP plays a vital role.[4] However, adherence to HEP is estimated to be lower than 50% in certain conditions like cerebral palsy which is highly influenced by parental/care giver adherence.[5]

Also the recent qualitative research evidences suggests that disabled patients and caregivers perform HEP activities that are vey easier for them rather performing the whole of HEP suggested by physiotherapist.[6-9]

REFERENCES

1. Sawhney N, et al. Disability: Prevention, Management and Rehabilitation. Jaypee Brothers Medical Publishers; 2020.
2. Sunder S. Textbook of rehabilitation, 3rd edition. Jaypee Brothers Medical Publishers; 2017.
3. Pruthvish S. Community-based rehabilitation of person with disabilities, 1st edition; 2006.
4. Pianta RC. Widening the debate on educational reform: Prevention as a viable alternative. Exceptional Children. 1990;56:306-13.
5. Bennett JW. A primer in genetics. In: Abroms KI, Bennett JW (Eds). Genetics and Exceptional Children. San Francisco: Jossey-Bass Inc; 1981. pp. 3-19.
6. Levy SR, Perhats C, Nash-Johnson M, Welter JF. Reducing the risks in pregnant teens who are very young and those with mild mental retardation. Mental Retardation. 1992;30:195-203.
7. Coleman M, Olson D. Medical conditions that affect learning. In: Knoblock P (Ed). Understanding Exceptional Children and Youth. Boston: Little, Brown and Co; 1987. pp. 69-97.
8. Fotheringham JB, Hambley WD, Haddad-Curran HÊW. Prevention of Intellectual Handicaps. Toronto, On: The Martin Group; 1983.
9. Helander E. Prejudice and dignity: An introduction to community-based rehabilitation. New York: United Nations Development Program Interregional Program for Disabled People; 1993.

CHAPTER 5

Home Exercise Programs for Various Classification of Disabilities

Shyam D Ganvir, Arijit Kumar Das

LEARNING OBJECTIVES

Through this chapter, the reader will be able to:
- To provide the necessity and importance of prescribing home exercise program to the disabled people
- To provide information about few recommended home exercise programs for different types of disabilities
- To understand the factors affecting compliance and performance of home exercise program
- To identify the factors affecting adherence and non-adherence to home exercise program
- To bring awareness on adapting effective technologies in home exercise program regime

■ INTRODUCTION

Disability and Physiotherapy Rehabilitation are the intertwined together to ensure the disabled person achieve maximum functional independence. Physiotherapy includes wide strategy of treatment maneuvers ranging from hands-on-skills to electrotherapy modalities which is usually offered by qualified and competent physiotherapists at a clinic, hospital, daycare centre. The disabled people are usually prescribed with home exercise program (HEP) by the treating physiotherapist with the objective of enhancing the functional potential of the disabled person considering their long-term disease condition. This HEP should be prescribed similar to that of a medicine drug dosage for an effective disability rehabilitation ensuring the importance of HEP in every disabled condition.

Main Content

The total disabled population in the world has been estimated around 1.2 billion persons accounting for 15% of the global population. In these 80% of persons with disabilities reside in low and middle-income countries (LMICS). All these disabled persons benefit from scientific and evidence-based physiotherapy and rehabilitation programs in clinics, hospitals, rehab centers, day-care centers and many other settings. Apart from these centers, almost all the disabled persons are prescribed with set of exercises to be performed at home by the treating physiotherapist. These sets of exercises are designed to address the physical and functional needs of the disabled person.

> Home Exercise Program is a subcategory of physical exercise which is planned, structured, repetitive, and purposive which can be performed at home settings with or without supervision leading to improvement or maintenance of bodily functions.

The Home Exercise Programs (HEPs) for any disabled condition are very important resource that contributes to significant functional improvements.[1] Usually these HEP's are individualized based on the patient's condition, disability level, types, and family goals.[2,3] The success of disability rehabilitation depends on various factors among which the HEP and adherence to HEP plays a vital role.[4] However, adherence to HEP is estimated to be lower than 50% in certain conditions like cerebral palsy which is highly influenced by parental/caregiver adherence.[5]

Also the recent qualitative research evidences suggests that disabled patients and caregivers perform HEP activities that are vey easier for them rather performing the whole of HEP suggested by physiotherapist.[6]

As discussed in previous chapters, there are many types of disabilities affecting a person's mobility, vision, hearing, thinking, memory, learning, communication, mental health, and social relationships.

Government of India has listed 21 types of disabilities under the Rights of Persons with Disabilities Act, 2016 (RPWD Act, also known as Divyangjan Adhikaar Kanoon 2016 in Hindi).

1. Blindness	11. Muscular dystrophy
2. Low vision	12. Chronic neurological conditions
3. Leprosy cured persons	13. Specific leaning disabilities
4. Hearing impairment	14. Multiple sclerosis
5. Locomotor disability	15. Speech and language disability
6. Dwarfism	16. Thalassemia
7. Intellectual disability	17. Hemophilia
8. Mental illness	18. Sickle cell disease
9. Autism spectrum disorder	19. Multiple disabilities
10. Cerebral palsy	20. Acid attack victims
	21. Parkinson's disease

In broadly disability can be classified into Physical, Sensory, Intellectual and Mental illness.

The commonly prescribed HEP for physical classification of disabilities are discussed in this chapter which are commonly encountered by physiotherapists/occupational therapists/healthcare workers in their clinical practice.

Ideal Home Exercise Program
- Should be recommended or advised by physiotherapist/occupational therapist
- Should be performed regularly if they are effective
- HEP routine should be developed at home
- Based on the needs of the disability condition
- Need the time of family/caregiver—a practical routine to suit the family's lifestyle.

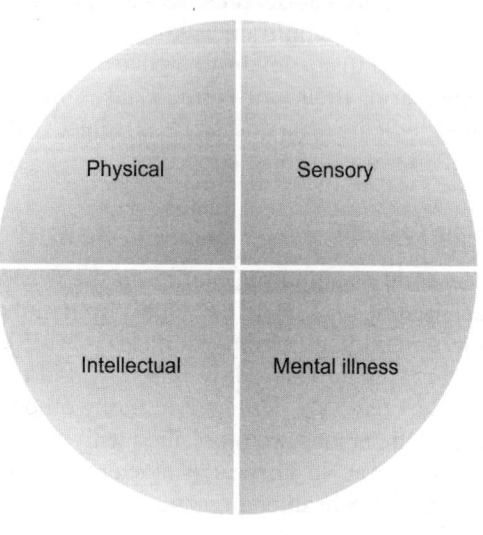

CHAPTER 5: Home Exercise Programs for Various Classification of Disabilities

Home Exercise Program for Cerebral Palsy

- Stretching (hamstring, glutes, TA, hip adductor)—10 sec hold/3 repetition, 2 sets a day
- AROM bilateral upper limb and lower limb—10 repetition/2 times day
- Bridging—10 sec hold/10 repetition
- Neck exercise—10–15 min hold/2 times a day.

This is a common HEP protocol for all the children with developmental disability like Cerebral palsy, Down syndrome. This includes a series of exercises usually performed by caregivers.[7] These protocols should be performed based on the child disability condition and proper assessment should be carried out to understand the child's physical and functional requirements.

Rolling: Place the child in side lying position. Shake a rattle above and behind the child's head and gently roll the child onto his or her back. Continue until the child begins to initial the movement independently. You can also use tactile cues by touching the child's back.	**Creeping:** Place the child on his or her stomach, resting the forearms on the floor, raise the child to a position on his or her hands and knees by supporting around the trunk. You can also place a towel under the stomach and trunk and pull up on both ends. Gradually use less assistance to get the child to raise onto all fours.
Raising to sit: Hold the child's hand and pull him slowly to a sitting position five times. The next five times pull until his or her arms are straight, pause, and say, "Get up". If the child does not pull after 3 sec, continue pulling him to a sitting position for the five attempts. Give the child your index fingers to hold, straighten his arms, then say, "Get up" and allow the child to pull to a sitting position.	**Sitting balance:** Place the child in sitting position and give some reach out activity (Forward and sideways reach). **Cruising:** While the child is standing at a couch/bench, place a toy just out of the child's reach and encourage him to get the toy.
Standing balance: Place the child in standing position next to stable supporting object, the child should free his body from support and maintain for 5 seconds.	**Walking (gait training):** Walking can be started with or without walker (walking frame) depends upon child's ability to walk.
Sits-ups: From back laying position, with feet flat on the floor and arm folded across the chest, the child should complete three to five sit-ups in 30 seconds.	**Push-ups:** Place the child in prone lying position and child will lift his chest and head with the extension both arms. Maintain this position for 30 seconds.
Positioning: Keep the child in long sitting position in which both leg should be straight, abducted and foot should be in neutral position. You should also promote prone position for your child.	

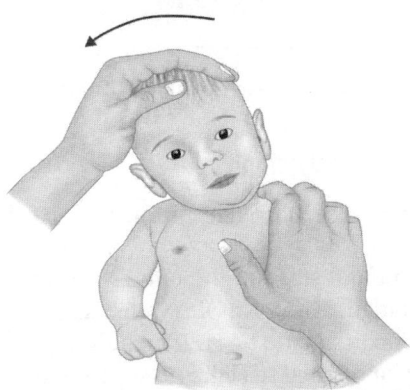

Figure 5.1: Child undergoing exercise with ear tilting towards shoulder.

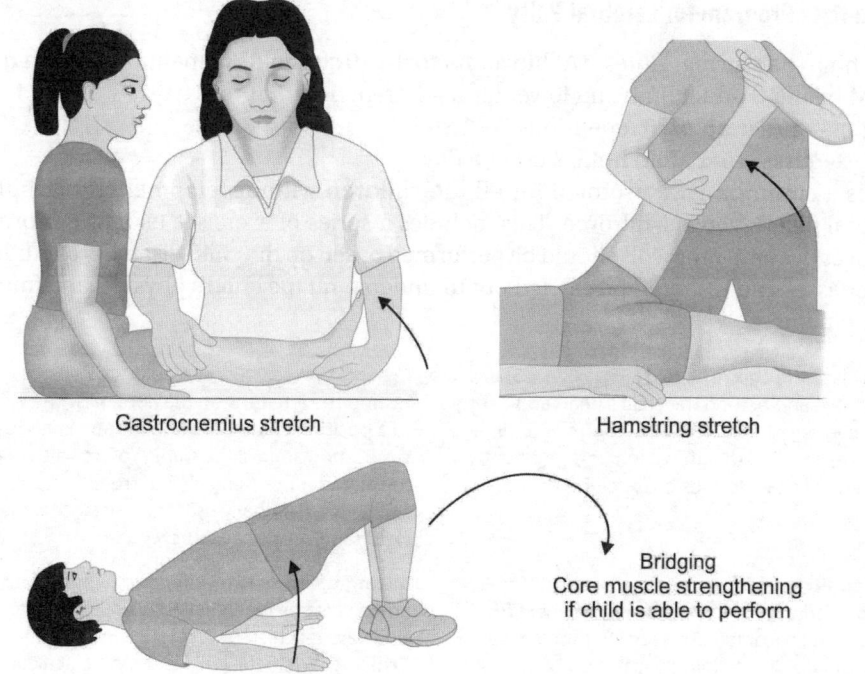

Figure 5.2: Simple exercises for children with CP.

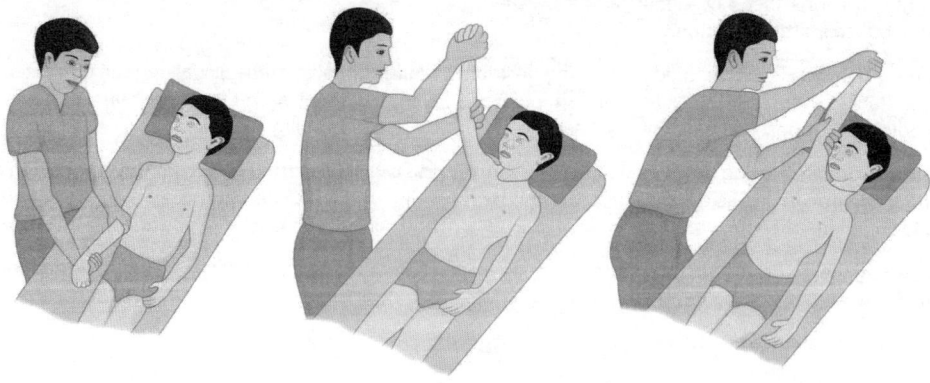

Figure 5.3: Active and passive range of motion exercise.

Home Exercise Program for Muscular Dystrophy

A child with muscular dystrophy will go through various stages of development, the HEP should reflect these changing needs.

During the early developmental stage of the child's it is important to encourage activity that does not cause extreme fatigue. Exercise with weights and eccentric muscle work such as trampolining should not be encouraged. The HEP includes.

* Regular stretches: Self and/or manual stretches as well as passive stretching—for the muscle groups that are tightening (tendo-Achilles, hamstrings and iliotibial band)

- Swimming, hydrotherapy
- Wearing orthoses (splints) at night to slow down contractures in the ankles
- Insoles—may be helpful for flat feet, used in ordinary lightweight footwear
- General games and fitness encouraging cardiovascular fitness.

In the later developmental stages, there will be a progressive loss of function. Although the child will be walking for periods of time, he or she will also require a wheelchair for mobility, specially over long distances. The HEP at this later developmental stage may include:

- Regular passive stretches for tendo-Achilles, hamstrings, hip flexor and iliotibial band muscles; some self-stretches may also be recommended
- Stretches to the upper limb muscles
- Swimming, hydrotherapy, wearing orthoses (splints) at night
- Prone lying and other good positioning
- Games to promote deep breathing including blowing bubbles and playing wind instruments.

The HEP at the wheelchair stage may include:
- Regular stretches to minimise the development of contractures in hips, knees and ankles and ensure comfort in bed, ease in dressing and positioning in wheelchair
- Use of ankle splints when sitting in wheelchair (instead of use of orthoses)
- Chest clearance techniques and assisted cough
- Stretches for the upper limbs to minimize contractures
- Using a standing frame
- Prone lying and other good positioning,
- Use of orthoses.

Tightening of muscles and tendons are very common in muscular dystrophy. Achilles tendon will be the first tendon to tighten followed by the muscles around the hips, knees, elbows and fingers can also be affected. Contractures can make some movements and activities more difficult. Hence regular daily stretches as HEP helps to maintain muscle length and keep joints mobile. The stretch can be passive, active-assisted and self-stretches.[8]

Home Exercise Program for Chronic Neurological Condition—Stroke

Stroke survivors lose physical abilities and cognitive skills or undergo behavioral changes because strokes cause temporary or permanent damage to the brain areas that control those functions. The brain has the ability to recover after stroke, whether initially or months to years later. While short-term recovery after stroke (called spontaneous recovery) is limited to the first six months, long-term functional recovery can occur at any point thereafter. Stroke survivors who continue to engage their affected side in daily activity and exercise can capitalize on functional recovery potential throughout their stroke journey.

HEP is very much essential for stroke survivors to enhance their physical and functional capacity though they are discharged from physiotherapy/rehabilitation services. The HEP for stroke depends on the brain lesion and gross structures involved. Hence the HEP is customized particularly meeting the patients' objectives. However, this chapter discusses the most commonly prescribed HEP for stroke survivors.

The HEP for stroke should incorporate both cardiovascular fitness and muscle strengthening to ensure the most effective outcomes among the stroke survivors.

Cardiovascular Fitness

Aerobic exercise is fundamental to building a healthy heart, improving endurance, and maintaining healthy lungs. Cardiovascular exercise can also improve the sensory perception and motor skills of stroke survivors. Brisk walking outside or on a treadmill, stationary cycling, recumbent cross training and many other forms of exercise that get the heart pumping are extremely beneficial for stroke recovery. Stroke survivors must get at least 20-60 minutes of light to moderate aerobic exercise (50–80% of your maximum heart rate) 3 to 7 days a week to improve the chances of stroke recovery.

Resistance Exercises for Strengthening Muscles

Resistance training or muscle strength training plays a crucial role in post-stroke recovery, as it helps to recover physical strength, stamina, stability, and improve range of motion.

Here are some commonly prescribed exercises for stroke recovery at home:

Upper limb stretching exercises	Lower limb stretching exercises
Upper limb muscular strengthening exercises	Lower limb muscular strengthening exercises
Upper limb functional exercises—hand functions	Lower limb functional exercises—mobility
Gait training exercises	Basic balance and coordination exercises
Advanced balance exercises—single leg stand, backward walking, Core exercises—bridging, pelvic floor, quadrupeds,	

Some of the simple resistance HEP for strengthening muscles in stroke survivors are:

Wrist curls by weight	Hand stretch by dumbbells
Shoulder openers	Table towel slide
Trunk bends	Knee rotations
Hip abduction/adduction	Standing knee raise
Sit to stand	Hip thrust

All these exercises can be performed at home with proper instructions and demonstrations from the treating physiotherapists.[9]

Home Exercise Program for Amputation

General Plan of Interventions

- Positioning to avoid contractures
- Standing balance and transfer activities
- Mobility training with crutches or a walker
- Residual limb care and protection; bandaging if
- Appropriate care of the remaining lower extremity (if circulation is compromised)
- Education on amputation and prosthetics.

CHAPTER 5: Home Exercise Programs for Various Classification of Disabilities

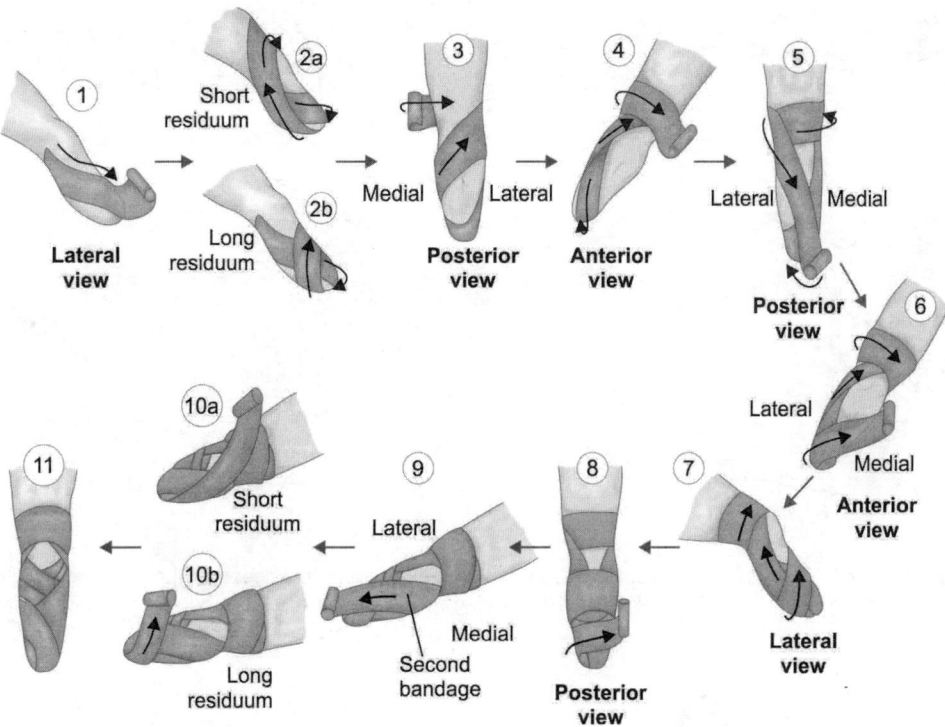

Figure 5.4: Transtibial residual limb bandaging.

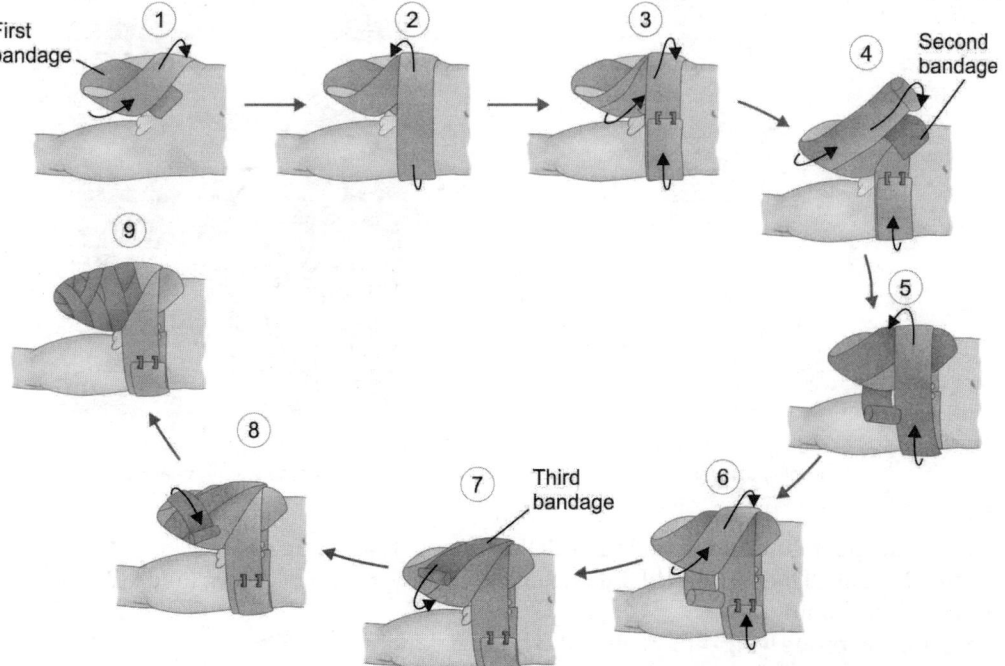

Figure 5.5: Transfemoral residual limb bandaging.

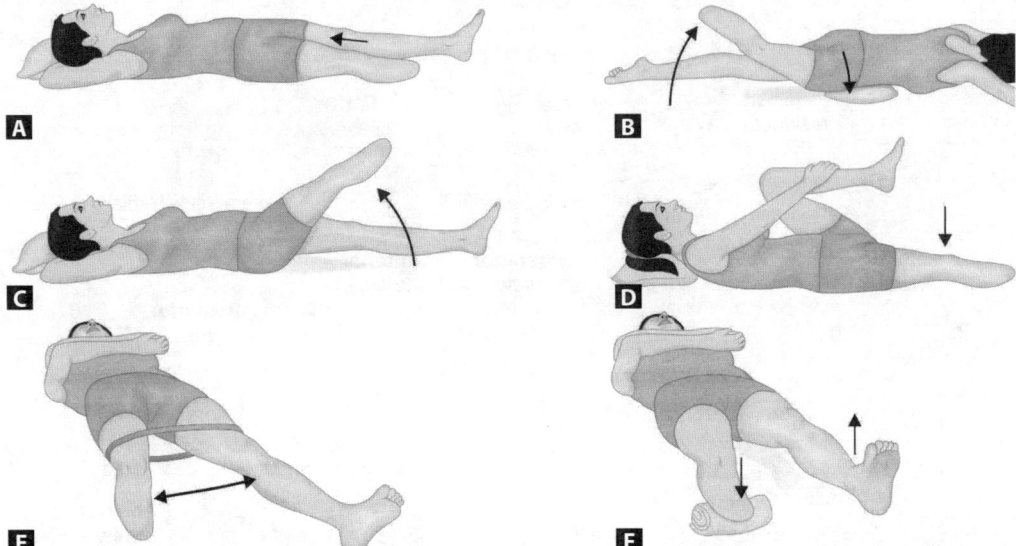

Figures 5.6A to F: Transtibial exercises. (A) Quad set; (B) Hip extension with knees straight; (C) Straight leg raise; (D) Extension of residual limb with the knee of the other leg against the chest; (E) Hip abduction against resistance; (F) Bridging.

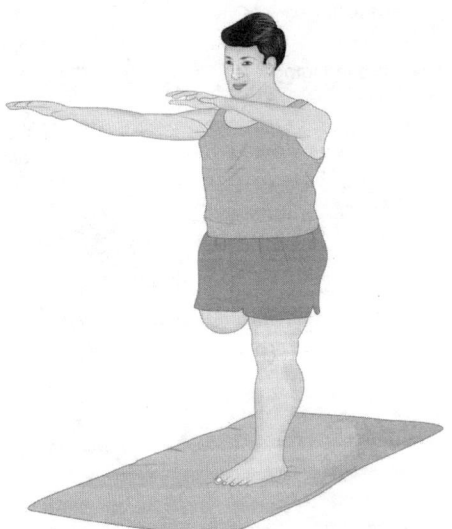

Figure 5.7: Standing balance exercises on a compliant surface.

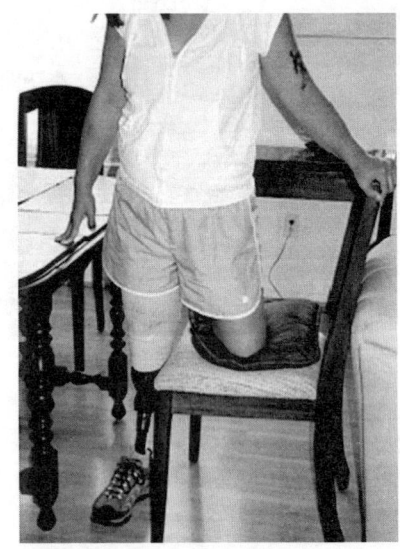

Figure 5.8: Kneeling on a pillow on a chair provides some weight bearing.

- Bilateral upper limb and lower limb AROM—20 repetition/2 times a day
- Stretching of all the muscles of the proximal joint of the stump—10 sec hold/ 10 repetition.
- Stump positioning
- Sleeping in prone lying—10-15 min/2-3 times a day
- Strengthening of upper limb and lower limb with the sand weights—10-20 repetition/2 times a day.

CHAPTER 5: Home Exercise Programs for Various Classification of Disabilities

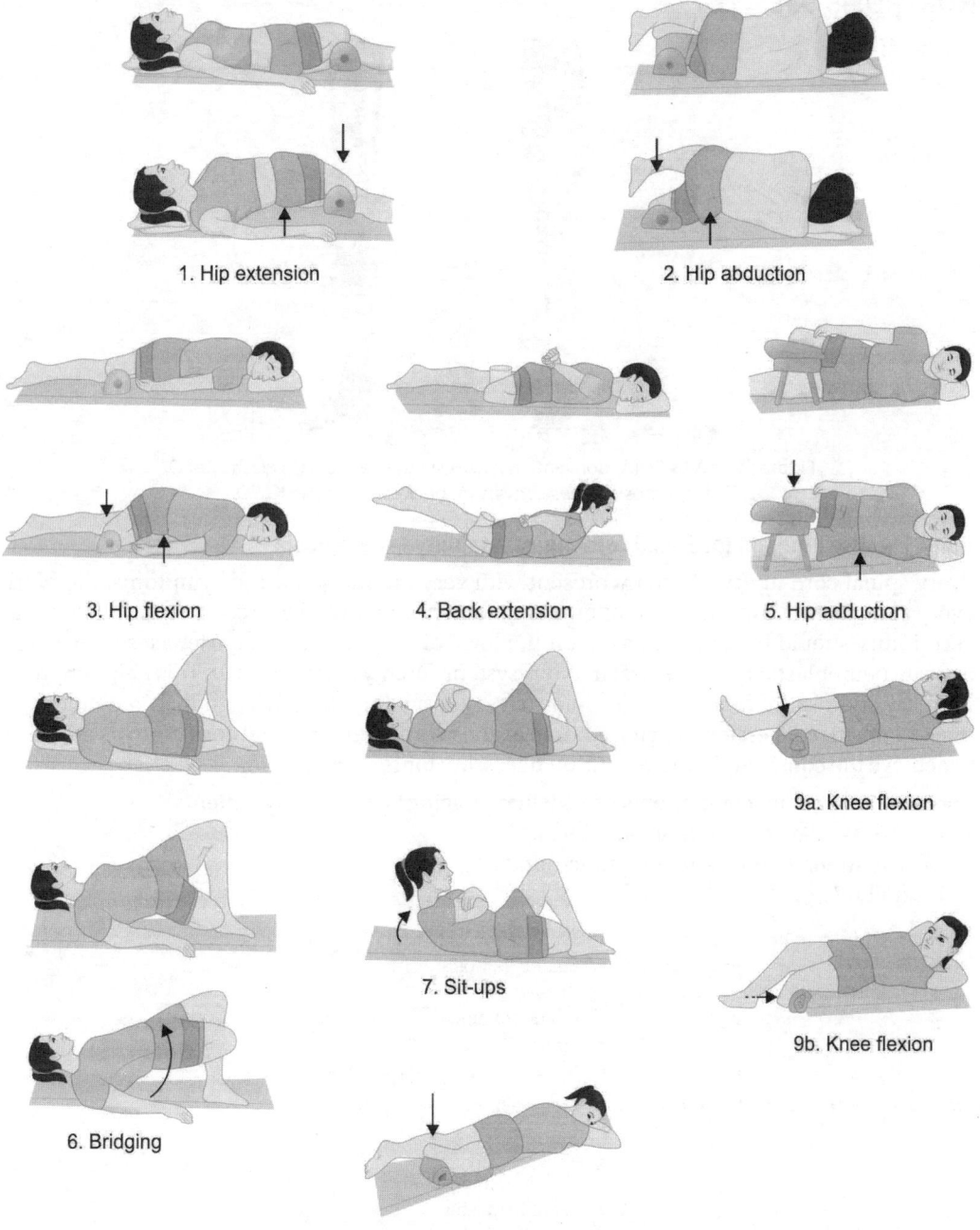

Figure 5.9: Prosthetic rehabilitation program exercises.

ORTHOSIS USE

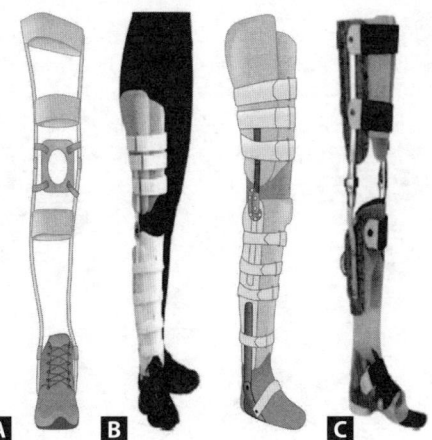

Figures 5.10A to C: (A) Conventional KAFO with knee cap; (B) Plastic KAFO; (C) This orthosis allows conversion between AFO and KAFO.

Home Exercise Program for Spinal Cord Injury Disability—Paraplegia

Every spinal cord injury disability present with very unique signs and symptoms, therefore every survivor will experience a different outcome. Every home exercise program for spinal cord injury should be tailored based on the level of injury. Practicing exercises daily helps activate neuroplasticity, the central nervous system's ability to rewire itself. This helps improve mobility and restore function. Neuroplasticity is best stimulated through high repetition, or massed practice. Therefore, having a home exercise program for spinal cord injury is essential to achieve the consistency and repetition necessary for recovery.

There are three main components of HEP in managing SCI disability patients
1. Cardiovascular conditioning (aerobics);
2. Muscle strengthening and endurance; and
3. Flexibility/stretching.[13]

Cardiovascular conditioning (aerobic exercises)	• Wheelchair pushing • Seated aerobics • Arm ergometer • Circuit training • Sports—rugby, basketball • Boxing or overhead punching
Muscle strengthening and endurance	• Free weights • Bands/elastics • Wall weights • Circuit training • Exercise machines • Labor/household tasks
Flexibility/stretching	*Upper body stretches—shoulder, upper arm, neck* • Assisted shoulder stretching exercises—posterior • Overhead shoulder stretch • Lateral stretch *Lower extremity stretches—hip, knee, ankle* • Passive range of motion for the legs (tetraplegia) • Self-range-of-motion program for persons with paraplegia

Respiratory Endurance and Strengthening

Depending on the level and completeness of injury, SCI can result in weakened respiratory (breathing) muscles and difficulty taking a deep breath. In these conditions, the HEP can include respiratory exercises which can improve the ability to breathe and bring oxygen into the body and brain.

The exercises include diaphragmatic breathing, forced expiratory technique, and incentive spirometry can be advised. Further proper wheel chair transfer techniques should be taught to the patient at home with minimal energy expenditure without harming the normal body parts.[10]

Home Exercise Program for Parkinson's Disease

Parkinson's is a progressive condition that can result in the loss of smooth and controlled movement of the muscles and joints, as well as causing problems in maintaining a good posture, and with balance, general mobility and confidence. This can limit some activities of daily living. Patients with parkinson's disease benefit greatly from HEP by maintaining the functional abilities, strengthening the muscles, increasing mobility in all joints and building up general fitness and health.

The Parkinson's Disease Society has recommended an unique HEP protocol which includes:
❖ HEP in lying position
❖ HEP in sitting position
❖ HEP in standing position.

HEP in lying position	Neck rolls, pelvic tilt, knee opening, knee lifts, leg stretches, arm reaching, arm and leg stretch
HEP in sitting position	Trunk rotations—lateral, free exercises of the upper limb in functional PNF patterns
HEP in standing position	Rocking sideways on foot, foot circling, sideways arm stretch, trunk rotation—lateral, forward, steeping, heel rise, wall squat

The exercises should be done in a paced relaxed manner and breathing exercise should be incorporated in between to ensure the patients are completely relaxed during the session.[11,14]

■ GERIATRIC HOMED-BASED REHABILITATION

Three sessions per week and a planned execution time of 40 min.

During each session, two to three sets will be performed with 5 to 15 repetitions for each exercise at a target effort rate of 13–15 ("a little difficult" to "difficult") on Borg's perceived exertion scale of 6 to 20 points.

Warm-up exercises: Active-free exercises of the upper and lower limbs, including extension, flexion, and rotation of the shoulders associated with breathing exercises.

Aerobic exercises: Displacement of a stick with both hands, from the knees to above the head and returning to the knees, and walking exercises with alternating thigh flexion and placing the hand on the opposite knee.

Resistance exercises: For the upper limbs: starting from the position with the elbow extended and the hand resting on the opposite thigh, movement of the whole member diagonally upwards and then returning the hand to the thigh. For the lower limbs: squatting exercise, starting from the sitting position on a chair and with arms crossed in front of the body, lifting to the orthostatic position and then returning to the sitting position.

Balance and coordination exercises: Walking on a straight line and walking while diverting from lined obstacles with progressively smaller distances. When possible, the exercise will evolve and the walk will be performed by touching the heel of one foot to the toes of the other foot (foot with foot).

Note: to ensure safety, these exercises will be performed close to fixed furniture in the house, making it possible to lean when necessary.

Stretching exercises: From the sitting position and with knees in extension, trying to reach the tip of the feet; from the sitting position on a chair and with the feet on the ground, performing rotation of the trunk to one side and elevation of the upper limb, on the same side, above the head, stretching as high as possible.

Disability and Health

Sedentary behavior is often associated with disability which leads to body deconditioning and health risk and even leads to Disability-associated Low Energy Expenditure Deconditioning Syndrome. Individuals with disabilities are 57% more likely to be obese than adults without disabilities. Obesity is an important risk factor for adults with disability with a 33% higher chance of having a chronic condition, such as heart disease, diabetes, stroke or cancer. The impact of these chronic diseases can be reduced by an effective HEP which includes aerobic physical activity.

Benefits of Home-based Physical Activity for Individuals with Disability

- Physical activity (PA) is essential for quality of life and act as a public health promoter.
- PA has amplified importance for cognitive, emotional and social difficulties.
- Psychological benefits such as enhanced self-perception through successful PA experiences.
- PA can reduce stress, pain, and depression. Activities of Daily Living (ADLs) are perceived to be easier.

Adherence to Home Exercises Program

Adherence to HEP by disabled patients in rehabilitation is a significant problem and challenging task to address because of multifactorial reasons, covering both psychological and situational factors that vary between each individual. This has to be considered by clinicians in the design of personalized home exercise programs.

- Providing a home exercise program (HEP) to patients is one of the most fundamental and important aspects of physiotherapy to ensure the patient achieve maximum independence.
- Patients who adhere to their prescribed exercises are significantly better at achieving their goals and demonstrate a greater increase in physical function and capabilities.
- Nonadherence of a HEP increases the risk of recurrent injury or flare-ups with less positive outcomes long term and can result in the physiotherapist believing that their current treatment is not effective leading to misconception about the therapy.
- Once designing the HEP, the therapist should identify the potential barriers to patient adherence to HEP and should also have right strategies that are effective at combating those barriers.

CHAPTER 5: Home Exercise Programs for Various Classification of Disabilities

Barriers for HEP

Despite the potential health benefits, there are barriers for HEP which pose immense challenges for the disabled individual. The barriers depends on age, type of disability, and barriers at an individual, social, environmental and policy level.

Individual Level Barrier

This barrier depends upon from individual to individual which includes:
- Lack of knowledge and fail to understand the HEP protocols during the initial demonstration
- Lack of accessible knowledge/information about optimal HEP for the disability, how much activity should one do, and how safe is HEP without supervision; fear of falling; the nature of the impairment producing pain during activity; lack of energy, lack of motivation, shame from being disabled; personal concerns about safety; apprehension of attracting unwanted attention.
- **Threat and beliefs:** The beliefs a patient holds regarding their condition and the decisions made by patients are based on their own beliefs, personal experiences, and the information they receive about the disability.
- **Pain:** Pain levels during exercise in musculoskeletal patients presented strong evidence as a barrier to adherence in few systematic reviews.
- **Psychological symptoms:** Depression as a barrier to adherence has strong supporting evidence.

Social Barriers

- Dependency of children with disabilities on parents;
- Over-protective attitude from caregivers, spouses, family;
- Caregivers lack professional preparation for HEP
- Negative societal attitudes about disability from others.

Environmental Barriers

- Accessibility (too narrow doorways for wheelchair access, no ramps, and inaccessible bathrooms or changing rooms)
- Architectural barriers in house and outdoor areas (e.g., poorly lit or congested house space, no railings).[12]

Embracing Health Technologies for Effective HEP

Health technologies, such as the use of mobile devices, mobile phones and tablets, software applications provides more opportunities to effectively monitor patients HEP, with a data-driven approach that incorporates features designed to increase adherence to exercise such as coaching, self-monitoring and education, as well as remotely monitor adherence rates more objectively.

Few Software applications exist on the market and may well change the way of many home exercise plans in clinics. These apps are easy to use with free access and features with beautifully designed instructional videos. The built-in efficiencies will reduce the workload and software motivates the patients and improves outcomes, with tracking tools and insightful analytics.

Combining the popularity of mobile devices with the on-going search for fitness, thousands of fitness applications (apps) are available for free or low cost. Apps allow users to set the exercise goals, track activity, gather exercise ideas, and share progress to the treating physiotherapists/clinicians. Physiotherapists should stay abreast with recent research and embrace this effective health technologies as they emerge.

■ SUMMARY

Home Exercise Program has much positive effect on various disabilities. The clinical significance of exercise intervention is worthy of affirmation. Compared with the huge cost of medicines and its side effects, home exercise intervention is an economic and safe way to prevent further complications of the disability and can reduce the economic burden on families and society.

However, following right HEP and avoiding injury is more important than engaging in exercise. Measures for preventing patient from injuries should be taken. When designing the HEP, a comprehensive assessment and evaluation of the patient should be taken to exclude all possible contraindications, and select the appropriate type and intensity of exercise.

■ WHEELCHAIR TRANSFER TECHNIQUES

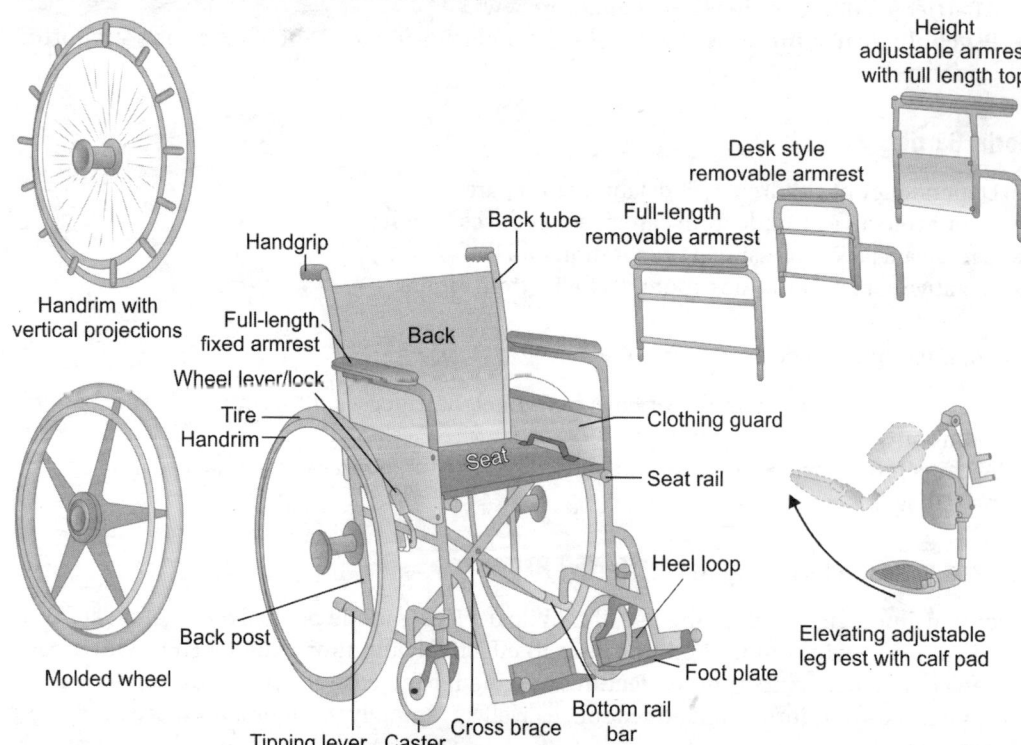

Figure 5.11: Foundation components of prescriptive wheelchair.

CHAPTER 5: Home Exercise Programs for Various Classification of Disabilities

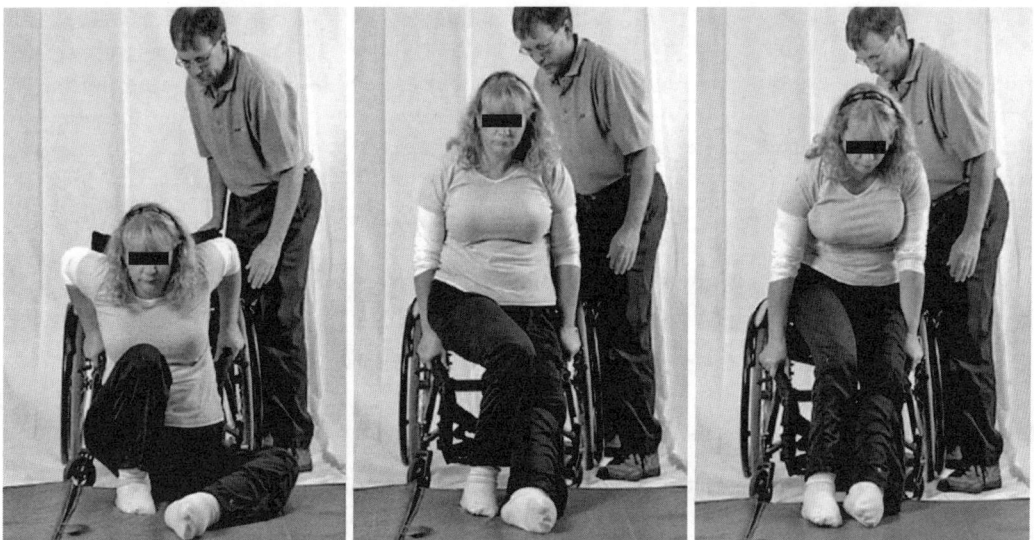

Figure 5.12: Floor to wheelchair transfer using backward approach.

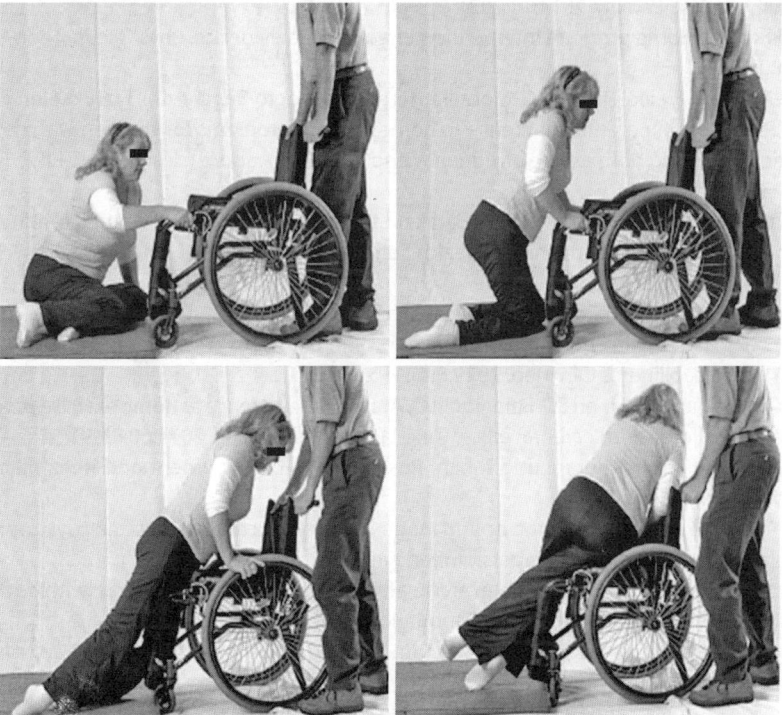

Figure 5.13: Floor to wheelchair transfers using a frontward approach.

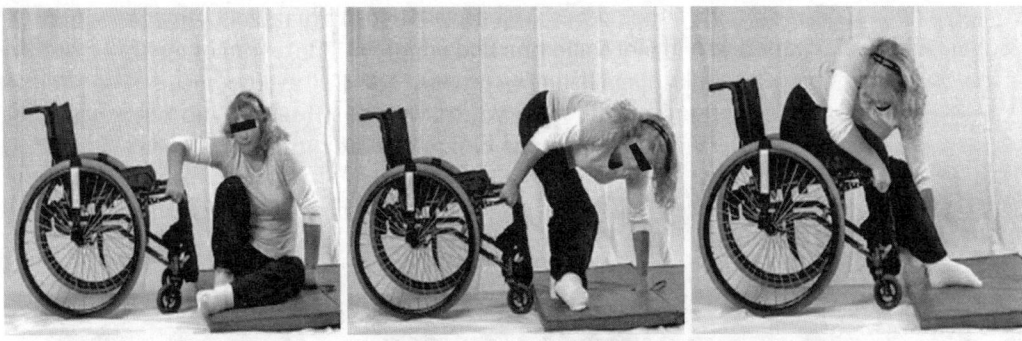

Figure 5.14: Floor to wheelchair transfers using sideways approach.

■ REFERENCES

1. Sunder S. Textbook of rehabilitation, 3rd edition. Jaypee Brothers Medical Publishers; 2017.
2. O'Sullivan SB, Schmitz TJ, et al. Physical Rehabilitation, 6th edition.
3. Pruthvish S. Community-based rehabilitation of person with disabilities, 1st edition; 2006.
4. Tinderholt Myrhaug H, Østensjø S, Larun L, Odgaard-Jensen J, Jahnsen R. Intensive training of motor function and functional skills among young children with cerebral palsy: A systematic review and meta-analysis. BMC Pediatr. 2014;14:292.
5. Novak, I Berry, J. Home program intervention effectiveness evidence. Phys Occup. Ther. Pediatr. 2014; 34:384-89.
6. Medina-Mirapeix F, Lillo-Navarro C, Montilla-Herrador J, Gacto-Sánchez M, Franco-Sierra MÁ, Escolar-Reina P. Predictors of parents' adherence to home exercise programs for children with developmental disabilities, regarding both exercise frequency and duration: A survey design. Eur J Phys. Rehabil. Med. 2017;53:545-55.
7. Psihogios AM, Fellmeth H, Schwartz LA, Barakat LP. Family functioning and medical adherence across children and adolescents with chronic health conditions: A meta-analysis. J Pediatr Psychol. 2019;44: 84-97.
8. Lillo-Navarro C, Montilla-Herrador J, Escolar-Reina P, Oliveira-Sousa SL, García-Vidal JA, Medina-Mirapeix F. Factors associated with parents' adherence to different types of exercises in home programs for children with disabilities. J Clin Med. 2019;8(4):456.
9. Başaran A, Karadavut KI, Üneri SO, Balbaloğlu O, Atasoy N. Adherence to home exercise program among caregivers of children with cerebral palsy. Turk. J Phys Med Rehabil. 2014;60:85-91.
10. Online Resources from Therapeutic Touch, Rosalin Child Development and Rehabilitation Centre, Lucknow, Uttar Pradesh, India.
11. A home exercise book—Physiotherapy Management for Duchenne muscular dystrophy, Muscular Dystrophy Campaign, Leigh Chambers, United Kingdom.
12. Hoessly M, Hedges K. Your Guide to exercise after stroke, A guide for people with stroke and their families. Margot Andrew. AH Somervill Foundation; 2017.
13. SCI Action Canada. Active Homes: Home Strength-Training Guide for People with Tetraplegia. Burlington, ON: Eagle Press; 2012.
14. Keep Moving—Exercise and Parkinson's by Richard Webber and Bhanu Ramaswamy, Parkinson's Disease Society of the United Kingdom; 2009.

Section 2 Community-based Rehabilitation

CHAPTER 6

Community Development

Shwetanjali Bhagra

LEARNING OBJECTIVES

Through this chapter, the reader will be able to:
- Community and its definition
- What is community development and its definition?
- Importance of community development
- History of community development in India
- Key values of community development
- What are the types of community development?
- Role of community-based organization in community development
- Various approaches for community-based development

■ INTRODUCTION

The concept of community development is coined from two words, i.e., community and development. To begin with, a common definition of community emerged as a group of people with diverse characteristics linked by social ties, sharing common perspectives, and engaging in joint action in geographical locations or settings.[1] The geographical community can be a town, a suburb, or even a small suburb section. There might be a few communities in the same town. There are other times when a town might be only part of a community, such as when the community includes the rural areas outside town or two towns are closely linked.[2] All communities are dynamic in nature. They act, interact, evolve, and change as a result of larger political and economic forces as well as internal and external forces.

Community development is a process in which community members take collective action to generate solutions to existing problems. Economic, social, environmental and cultural welfare of the community often evolves from this type of collective action. Community development actions can be either the initiatives within a small group or broader community. Community development is a broad term that defines the practices of civic leaders, activists that are aimed at involving citizens and professionals in the various aspects of community life to build stronger and more stable local communities. Community development is a professional discipline, and a practice-based profession focused on promoting participative democracy, sustainable growth, increasing the number of economic opportunities, improving social justice, through the organizing, educating and empowering people in the urban and rural communities.

■ DEFINITION OF COMMUNITY DEVELOPMENT

A few definitions of community development are:
- Community development is a process where community members come together to take collective action and generate solutions to common problems. Community wellbeing (economic, social, environmental and cultural) often evolves from this type of collective action being taken at a grassroots level. Community development ranges from small initiatives within a small group to large initiatives that involve the broader community work.[3]
- Community development is a group of people in a community deciding to initiate a social action process to change their economic, social, cultural and environmental situation.[4]
- Community development is a movement designed to promote better living for the whole community with the active participation and on the initiative of the community.[3]
- Community development is a balance program for stimulating the local potential for growth in every direction. Its promise of reciprocal advance in both wealth and welfare, not on the basis of outside charity but by building on the latent vitality of the beneficiaries themselves with the minimum of outside aid.[3]
- Community development is technically-aided and locally organized self-help.
- The term "community development" has come into international usage to denote the process by which the efforts of the people themselves are united with those of governmental authorities to improve the economic, social and cultural condition of the communities to integrate these communities in the life of the nation and to enable them to contribute fully to national progress.[5]

■ THE HISTORY OF COMMUNITY DEVELOPMENT

The Community Development Programme (CDP) was launched in India on 2nd October, 1952 with 55 community development projects (CDPS). Each project had about 60 multi-purpose village level workers (VLWs), one for each group of 5–10 villages. The people in all the project area responded enthusiastically and the need for a rapid expansion of the program to other parts of the country was urgently felt. In 1956, by the end of the first 5-year plan period, there were 248 blocks, covering around a fifth of the population in the country. By end of the second 5-year plan period, there were 3,000 blocks covering 70% of the rural population. By 1964, the entire country was covered.[6]

■ PRINCIPLES OF COMMUNITY DEVELOPMENT

Community development is a holistic approach grounded in principles of empowerment, human rights, inclusion, social justice, self-determination and collective action.[7]
- Self-help and self-responsibility are required for successful development.
- Participation in public decision-making should be free and open to all citizens.
- Broad representation and increased breadth of perspective and understanding encourage effective community development.
- Methods that produce accurate information about the community are vital to the process.
- Understanding and the general agreement is the basis for community change.
- All individuals have the right to be heard in open discussion, whether in agreement or disagreement with community norms, and the responsibility to respect opposing viewpoints.
- Trust is essential for effective working relationships.

CHAPTER 6: Community Development

■ VALUES OF COMMUNITY DEVELOPMENT

Community development is fundamentally based on the values of human rights, social justice, equality and respect for diversity. The principles which underpin its practice are: self-determination—people and communities have the right to make their own choices and decisions.[7]

- All people have basic dignity.
- People have the right to participate in decisions that affect their current and future well-being.
- Participatory democracy is the superior method of conducting the civic business of the community.
- People have the right to strive to create an environment they desire.
- People have the right to reject an externally imposed environment.
- Maximizing purposeful interaction and dialogue within a community will increase the potential for learning and development.
- Implied within a process of purposeful interaction is an ever-widening concept of community.
- Every discipline and profession is a potential contributor to a community development process.
- Motivation is created through interaction with the environment.

■ CHARACTERISTICS OF COMMUNITY DEVELOPMENT

There are characteristics that community development possesses, according to Driu (2014), that make it distinctive,[2] and these include:

- Community development is about people's active involvement in the issues that affect their lives. It is a process based on sharing power, skills, knowledge, and experience.
- The community development process is collective. Still, the experience of the process enhances the integrity, skills, knowledge, experience, and equality of power for each individual involved.
- Where community development takes place, certain principles are central to it. The priority of the community development process is the empowering and enabling of those who are traditionally deprived of power and control over their common affairs.
- It claims as important the ability of people to act together to influence the social, economic, political, and environmental issues which affect them. Community development aims to encourage sharing and create structures that give genuine participation and involvement.
- Community development is crucially concerned with the issues of powerlessness and disadvantage. As such, it involves all members of society and offers a practice that is part of a process of social change.

Summarily, effective community development must be "well-planned, inclusive and equitable, initiated and supported by community members, a long-term endeavor, holistic and integrated into the bigger picture, of benefit to the community and grounded in experience that leads to best practices".[8]

■ OBJECTIVES OF COMMUNITY DEVELOPMENT

Having stated the characteristics of community development, as known that every field of profession and study has objectives behind them; the following are the objectives of community development:[2]

- Community development seeks to enable individuals and communities to grow and change according to their own needs and priorities and at their own pace, provided this does not oppress other groups and communities or damage the environment.

- Community development seeks to enable individuals and communities to grow and change according to their own needs and priorities and at their own pace, provided this does not oppress other groups and communities or damage the environment.
- Community development should seek to develop structures that enable the active involvement of people from disadvantaged groups, particularly people from Black and minority ethnic groups.

Also, according to Enugu and Oyitso (2005), cited by Olajide, the objectives of community development are:
- To contribute to the process of building democracy and human development.
- To promote the human development of the groups with which it works.
- To promote the popular sectors in developing and reinforcing social and political awareness and make community members become conscious protagonists of their lives.
- To promote popular culture and education and assert the values and attitudes required to change and develop locally and nationally realities.

Summarily, community development is both a practice-based profession and an academic discipline geared towards allowing all community members and developmental agents to come together as a collective body to take actions and "generate solutions to a common problem."

COMPONENTS OF COMMUNITY DEVELOPMENT

Community development covers a wide range of activities and programs. These differ from one community to another and depend on the priorities, issues, plans, problems and solutions of a society. The following are the significant components of community development:[8,9]
- Active participation against unhealthy social taboos and social isolation
- Development of self-esteem, sympathy, empathy and confidence building
- Creative thinking and practical action
- Social adjustment and mutual support
- Involvement in the practice of community development
- Mobilizing funds to meet emerging needs
- Identification of priority areas by the community.

The following are the major community development programs:
- Child development programs
- Adolescent development programs
- Youth development programs
- Women development programs
- Welfare of the senior citizens
- Health and family welfare programs
- Family life education
- Agricultural and allied activities
- Cooperative service society
- Education
- Communication

THE METHOD AND PROCESS OF COMMUNITY DEVELOPMENT

Community development is considered to be method as well as process. It is the method of helping local communities to become more aware of there needs to assess their resources more

CHAPTER 6: Community Development

realistically, to organize themselves and resources in such a way as to satisfy some of their needs through occasional projects so that villagers are unable to their own efforts to move steadily towards the goal of self-improvement.

Community development is not easy and requires people with specific knowledge and skills to facilitate the process. It is a process through which people develop the ability to collectively help themselves and reduce reliance on external resources. It includes a set of steps to guide problem-solving, program planning and task completion. Community development practitioners subscribe to a basic process but with minor differences.[10]

Seven Process of Community Development

A. **Organize:**
   1. Establish the organizing group
   2. Create a Mission Statement
   3. Identify Community Stakeholders
      a. Do we create a new organization or use an existing one?
      b. Who will lead the charge?
      c. Do we need a professional developer?
      d. What is our mission? Who are the stakeholders?

B. **Analyze**
   4. Collect and analyze information
      a. What information do we have, and what do we need?
      b. Who can analyze the information and use it to describe the condition of the community and engage the public?
      c. Is the data complete, accurate, valid and reliable?

C. **Communicate:**
   5. Develop an effective communications process
      a. How will we obtain input from citizens?
      b. How will we keep citizens informed about the process?
      c. Are all available methods used, especially those that reach disenfranchised citizens?
      d. How can local media be involved?

D. **Plan:**
   6. Expand the community organization
   7. Identify the leadership and establish a plan
   8. Create a vision statement
   9. Create a comprehensive strategic plan
      a. Who else and what other groups need to be included?
      b. What is the shared vision of the stakeholders for a common future?
      c. What goals and objectives are required to achieve the vision?
      d. Who will champion and lead the effort?

E. **Implement**
   10. Implement the plan
       a. What activities will produce early results?
       b. What activities will be prominent?
       c. What activities are most popular among citizens?
       d. What activities can be accomplished with few resources?
       e. What will build/sustain momentum?

F. **Evaluate:**
   11. Review and evaluate the planning outcomes
      a. How often will the plan be reviewed, and are "plan, do, check, and adjust" elements built into the process?
      b. What is working needs to be changed, eliminated or added?
      c. Have community conditions changed?
G. **Celebrate:**
   12. Celebrate the successes
      a. How can we publicly celebrate success?
      b. What should we do periodically and annually to celebrate?
      c. How do we recognize the efforts of citizens?
      d. How do we assure that all stakeholders of all generations are included?
      e. What activities will continue the momentum?
   13. Create new goals and objectives as needed
      a. What goals were expressed by citizens not included in the original plan?
      b. Can these be incorporated as new goals and objectives?
      c. How can fresh input be gained to keep the plan relevant?
      d. Are resources adequate for continued work?

■ STEPS FOR INITIATING COMMUNITY DEVELOPMENT

Each community has unique characteristics, making it different from other communities. The differences may include availability and utilization of resources, culture, attitude, behavior and social development needs. The following are the significant steps for initiating community development.[11]

Step 1: Goal setting: Goal setting is the first step in initiating community developmental activities. It comes before planning and implementation. During goal-setting, the CDW should consider the community's socio, economic, cultural, and demographic aspects. In addition, they should also look at the availability of resources like manpower, planners, and implementers. The goal should be "simple" in nature.

Step 2: Understanding the people in the community: Before planning and implementing a community development program, it is essential to learn about the people in the community. You can do this by finding out the information:

Their needs, educational levels and requirements, cultural and religious compositions, The problem and issues they face, their history, political setup and political leaders, attitude of the society, issues relating to health, quality of life, socioeconomic situation, employment opportunities, availability of cooperative sectors, self-help groups, etc.

Step 3: Identify the opportunities, problems and issues on community development: The information you gather about the community will also help you identify the opportunities, problems and issues related to community development. It is vital to list them before planning and implementing developmental activities.

Step 4: Prioritize issues and problems: Once you prepare a list of topics and cases in the community, the next step is to identify the ones that need to be tackled first. This should be done in consultation with the community. The issues that demand urgent attention should be addressed first. Thus, prioritizing the needs and problems of the community according to their necessity and urgency is an essential step in community development.

Step 5: Resource mapping: Once you have identified and prioritized the needs and issues, the next step is resource mapping. What is resource mapping? It identifies all the available resources, such as manpower, material and finance, required for particular development plans. It is essential to analyze the quality and quantity of each resource and how it can be used to address community development needs.

Step 6: Plan and prepare the activity: Once the goals have been set, the needs identified, and resources mapped, the CDWs should plan and organize activities to achieve the goals. They can do this with the help of social workers, decision-makers, policymakers, implementers and organizers, who are supposed to play an active role in the planning and preparing of community development activities.

Step 7: Prepare the design for implementation: This process will help the planners and implementers to understand the theory and practicability in implementing the activities/programs. Particular focus is given to the implementation strategies while preparing the design. Environment creation, resource support and people support will become part and parcel of the design.

Step 8: Prepare time and cost estimates: Time and cost estimates are two essential aspects you should consider when planning and implementing community development activities. A reasonable timeframe should be given for each sub-activity and main activity. The cost estimate should be prepared carefully, and you can seek help from people who have the expertise and experience. By utilizing community support and other resources, the cost of implementation can be reduced to the maximum.

Step 9: Implementation of community development activities and programs: After planning, preparing activities, designing and preparing your work plan and budget, the next step is implementation. This step aims to tackle the priority problems and issues you have identified. This requires effective coordination and preparation of the essential activities in implementation. The process of performance should be systematic, scientific and time-bound.

Step 10: Documentation of the activity: Documentation simply means creating a record of all the processes involved in the program, from the beginning to the end. You should remember to document the successes and challenges of the program as clearly as possible. This will be circulated to community people and experts for collecting feedback and opinion. It will help you get the people's support and develop a positive attitude among community members.

Step 11: Monitoring: Monitoring is another essential step in community development. During monitoring, you continuously track the progress of the activities you are implementing to ensure that they are going as planned. Monitoring enables you to analyze the challenges and successes of the activities you are implementing to take corrective measures in good time. Monitoring involves the following tasks:

- Recording what is happening as well as what is not happening
- Checking or observing the activities
- Collecting facts and figures on activities and results
- Assessing whether implementation is going in the right direction or is achieving the desired results.

Step 12: Evaluation: Evaluation allows you to judge a project's achievements. It measures how well the program's activities have met its aims, goals, and objectives. Proper evaluation demands:
- Accuracy and attention,
- An external—outside agency, the external evaluation is nothing but the review carried out by someone not directly involved in the process implementation.
- The internal—implementing agency, the evaluation carried out by some from the actual project team.

Step 13: Recycle the planning and implementation processes: The feedback you receive from monitoring and evaluation. During this step, you use data from monitoring to address those activities that need adjustment to achieve the intended outcomes. Similarly, you use data from evaluation to help you improve the design, planning and implementation of subsequent programs.

TYPES OF COMMUNITY

There can be four types of communities, as defined by Brown & Hannis (2012):[12]
1. A geographic community is a group of people living in the same physical area. The three main types of communities are rural, urban, and suburban.
   a. **Rural:** Rural communities are placed where the houses are spread very far apart.
   b. **Urban:** Urban communities are located in cities.
   c. **Suburban:** The suburban areas are the mix of the urban and rural.
2. A group of people "who share or possess a common and essential factor such as gender, race, religion, or socioeconomic status"
3. A group of people "who come together to address a common interest or concern". This category would include professional associations, trade unions, and social action groups, for example.
4. A virtual community that comes together to learn about work and "share their passion and hobbies".[12]

TYPES OF COMMUNITY DEVELOPMENT PROGRAMS

They are classified into three types:[13]
1. **Integrated-type:** It has a countrywide scope and emphasizes technical services' development and coordination. Based on the need of people, the objectives are set. The relevant departments and programs are incorporated into the programs and implemented through a readily available department to achieve these objectives. This department coordinates the efforts of both governmental and non-governmental organizations at every level. In some cases, new administrative areas are created into the traditional ones to coordinate technical services closer to people.
2. **Adaptive type:** It was designed to be countrywide, emphasizing community organization self-help and involves a change in government administrative organizations. They can be attached to any department and adjusted to the prevailing administrative organization of government.
3. **Project type:** These are of geographical scope, emphasizing development. They cannot be implemented without the interference of local government organizations.

EFFECTIVE APPROACHES TO COMMUNITY DEVELOPMENT

Community development is a holistic approach grounded in principles of empowerment, human rights, inclusion, social justice, self-determination and collective action (Kenny, 2007).[14] Community development considers community members to be experts in their lives and communities, and values community knowledge and wisdom. Community development programs are led by community members at every stage—from deciding on issues to selecting and implementing actions, and evaluation. Community development has an explicit focus on the redistribution of power to address the causes of inequality and disadvantage.[2]

Through community development initiatives, community members can become more empowered. This enables them to increasingly recognize and challenge conditions and structures which are leading to their disempowerment or negatively impacting their wellbeing (Ife, 2016).[15] At the community level, community development and empowerment initiatives can achieve long-term outcomes such as stronger and more cohesive communities, evidenced by changes in social capital, civic engagement, social cohesion and improved health (Kenny, 2007; Ife, 2016; Campbell, Pyett, & McCarthy, 2007)[14-16]

The community development approaches involves different methods and techniques of operation and functioning with communities for conventional programs and organization. Community development approaches include: needs-based approach, problem-solving approach, participatory approach, asset-based approach, community-based approach, the power-conflict—approach, welfare approach and rights-based approach.[10,17]

- **The needs-based approach** focuses on the community's needs, deficiencies and problems. It focuses on identifying needs in a deteriorating community and creating external inputs to meet those needs. As a traditional approach, is generally understood as a deficit model which focuses on the community's needs, deficiencies and problems.
- **The problem solving approach** focuses on different methods approaches that can be used in creating different solution for the problems that are faced by communities.
- **Participatory approach** focuses on ensuring that people are educated and encouraged to participate in the development process. People should participate in every step from initiation to evaluation on every development project and program.
- **The asset-based community development** is an approach to sustainable community-driven development. Asset-based community development's basis is that communities can drive the development process themselves by identifying and mobilizing existing, but often unrecognized assets.
- **The power conflict approach** concentrates on creating a peaceful community. The process deals with solution that will deal with conflicts that slow the progress and hamper development process.
- **Welfare approach** is an approach that deals with working communities to build their capacity that improves their wellbeing, happiness and eventually their prosperity.
- **Right-based approach** focused on ensuring that people's human rights are by themselves and the leaders. The process deals with human rights abuses which especially have kept people in suffering and poverty.

IMPORTANCE OF COMMUNITY DEVELOPMENT

Community development emphasizes self-help, mutual support, the building up of neighborhood integration, the development of neighborhood capacities for problem-solving and self-representation, and the promotion of collective action to bring a community's preferences to the attention of political decision-makers.

Community development is essential because it serves as the foundation upon which a city can build to improve the lives of its citizens. It builds strong, diverse communities capable of attracting and retaining talent, starting and growing businesses, and overcoming challenges. Citizens will be happier, healthier, and wealthier, living longer lives. Companies will have a more extensive customer base from which to sell their goods and services, and the city will earn tax revenue to support essential programs and reduce debt.

When community development is effective, there is less crime, less disparity among citizens, more jobs available, a more talented workforce, and fewer overall issues affecting residents. Community development does not necessarily solve problems in cities; instead, it reduces issues and expands growth opportunities. Both economic and business development suffers significantly in the absence of community development.

Community development helps build community capacity to address issues, take advantage of opportunities, find common ground, and balance competing interests. It does not just happen—capacity building requires both a conscious and a conscientious effort to do something (or many things) to improve the community. It recognizes:
- The connection between social, cultural, environmental and economic matters;
- The diversity of interests within a community; and
- Its relationship to building capacity.

Community development seeks to improve the quality of life. Effective community development results in mutual benefit and shared responsibility among community members. Community development ranges from small initiatives within a small group to large initiatives that involve the broader community. Community development produces self-reliant and self-sustaining communities that mobilize resources to benefit their members.[18]

■ ROLE OF COMMUNITY DEVELOPMENT WORKER/COMMUNITY DEVELOPER

Currently, few positions are explicitly named "community developer". It is increasingly more common for managers and employees in various settings to be expected to take a community development approach to their work. There are many opportunities for anyone involved with community members to incorporate a community development role into their practice.

A community developer may take on various roles, and he/she works with the community. However, in all the functions, the worker always respects the autonomy and self-determination of the community members and does not impose an externally directed agenda upon them. Their work conforms to professional standards and ethics and is comprehensive and systematic in its approach.[19] The roles commonly ascribed to community development workers are enablers, guides, technical experts, and liaisons in community development literature.
- **Guide:** As a guide, the worker helps the community identify their goals and find the means to achieve them.
- **Enabler**: The worker can enable the community in a variety of ways. He/she might facilitate a problem-solving process with the community, including helping them articulate dissatisfaction and identify their causes. The worker could also help them organize and plan their activities and encourage positive interpersonal relationships. The enabler role is most associated with locality development strategies.
- **Technical assistant:** This "expert" role is most associated with social planning. However, in all forms of community development, there is usually some need by the community to

access technical support in areas such as community assessment, media relations, accessing information or project development.
- **Liaison/advocate:** Depending on the nature of the community and the type of community development initiative it has taken on, the worker may need to assume a liaison or advocacy role. He/she may be the intermediary between the community and other bodies such as government, institutions or other community factions. The community may ask the worker to present their views, access information, or negotiate an agreement.

Community developers do not promote specific programs, remedies, or actions. Instead, the community developer focuses on the processes that increase civic capacity, open doors for increased citizen participation, and develops in people the ability to give purposeful direction to their own future.[19]

■ THE ROLE OF PHYSIOTHERAPISTS IN COMMUNITY DEVELOPMENT

Phase 1: Education Phase

- Establishing rapport and initiating observations to assess the community context.
- Hold several group meetings organized for persons with disabilities and their families, members of subdistrict administrative organizations, community leaders (e.g., sub-subdistrict headman, monks), representatives of various community groups (e.g., the elderly, women, and adolescents groups), and local civil servants.[2]
- The purposes of the meetings should be to introduce the CBR strategy as well as the objectives, and to mobilize communities in sharing their experiences on issues regarding persons with disabilities.
- Finally, a core organization that would be the leader of the CBR program in each subdistrict should be organized.[20]

Phase 2: Empowerment Phase

- The core organization of the CBR program to be facilitated to arrange group meetings among persons with disabilities and their families, subdistrict administrative organization's members, community leaders, representatives of various community groups, local civil servants, and other relevant sectors.
- To create an atmosphere for open dialogues and reflection during the meetings.
- An analysis of the persons with disabilities' current situation to be discussed collaboratively among the participants.
- They were encouraged to discuss problems as well as barriers and limitations of the current rehabilitation services for persons with disabilities.[2]
- The problems should be prioritized, then strategies and action plans to manage such problems should be established by the participants.[20]

Phase 3: Implementation Phase

- The participants should implement their action plans in order of priority according to the problems' perceived importance.
- Arrange regular visits to observe and record its activities.
- To encourage the core organization and the participants to keep processing the program, and to offer any necessary advice and help.

❖ The core organization should regularly arrange group meetings among the participants to evaluate the program, and to review and modify the action plans.[20,21]

REFERENCES

1. MacQueen KM, McLellan E, Metzger DS, Kegeles S, Strauss RP, Scotti R, et al. What is Community? An Evidence-Based Definition for Participatory Public Health. Am J Public Health. 2001;91(12):1929-38. doi:10.2105/ajph.91.12.1929.
2. DRIU A. Basic Concepts of Community Development, Centre for Vocational and Continuing Education. The University of South Pacific, Suva, Fuji; 2014.
3. Definition of CD. *Community Development Exchange. Archived from* the original *on 2010-07-14*.
4. Christenson JA, Robinson JW. Community Development in Perspective. Lowa: Lowa State University Press; 1989.
5. Community development. *UNTERM*. Archived from the original on 14 July 2014. Retrieved 7 July 2014.
6. Siddiqui HY. Working with communities: An introduction to community work. New Delhi: Hira Publications; 1997.
7. Pawar M. Values and Principles for Community Development. Community Development in Asia and the Pacific. 1st edition. First Published 2009 Imprint Routledge; 2009.
8. Robinson J Green G. Introduction to Community Development: Theory, Practice, and Service-Learning. SAGE Publications; 2010.
9. Ghazala M, Vijayendra R. Community Based (and Driven) Development: A Critical Review. SSRN Electronic Journal; 2004. 10.2139/ssrn.501663.
10. Maria A, Quimbo T, Erinorio J, Perez M, Tan FO. Community development approaches and methods: Implications for community development practice and research, Community Development. 2018;49:5, 589-603.
11. Tyler N, Ward R. Planning and Community Development: A Guide for the 21st Century Paperback— Illustrated. WW Norton and Company; Illustrated edition; 2010.
12. Brown JD, Hannis D. *Community development in Canada*. Pearson; 2012.
13. Phillips R, Pittman R. An Introduction to Community Development, 2nd edition. Routledge; 2014.
14. Kenny S. *Developing Communities for the Future, 3rd edition*. South Melbourne: Thompson; 2007.
15. Ife J. *Community development in an uncertain world: Vision, analysis and practice,* 2nd edition. Port Melbourne: Cambridge University Press; 2016.
16. Campbell D, Pyett P, McCarthy L. Community development interventions to improve Aboriginal health: Building an evidence base. *Health Sociology Review*. 2007;16;304-14.
17. Institute of Medicine and National Research Council. Community Development Approaches: Overcoming Challenges, Striving for Change. Focusing on Children's Health: Community Approaches to Addressing Health Disparities: Workshop Summary. Washington, DC: The National Academies Press; 2009. doi: 10.17226/12637.
18. Willetts J, Asker S, Carrard N, Winterford K. (2014). The practice of a strengths based approach to community development in Solomon. Islands, Development Studies Research. An Open Access Journal. 2014;1(1):354-67. doi: 10.1080/21665095.2014.983275.
19. Chakrabarti V, Popli UK. Community Organization and Development in the context of Literacy. Module-5.13. Basic roles of community worker; 2007.
20. World Confederation for Physical Therapy Keynotes Community-based Rehabilitation. *Changing concepts of CBR 2? Implications for physical therapists.* http://www.wcpt.org/common/docs/ wcpt_keynote_CBR2.pdf.
21. Bury T. Primary health care and community-based rehabilitation: implications for physical therapy. Asia Pacific Disability Rehabilitation Journal. 2005;16:29-61.

CHAPTER 7

The Link Between Institution-based Rehabilitation and Community-based Rehabilitation

Shwetanjali Bhagra

LEARNING OBJECTIVES

Through this chapter, the reader will be able to:
- Institution-based rehabilitation and the strategies of institution-based rehabilitation
- Institution-based rehab programs
- Switching from institution-based rehabilitation (IBR) to community-based rehabilitation (CBR)
- Role of community-based rehabilitation
- Approaches of community-based rehabilitation
- Links between IBR and CBR
- Role of physiotherapist as a link between IBR and CBR

■ INTRODUCTION

- ❖ The institution-based rehabilitation also known as the rehabilitation taking place under guided supervision. The care framework in the rehabilitation aims to guide and support the patients at every step, from the homes to their re-entry into the society.
- ❖ This supervision-based treatment protocol undeniably plays a major role in the treatment schedule, period and prognosis of the patient condition.
- ❖ Institutional-based rehabilitation sets the policy and directions with care standards of homes for children and young persons with rehab or disability-related cases. Rehabilitation is acknowledged as an opportunity when self-care, family support arrangement, and community options are not enough.

■ INSTITUTIONAL REHABILITATIVE STRATEGIES

Two key strategies are part of this service.
1. First is the holistic assessment. This strategy assesses the patient in three areas such as education, personal mastery, and socio-emotional development. With the use of the relevant tools, these services objectively and efficiently identify the needs and risk factors of the patient. These set of tools are supervised timely with specific interventions through the creation of individual care plans in every core area that need assessment.
2. The second strategy is the individual family and work. The family members are brought together with the patient to conduct a formal conference. This strategy allows both sides to address their behaviour that needs to be altered to adjust their relationship for the better.

■ INSTITUTIONAL REHABILITATION PROGRAMS

- ❖ This program primarily focuses on essential factors such as therapy, holistic education, personal mastery of habits and self-discipline.
- ❖ In the therapeutic program, the service motivates the patient to rethink everything, assess reasoning, react to sessions and manage relationship building.
- ❖ For the education program, the service provides sessions for restoring self-belief and strengthening the foundation for future learning.
- ❖ The personal mastery of habit focuses on strength and weaknesses. It broadens horizon, adapts to skills, and explore opportunities.
- ❖ And self-discipline manages to evaluate the person's overall capability to adjust to stressful situations.

Switching between the Institution-based Rehabilitation and Community-based Rehabilitation

- ❖ Let's take an example of a stroke patient. An acute stroke patient admitted in the hospital with hemiplegia will be treated in the hospital or we may call it as treating under the institution-based supervised rehabilitation. The treatment may take up to 4 weeks. The condition of the patient improves and the patient should be discharged under home supervision.
- ❖ Sometimes due to certain obligations of the institution or the organisation, or due to the patient himself, he needs to be discharged. If the treatment should continue as part of his rehabilitation, then the institution-based rehabilitation should shift from IBR to CBR.
- ❖ Therefore, this establishes the link and shifts the services from IBR to CBR
- ❖ Although, this program focuses on restoring lives empower transformation and recreate the patient's future. It possesses a multidisciplinary approach.
- ❖ Once the institution-based rehabilitation is over the patient is shifted to community with his existing disabilities.
- ❖ The disabilities are not only physically demolishing but also emotionally draining. Community rehabilitation plays a significant role towards re-establishing the life of its patient back to the society. It provides a safe environment for improvement and a foster care program during the rehabilitation process. The community has to maximize the strength and potential of its patient, not only for himself but also for his families and the community.
- ❖ Therefore, Community-based Rehabilitation is a strategy within community development for the rehabilitation, equalization of opportunities and social integration of all people with disabilities.
- ❖ CBR is implemented through the combined efforts of disabled people themselves, their families and communities and the appropriate health, education, vocational and social services (ILO, WHO 1994).

What is the role of community-based organization?

- ❖ Community-based organizations (CBOs) are not for profit, organizations on a local and national level, facilitating community efforts for community development. The purpose of CBOs is to plan, implement, and monitor social and economic development programs and provide technical and financial help to the communities.
- ❖ Community development approach: There are various approaches to the idea of community development.
- ❖ While some of them focus on the processes taking place in the communities, others focus on the outcomes/objectives.

CHAPTER 7: The Link Between Institution-based Rehabilitation and Community-based Rehabilitation

These approaches include:
- **Community engagement:** This approach is focused on facilitating understanding, exchange of information to build social capital and enhance social outcomes through a decision-making process.
- **Women self-help group:** It is focused on the contribution of women in the community's development.
- **Community capacity building:** It is concerned with helping communities in obtaining, strengthening, and maintaining the ability to set and achieve their own development goals.
- **Large group capacitation:** This approach is related to an adult education and social psychology development. It is aimed at the increase of activity of the large groups of unemployed or semi-employed citizens, often with Lower Levels of Literacy (LLL).
- **Social capital formation:** An approach focused on the cooperation between individuals and large social groups.
- **Nonviolent direct action.** This kind of action is aimed at revealing an existing problem, highlighting an alternative, and demonstrating a possible solution to an existing social problem.

■ LINKS BETWEEN CBR AND IBR

The role of various organizations to link CBR and IBR
- The role of these organizations includes providing a voice of their own, identifying needs, expressing views on priorities, evaluating services and advocating change and public awareness.
- As a vehicle of self-development, these organizations provide the opportunity to develop skills in the negotiation process, organizational abilities, mutual support, information sharing and often vocational skills and opportunities. In view of their vital importance in the process of participation, it is imperative that their development be encouraged.
- It is recognised that NGOs have played a significant role in the development of rehabilitation services for persons with disabilities worldwide. This has been done regularly in the absence of Government involvement and initially took an institutional, charity-based approach.
- Present day developments, however, favour a participatory, community-based approach, complementing and liaising with Government plans and services, and working with all the stakeholders' groups. NGOs and governments vary in their capacity to change their working practices to achieve these aims.
- Organisations for persons with disabilities tend to be focused on specific impairment groups and are charity-based. Their membership often has a common denominator such as:
  - Local community members living in the same geographical areas such as traditional organisations.
  - Religious organisations/associations.
  - Professional membership.
- **Organisations of people with disabilities (PWDs):** Organisations of people with disabilities were also established on the premise of uni-disability, for example, organisations dealing with the blind, the deaf.
- The emergence of organisations of persons with disabilities, is a relatively new development that is timely and in line with a slogan of, "nothing about us without us".

■ GAPS TO BE FILLED BY LOCAL NGOS[3]

Local NGOs have endeavoured to fill up gaps left by governments in promoting participation of the identified stakeholders; to redress issues of access to community-based rehabilitation services for people with disabilities, through various strategies that may include:
- Resource mobilisation
- Community mobilisation and sensitisation
- Community education and training
- Attitude and behaviour change
- Capacity building
- Mechanisms for social economic empowerment
- Research and information dissemination
- Networking, lobbying and advocacy.

Role of physiotherapist as a link between CBR and IBR: Bridging the gap
- A physiotherapist works with a patient in the institution but it is equally important that the PT enables the patient to take care of him/herself in the community. The disabled should be made as much as possible independent to take care of themselves physically, emotionally and socially.
- Patient education and awareness in the field of disability and its effects on home environment are solely the responsibility of a physiotherapist.
- The following programs can be used to by the physiotherapist to know/check whether the patient is complying to the treatment protocol or not:
  - *Home-based exercise program:* A home-based exercise program can be taught to the patient, one family member, or the caretaker to ensure that the rehabilitation continues at home as well. It can be in the form of verbal instructions or a written format whatever the patient is comfortable with.
  - *Maintaining a diary:* A small diary can be asked to fill by the patient or regular checks with dates in the diary to ensure that all days the treatment was followed. The patient can be given the responsibility of ensuring to fill up the diary, this gives a sense of assurance of well-being to the patient.
  - *Hand-written notes/pamphlet:* A common pamphlet in the form one page note for common ailments such as back pain, knee pain in the form of a handout can be helpful to elaborate on the dos and don'ts of certain conditions. Such for knee pain can be given instructions for not to sit cross leg or squat.

As a physiotherapist, it is essential to educate the person with disabilities about the rights and many concessions given to person with disabilities under the government legislature. Therefore, every person with disability should be given the right direction and knowledge about such laws and benefits provided by the government for PWD. A PWD should be empowered socially, physically and emotionally in equality.

CHAPTER 7: The Link Between Institution-based Rehabilitation and Community-based Rehabilitation

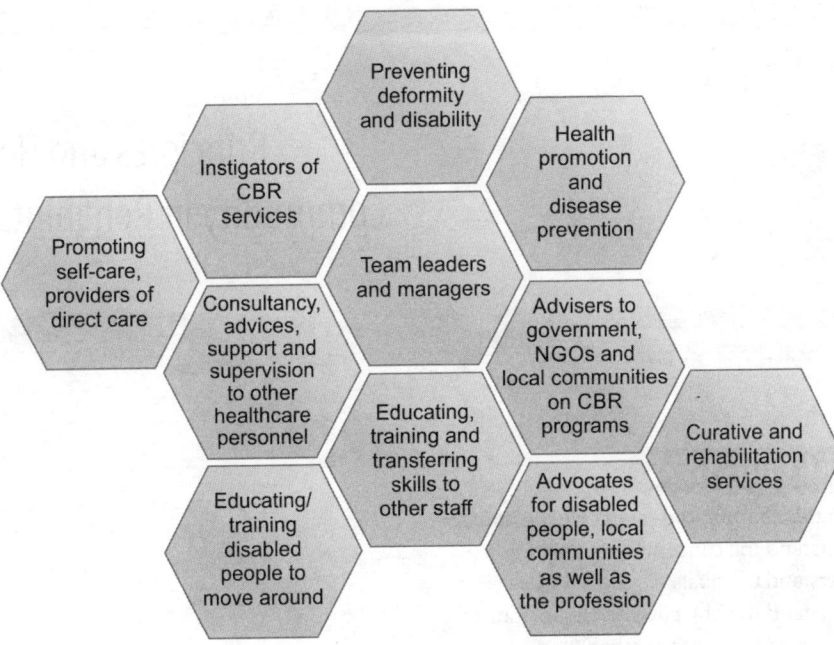

Figure 7.1: Roles of physiotherapists in CBR.

■REFERENCES

1. Khasnabis C, Heinicke Motsch K, Achu K (Eds), et al. Community-Based Rehabilitation: CBR Guidelines. Geneva: World Health Organization; 2010.
2. Frank B. "Who Represents Disabled People?" In 1980 World Congress Plenary Session Papers. Edited by Rehabilitation International, New York: Rehabilitation International; 1980. pp. 13-5.
3. Boyce W, Johnston C. Collaboration in community-based rehabilitation. International Journal of Rehabilitation. 1998;21:1-12.

CHAPTER

Principles and Role of Community in Rehabilitation

Shubhangi Patil

LEARNING OBJECTIVES

Through this chapter, the reader will be able to:
- Understand the concept of rehabilitation
- Understand the goals of rehabilitation
- Understand the objectives of rehabilitation
- Understand the types of rehabilitation
- List the members involved in rehabilitation team
- Understand various approaches for effective rehabilitation
- Discuss principles of rehabilitation
- Understand the role of community in rehabilitation

■ INTRODUCTION

Rehabilitation is an important part of universal health care system which is patient centered, goal directed and aims to promote patients function and quality of life, prevent complications and increase community participation (WHO). Rehabilitation is a problem-solving educational process for promotion of good health, prevention and treatment of diseases and care of terminally ill patients and their families.[1]

Rehabilitation helps everyone to achieve highest level of function in everyday activities and enable participation in education, work, recreation and meaningful life role such as taking care of family. Fundamentally, rehabilitation is based on the principle that every person has the inherent tendency and right to be an expert in their own health care.[2] This indicates the difference between acute care and rehabilitation, where acute care is concerned with an individual's survival, while rehabilitation is concerned with the education and training of individuals to be able to carry out activities of daily living by themselves, thus promoting self-care and functional independence.[3] Rehabilitation in the health system requires strengthening in low and middle income countries so that high quality, affordable services are available to all who need them. Such strengthening will not only ensure respect for human rights but also improve health and provide social and economic benefit.[4] Globally an estimated 2.4 billion people are currently living with a health condition that benefits from rehabilitation. Despite this, currently there is no universal definition or understanding of rehabilitation present. Different authorities used different definitions for rehabilitation.

■ DEFINITION OF REHABILITATION

Rehabilitation is defined as a set of interventions (medical, social, educational and vocational) designed to optimize functioning and reduce disability in individual with health condition in interaction with their environment (WHO). Rehabilitation refers to the action or set of measures taken to assist an individual to restore health who have experienced any trauma or illness that result in an impairment and disability and loss of function (physical, psychological, social and vocational).[1]

The National Cancer Institute (2007) defines rehabilitation is a "process to restore mental and/or physical activities lost due to injury or disease, in order to function in a normal or near normal way".[5]

Examples of rehabilitation:
- Exercises to improve balance and coordination in elderly for prevention of fall
- Training with prosthesis for a person with amputation of lower limb. Rehabilitation is a person-centered approach meaning that the person is placed at the center of services.

The focus of rehabilitation is on the persons abilities, not on their condition or disability. Rehabilitation involves identification of persons problem and needs, relating the problem to relevant factors of the person and the environment, defining rehabilitation goals, planning and implementing the measures and assessing the effect.

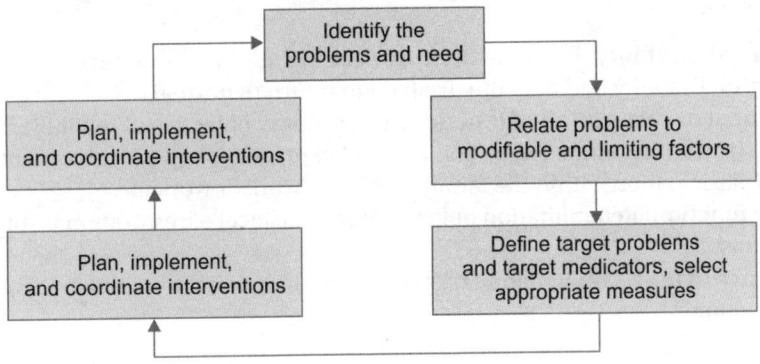

Figure 8.1: Rehabilitation cycle.[6]

■ GOALS OF REHABILITATION

In rehabilitation, interventions and approaches selected for each individual depends on their goals and preferences. Professionals and other personnel involved in the rehabilitation of persons with disabilities may plan and develop rehabilitation programs for individuals based on these essential goals. Habel stated that "rehabilitation goals are the desired outcome for each rehabilitation client. All members of rehabilitation team, although concentrating on a particular area, share similar goals for the client. These include promoting self-care, mobility, maximizing independence, maintaining and restoring functions, preventing complications and restoring functions, preventing complications and encouraging adaptation. **Table 8.1** list the common goals of rehabilitation.[7]

Table 8.1: Common goals of rehabilitation.

- **Self care:** Set of interventions that helps the person with disability to carry out activities of daily living independently
- **Mobility:** Set of interventions that helps the person to move freely
- **Functional independence:** Set of interventions to improve the person's ability to carry out the activities of daily living safely and independently
- **Social participation:** Set of intervention that helps the person with disability to participate in activities that provides interaction with others in society or in the community, e.g., participating in community events or activities
- **Education:** Interventions that helps the disabled person to be independent in their life and enable their participation in education
- **Work:** Interventions that helps the person with disability to maximize their function and work

■ OBJECTIVES OF REHABILITATION

The main aim of rehabilitation is to allow every single person to lead a normal life as far as possible. The objectives of rehabilitation can be achieved by focusing on the improvement of the abilities of the person with disability which subsequently foster the independence of the patient and family or caregiver.

Rehabilitation Objectives

- ❖ **Prevention of disability:** Rehabilitation services includes all those measures that helps in prevention of disability and help the disabled to return to normal
- ❖ **Improvement or restoration of function:** The primary objective of rehabilitation involves restoration (to the maximum degree possible) either of function (physical or mental activities) or of role (participation within the family, social network or work force).
- ❖ **Maximize function:** Rehabilitation helps to maximize level of restoration through different interventions
- ❖ **Maintenance of function:** Rehabilitation helps the individual to maintain his/ her present level of function.

■ TYPES OF REHABILITATION

The various problems encountered by the persons with disabilities are physical, psychological, social and vocational. Rehabilitation measures includes training to increase independence in self-care, educational and vocational measures aimed at achieving economic independence and social measures to ensure full integration and acceptance in community. Rehabilitation can be divided into:

1. Medical Rehabilitation

Medical rehabilitation is defined as the process of complete physical restoration of functions, activities and potentials of a person with disability by using standardized modalities of interventions like therapies, aids and appliances, training, counselling, drug therapy and surgery so that the persons with disabilities are made physically fit for integration into all developmental activities of society. Medical rehabilitation is the process targeted to promote and facilitate the recovery from physical damage, psychological and mental disorders, and clinical disease. The medical rehabilitation involves compulsory assessment of all clinical syndromes and correction with different methods of rehabilitation. Medical rehabilitation should be started from the acute phase of the disease and continue to get maximum results in elimination of physical, psychological and professional disturbances. In medical rehabilitation, complex measures can be carried out in hospitals, policlinic or organisations.[8]

2. Social Rehabilitation

Social rehabilitation offer rehabilitation services to the people with disabilities in order to decrease the impact of disability and promote independence and full participation in society. Social rehabilitation includes:
- The promotion of independence in personal care skills
- Recreational activities
- Family and carer training
- The facilitation of general reintegration into society.

3. Vocational Rehabilitation

Vocational rehabilitation is defined as enabling individuals with either temporary or permanent disability to access, return to, or remain in, employment. This definition is similar to that proposed by the International Labour Organisation and based on the objective: "to enable a disabled person to secure and retain suitable employment" a job". The purpose of vocational rehabilitation program is to empower individuals with disabilities to achieve high quality employment outcomes to which they aspire and that are consistent with their unique strength, resources, priorities, concerns, abilities, capabilities, interests and informed choice. Vocational rehabilitation deals largely with vocational assessment, work re-training, education and counselling, work guidance and ergonomic modifications, and psychosocial interventions (including vocational orientation and all other forms of preparation for returning to work).[9,10]

4. Psychosocial Rehabilitation

The process of rehabilitation is never complete unless the psychosocial aspects are duly taken care of. Psychosocial, social and economic rehabilitation of patients with disabilities are in timely interrelated. Together, they provide the crowning glory to the entire success story of a patient's ultimate rehabilitation. The benefit from such treatment occurs only when it is conceived and planned from the outset with the effect on the patients working capacity and his home life in mind. The likely residual disabilities, their effect on his work/occupation and the need for retraining must be assessed. Illness and injury always induce some anxiety in the patient and relatives, and the response to incapacity depends on the patient's personality, education and social and economic situation. Motivation may be described as the expression of the patient's personality when striving to overcome adversity, and thus, it is also an expression of his response to rehabilitation. Evaluation of the premorbid personality and adequate assessment of the social, educational and economic circumstances are as important in rehabilitation as a realistic delineation of the prognosis and likely functional handicap. Specific psychological problems of patients with disabilities include—depression, anxiety, feeling of insecurity, loneliness, behavioural disorders, affective disorders, personality disorders, suicidal tendencies, dependence, low self-esteem, irritability, impaired psychomotor coordination, malingering and hysteria.

The clinician, besides his role in the diagnosis and cure of patients has to carry out the sacred duty of explaining and reassuring his disabled patient about his disabilities, their effect on his work and its possible solutions. This may not necessarily require the services of a specialized rehabilitation unit or an expert psychiatrist. A little change in the attitude of the treating doctor can easily accomplish this supposedly difficult task. A genuine interest in the patient's welfare is the key to success in this hallowed work.[11] **Table 8.2** shows the overview of different types of rehabilitation.

Table 8.2: Types of rehabilitation.
- Medical rehabilitation means restoration of function.
- Vocational rehabilitation means restoration of the capacity to earn livelihood.
- Social rehabilitation means restoration of family and social relationship.
- Psychosocial rehabilitation means restoration of personal dignity and confidence of the disabled person

THE REHABILITATION TEAM

The rehabilitation team work together with the patient and family to help a person with disability to reach maximum potential.

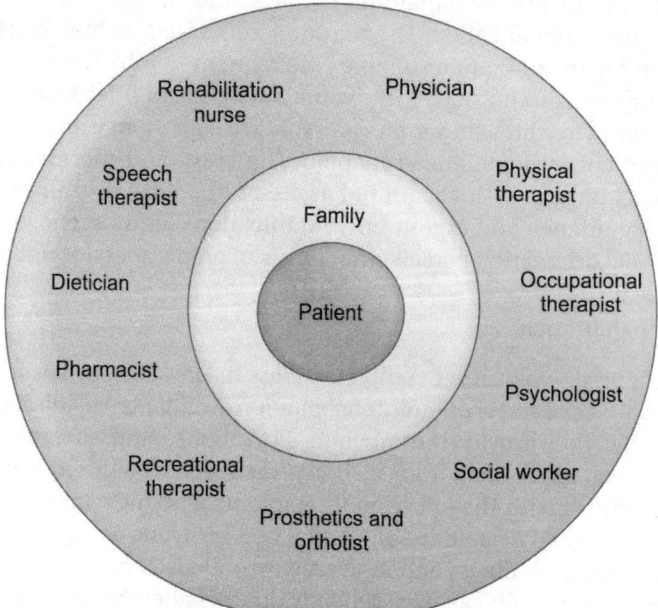

Figure 8.2: Rehabilitation team.

Team Members Role

- **Patient:** The individual accessing rehabilitation services are and always should be a key member of the team throughout each phase of the rehabilitation process. They are key in the development of rehabilitation goals and should always have the opportunity to question the process and direct their rehabilitation needs in order to optimise their function.
- **Family:** Family members, friends and caregivers play an essential role and provide key emotional support to the individual and should be an important and integral part of any rehabilitation program.
- **Physician (psychiatrist or other type of medical doctors):** The doctors who lead the team will decide what diagnostic tests should be done and what treatment should be prescribed
- **Physical therapist:** The physical therapist is primarily involved in helping the client to recover strength, flexibility, endurance and mobility. They also treat the pain and manage conditions such as lymphedema. Many physical therapist specialize in certain type of medical problem such as orthopedic and neurologic.
- **Occupational therapist:** The primary goal of occupational therapy is to help someone to resume doing his or her usual daily activities such as bathing, dressing and even returning to work. Occupational therapists devote considerable efforts to improving the functional use of the arm including helping to improve arm strength, coordination and range of motion. They can also treat pain and some are certified in lymphedema therapy.
- **Speech and language pathologist:** This type of therapist concentrates on problems that have to do with language comprehension or expression as well as swallowing issues.
- **Rehabilitation nurse:** These healthcare specialists are always available in inpatient rehabilitation settings but often work in outpatient settings as well. Rehabilitation nurses perform all of the usual nursing functions but also focus on helping patients with bowel and bladder function, sexuality issues, and providing education and support for the family. Rehabilitation nurses can also help people to regain the ability to move, speak and swallow by reinforcing what the therapy team is working on.
- **Vocational rehabilitation specialist:** This professional evaluates whether someone can return to work and if so how best to accomplish this. This may involve the use of special equipment such as a one-handed computer keyboard. If it is necessary for the cancer survivor to work in an entirely new occupation, vocational retraining may be offered
- **Therapeutic recreational therapist:** These therapists are not always found in rehabilitation settings, but many hospitals have at least one therapeutic recreational therapist on staff. This specialist helps people to embrace leisure and educational activities that are part of having a good quality of life. These activities may include cooking, gardening and playing sports.
- **Dietician:** A registered dietician helps to figure out the best diet for someone going through cancer treatment and/or rehabilitation. A dietician can offer guidance as to how to gain or lose weight and improve energy through nutrition
- **Orthotist:** This is a professional who has training in how to fit and make braces. Braces are sometimes necessary for people who have some weakness or paralysis.
- **Prosthetist:** This is a rehabilitation professional who is an expert at making and fitting artificial limbs—usually after an amputation.

Approaches to rehabilitation: There are two main approaches to carry out rehabilitation and these are as follows:
- Institution-based rehabilitation
- Community-based rehabilitation
- Outreach program for rehabilitation

Institutional-based rehabilitation: Institutional Rehabilitation (IBR) provides excellent services in hospital for people with disabilities (PWDs). It is usually available only for a small number at a very high cost and located in urban centres. In institutional-based rehabilitation, patients receive treatment for short-term and the treatment usually starts from the acute phase of disease.

Moreover, an attempt to rehabilitation of disabled in an institution, is often different from the felt needs of the disabled person, and thus falls short of their expectations.

In an institutional rehabilitation program, the community is not linked with the process. Hence, when the disabled person returns home, it may become difficult for them to integrate into their community. Institutional services, including medical and vocational rehabilitation centres, residential homes, special schools with therapy and nursing care, sheltered workshops and day centres have formed the backbone of rehabilitation services in developed countries.

Rehabilitation in institution can provide a basic care service but it is little effective in providing psychological, social, educational or vocational rehabilitation. Governmental organisations provide some economic support to rehabilitation institutions in the private sector, they cannot afford to build or finance rehabilitation institutions for all the disabled in need of rehabilitation or long-term care. Along with acute medical rehabilitation, long-term therapy, accommodation, education, vocational training and employment are the most critical for the successful integration of people with disabilities. In developed countries long term institutional care is now widely seen in a very negative light.[12]

Studies done by Miller and Gwynne (1974), Shearer (1981), and many others highlight the risks of institutionalisation such as dependency, boredom and under-achievement, low self-esteem, stigmatisation and loneliness. In many developing countries it is commonly believed that institutions can provide better services than can home care, because they have specialist staff, specialised facilities and equipment, special education or vocational training on the premises which is lacking in rural areas or in community-based rehabilitation.[13]

Institutional-based rehabilitation also removes the burden of responsibility and the stigma of disability from the family, particularly among less educated, poor, rural families where the disability can be an intolerable economic burden to the family, and the cause of severe social and family problems because of the widespread stigma attached to disability and suspicion as to its causes (WHO, 1984). But the reason behind the failure of institutional based rehabilitation is that it separates the disabled person from the family, community and normal home environment. Institutional-based rehabilitation removes responsibility of family and community for the disabled person and the development of understanding of the disabled person's needs and of her/his capacity to contribute to society.[14]

Institutions do not play any role for reduction of cultural fears and beliefs about disability. Institutional rehabilitation do not create a climate of acceptance for the disabled person's return to community and the family learns to live without the disabled person. Removal from the family also reduces the chances of the disabled people themselves learning to cope with their disability. In short, long-term institutional care is probably the worst possible strategy for promoting integration of the disabled into their communities. And for this reason, the demand for community-based rehabilitation is continuously growing.

Table 8.3: Advantages and disadvantages of IBR.[15]

Advantages	Disadvantages
Skilled person available	Cost of care is expensive
Application of advanced techniques are possible	Only few institutions are accessible to all
Good quality of service	Extension of services are not possible
Evaluation is possible	Social rehabilitation is not possible as the patient is away from the family
Research program can be carried out	Psychological rehabilitation is not much possible
Complicated problems are easy to tackle	Active participation is not possible
Service providers are decision maker	Socioeconomic status is not considered
Statistics can be generated	Promotion of awareness is not possible
Rare conditions can be treated	Community interaction is not possible
Excellent infrastructure available	No follow up when the patients are discharged
	Delayed intervention

■ COMMUNITY-BASED APPROACH

Community-based rehabilitation (CBR) is the main way in which disabled people in most of the world have any chance of accessing rehabilitation services.[16] CBR was first promoted by WHO in the mid-1970s to address the shortage of rehabilitation assistance by providing services in the community with use of local resources.[17] The strategy drew on the principles of primary health care, accepted international rehabilitation practices of the time, and also existing local practices.[18]

Community based rehabilitation is a community action to ensure that the people with disability have the same rights and opportunities as all other community members. This includes for example equal access to health care, education, skill training, employment, family life, social mobility and political empowerment. Community Based Rehabilitation (CBR) is an accepted model to improve the delivery of rehabilitation in the community.

Definition of CBR

CBR was initiated by WHO following the declarations of Amla Ata in 1978 in an effort to enhance the quality of life for peoples with disabilities and their families, meet their basic needs and ensure their inclusion and participation in community.[19]

Over the decades, development of CBR has been influenced by concerns of disabled people at the community level and by disabled people's organisations. These concerns have contributed importantly to the evolution of the CBR concept and resulted in increased recognition of discrimination and exclusion and the need to address social and political aspects of disability. As a result, the medically oriented individualised model, on which CBR was originally based, has expanded and now includes socially oriented rights-based approaches. This process of change caused confusion over the definition of CBR but in 2004 it was clarified as **"a strategy within general community development for rehabilitation, equalization of opportunities, and social inclusion of all people with disabilities implemented through the combined** efforts of people with disabilities themselves, their families and communities, and the appropriate health, education, vocational, and social services".[20]

Objectives of CBR

The objectives of CBR are not only to maximize physical and mental ability but also to support access to regular services and opportunities, and to assist people with disabilities to become active contributors to the community and society at large as well as encouraging communities to promote and protect the human rights of people with disabilities through changes within the community, for example, by removing barriers to participation.

Components of CBR

- Creation of positive attitude towards people with disabilities
- Provision of rehabilitation services
- Provision of education and training opportunities
- Creation of micro and macro income generating opportunities
- Provision of long-term care facilities
- Prevention of cause of disabilities
- Monitoring and evaluation.

Principles of Community-based Rehabilitation[21]

- **Inclusion:** Inclusion means the removal of all kinds of barriers which block people with disabilities from access to the mainstream. Inclusion means placing disability issues and people with disabilities in the mainstream of activities, rather than as an after-thought or 'bolt-on'. Inclusion also means 'convergence' – that is, the involvement of people with disabilities in the campaigns, struggles and activities of other oppressed groups which are not centred exclusively on disability issues, such as children living on the streets, farmers, land rights and environment, women's groups. It means including all forms of impairment and disability such as physical, sensory, communicative, mental health and illness, and intellectual and developmental disabilities. It also includes rehabilitation of young people particularly children, their care and protection from violence and abuse and it includes older people and their care and protection from abuse too. It means the inclusion of those groups in society who are traditionally excluded and discriminated against such as women, people with multiple and severe disabilities, people of particular religious beliefs, ethnic, caste or community background, refugees, and people who are HIV+ or have AIDS. It also includes people with disabilities living in extreme poverty, and people suffering from conflict and war and its aftermath. Inclusion also means access, that is, the removal of any barriers which disable people encounter. These barriers can be environmental, physical or technological, social or cultural.
- **Participation:** Participation means the involvement of disabled people as active contributors to the CBR program from policy making to implementation and evaluation. Participation also means people with disability being a critical resource within any CBR program for providing training, making decisions etc. It covers the participation of women in all processes and decision-making and that of other groups who are typically not listened to or excluded. Likewise children and young adults can and should be part of the processes and decision-making.

- **Sustainability:** Firstly, the benefits of the program must be long lasting. Secondly, the CBR activity must be sustainable beyond the immediate life of the program itself. Strong links between government organizations, NGOs, community-based/development organizations and disabled peoples organizations will contribute towards sustainability. This means that disabled people's organizations and self-help groups are the hub of any CBR activity.
- **Empowerment**: Empowerment means that local people and specifically people with disabilities and their families make the program decisions and control the resources. It means people with disability taking leadership roles within programs. It means CBR workers, service providers and facilitators are people with disabilities and all are adequately trained and supported. The empowerment of women is central to any program. Empowerment necessitates capacity building that is, the developing and using of the skills necessary to act with authority and responsibility, independent of the initiating agencies and CBR program managers. The skills of CBR workers and their managers are crucial too. They need to be empowered by ensuring they have a range and depth of skill appropriate to the complexities of the work. Their training should include an understanding of the causes and effects of poverty and the contribution the CBR program can make to poverty alleviation.
- **Self-advocacy:** Self-advocacy means the central and consistent involvement of people with disabilities defining for themselves the goals and processes for poverty alleviation. Family members will also play a key role. Self-advocacy is a collective notion, not an individualistic one. It means self-determination. It means mobilizing, organising, representing, creating space for interaction and demands.

Table 8.4: Advantages and disadvantages of CBR.[22]

Advantages	Disadvantages
Cost of treatment is cheap and affordable	Improper care due to lack of specialized trainee
Accessible to all	Application of advanced techniques are not possible
Social rehabilitation is possible as the patient is with family	Good quality of service is not available
Psychological rehabilitation is possible as they have full family support	Difficulties with evaluation
Extension of services are possible	Research program cannot be carried out
Active participation is possible	Complicated problems are difficult to tackle
Community interaction and empowerment is possible	Statistics cannot be generated
Wide use of local resources	Rare conditions cannot be treated
Family and PWD are decision makers	
Guarenteed follow up	
Early intervention	
Promotion of awareness is possible	

Multisectoral Support of CBR

The goal of CBR is to contribute towards the empowerment of persons with disabilities, facilitating an independent lifestyle in which they participate in all aspects of community life.

Multisectoral collaboration is therefore imperative if such a goal is to be achieved, as no one sector alone, can achieve such a broad objective. The breadth of the challenge necessitates a partnership between all the various sectors, i.e., social sector, health sector, education, labour, vocational, housing, welfare, sports and agriculture sector in collaboration with NGOs, Disabled Peoples Organisations (DPOs), and the traditional and religious leaders within the community.

1. Support from Social Sector

Although the allocation of responsibility for social affairs varies from country to country, matters commonly addressed include disability pensions, technical aids and adaptations, housing, vocational training and employment and coordination of referrals for individuals who require services from other sectors. If the social affairs ministry initiates CBR, social welfare officers may be managers of the program. A ministry for social affairs may not have personnel at local level, but it is common that personnel posted at district/intermediate level are familiar with social and economic conditions and knowledgeable about resources within the district/intermediate level including those in the non-governmental sector. This information is very useful in a CBR program, particularly for identifying vocational skills training and work opportunities for women and men with disabilities. Personnel from the social affairs ministry can advise individuals with disabilities and family members as well as personnel from other ministries regarding community resources.

2. Support from NGOs and Local Community

Most communities have a variety of non-governmental organizations (NGOs) and groups that can contribute to a CBR program. These may include relief and development organizations, faith-based organizations, and service clubs as well as women's and youth groups. Some of these may provide services to people with disabilities, while others can make special efforts to include them in their activities. In the framework of governmental policy, national and international NGOs can also make significant contributions to the development of CBR, by initiating programs in local communities and then scaling it up, by training CBR program managers and other personnel, and by helping to strengthen the services within the various sectors that contribute to CBR.

3. Support from Health Sector

The Declaration of Alma Ata (1978) states that Primary Health Care (PHC) is the key to attaining health for all. It also states that PHC needs to address the main health problems in the community, providing promotive, preventive, curative and rehabilitative services. The health care system is usually responsible for providing medical care and rehabilitation services including assistive devices. Most basic rehabilitation activities can be carried out in the disabled person's own community using local resources. PHC can play a major role in this context both as a provider and supporter. Many people with disabilities need to be referred to specialised rehabilitation services outside their own communities. PHC personnel can facilitate links between people with disabilities and specialised services such as physical, occupational and speech therapies; prosthetics and orthotics and corrective surgeries. PHC also supports CBR activities. At community level, there are usually no specialised personnel in either health or rehabilitation. Therefore, PHC personnel are responsible for carrying out the early identification of impairments and providing basic interventions for people with disabilities. In addition, they can transfer basic knowledge and skills in rehabilitation to the community, especially to CBR workers.

The health sector needs to make serious efforts to ensure that rehabilitation is part of PHC and to provide training to PHC personnel on disability and rehabilitation. The health sector can also strengthen specialised services so that they are a better support to PHC personnel and CBR workers. To be most effective, the rehabilitation services must collaborate with all the other services within the health care system.

4. Support from Educational Sector

Good cooperation between communities and the education sector is imperative if the goals of Education for All are to be met. With more than 90 per cent of children with disabilities in developing countries not attending school. It is evident that steps must be taken to ensure access to education for all of these children. The community school plays a central role in this work.

The educational sector can make an important contribution to CBR by assisting community schools within the regular school system to become more inclusive. Schools may require assistance to change their methods of teaching in order to provide quality education for all children. Within the school system there are many people with knowledge and skills that could be shared with community schools. For example, there are schools that teach only children with special needs and the teachers from those schools can serve as resources to teachers in community schools. Schools that are already inclusive can help other schools learn how to respond to the needs of all learners, treat all children with respect, and be model schools.

The regular school system must take responsibility for the education of all school-aged children. Children with multiple or severe disabilities who require extensive additional support may be taught within special units, depending on the existing level of external support being provided. Special schools are important partners in the school system and may be used as a resource for regular schools in promoting inclusive education.

To promote Education for All, the educational sector should adapt the initial and in-service training of both regular and specialised teachers in response to the new roles in the inclusive school, as well as ensure that classrooms, facilities and educational materials are accessible. The education sector must take responsibility for the quality of education and for the educational assessment of children with disabilities. It must be emphasised that children with disabilities should not be treated as sick children. Their needs and aspirations are the same as those of all children.

5. Support from the Employment and Labor Sector

Productive and decent work is essential for the social and economic integration of individual women and men with disabilities. A gainful livelihood provides an individual with income, self-esteem and a sense of belonging and a chance to contribute to the larger community. Collaboration between a CBR program and the employment and labour sectors is essential to ensure that both youth and adults with disabilities have access to training and work opportunities at community level. The employment and labour sectors promote vocational training, employment and good working conditions. Ministries responsible for vocational training, employment, labour as well as social services can facilitate social and economic integration by providing vocational rehabilitation services, vocational guidance and skills training through both mainstream training institutions and through specialised training centres and programs. The employment and labour sectors encourage equal employment opportunities through national policies and legislation. Employment services organized by the sector help job seekers with disabilities to find employment opportunities in the open labour market. In addition, the civil service can set a good example by employing workers with disabilities.

At community level, informal apprenticeships with master trainers or local businesses can provide individuals with disabilities opportunities to learn employable skills and gain practical experience. The business community can provide valuable support to CBR by providing on-the-job training, hiring workers with disabilities, mentoring entrepreneurs with disabilities and providing advice on current and emerging skills requirements to vocational training centres. Micro and small enterprise development programs can provide business skills training and advisory services. They can provide access to credit to assist women and men, including people with disabilities, to start their own businesses and become self-employed. Such programs are often operated by the ministry responsible for trade and industry or by a separate government agency, as well as by NGOs. Special efforts are often required by a CBR program to ensure the inclusion of youth and adults with disabilities in such programs.

6. Support from the Media

Newspapers, radio, television and the internet can provide the public with information about disability issues, and also present a positive image of individuals with disabilities at school, work or in social settings. All CBR stakeholders should work closely with the media to identify priorities and to provide relevant information.

■ OUTREACH PROGRAM FOR REHABILITATION

This is one in which the professionals in the rehabilitation field provide services to people with disabilities, who visit the community or the homes of people with disabilities. The purpose of the community outreach campaign is to provide professional, compassionate, interdisciplinary health services to the underserved at their door step. Outreach services will play an important role in systematically delivering various benefits of health services to those who need them the most and find it difficult to access the center based services. Outreach services mainly target the rural population and slum dwellers and other vulnerable groups in towns and cities. Advice is given on how to improve in specific activities such as self-care, moving around or communication. The outreach services could either form an extension of the institution to the neighbouring area or by organising camps in the neighbouring area from time to time.[23]

■ PRINCIPLES OF REHABILITATION

There are several principles of rehabilitation, some are general principles which reflects the general approaches and there are specific ones that explain the underlying mechanism of recovery. Mauk (2012) outlined the following principles of rehabilitation.

- ❖ **Promote adaptation, not just recovery:** Recovery of functions impaired by disability or injury can only be completed to the maximum extent by simultaneously creating an environment for adaptation. In fact the prime aim of rehabilitation is to help the individual to adapt to the day-to-day demands of life, which at times require a change in the life-style of the client. Therefore, it is important for the rehabilitation professionals to prepare the client for this change. People with developmental disabilities often would not be able to return to a normal level like that of their normal counterparts. The client and family member must accept this, instead of nurturing false hopes for normalcy. In case of acquired disability, however the focus is primarily on adaptation to the life altering situation. Expressed emotion such as anxiety, depression or anger of the family member because of the disability often complicate the process of rehabilitation. Hence, they should be taught to manage them effectively.
- ❖ **Emphasising ability:** This is one of the key principles of rehabilitation. Most people with disabilities whether due to a traumatic incident and those acquired during childhood might have disabilities in certain areas of functioning whereas other areas of functioning may remain intact. For instance, a person having locomotor disability may have his speech and intellectual

functions intact. Rehabilitation professionals should train these people in developing these functions to the fullest extent and make maximum use of them to compensate the functions affected by disease or disability. This may give the client a sense of accomplishment.

- ❖ **Treat the client as a whole person:** In rehabilitation we treat a person and not a 'disease'. The person with disability should be treated as a holistic being. Denial and non-acceptance of limitations cause anger and depression in the client. Unconditional regard for the individual with disability plays a crucial role in enhancing psychological well-being of such clients. Attempt should be made to enhance a sense of self-efficacy in people with disability. It restores confidence and determination in overcoming many obstacles both physical and psychological.
- ❖ **Disability affects the entire family:** Disability in a member in any family affects the entire family, as the trauma, physical cost and psychological burden is shared by all members of the family. This is not only because of close interpersonal ties between the family members but also due to demand for their involvement in care of the person with disability. Hence, in a way treating a person with disability is also like treating his family members as well. Hence, time should be spent with the family members in listening to them and advising them and helping them to overcome their negative overwhelming emotional feelings and bolster their abilities to cope with such family stresses effectively.

ROLE OF COMMUNITY IN REHABILITATION

Community means a group of people with common interests who interact with each other on a regular basis; and/or a geographical, social or government administrative unit. According to E Helander (1992): "A community consists of people living together in some form of social organization and cohesion. Its members share in varying degrees political, economic, social and cultural characteristics, as well as interests and aspirations, including health. Communities vary widely in size and socioeconomic profile, ranging from clusters of isolated homesteads to more organized villages, towns and city districts."[24]

In rehabilitation, community is considered as "Disabled people, their families and the organisations working for the disabled. However, the effectiveness of rehabilitation and the long-term development and sustainability of any rehabilitation program will require the coordination, involvement and collaboration of all community members. The community members and their suggested roles are as follows:

- ❖ **People with disabilities:** People with disabilities can and should contribute to all levels of rehabilitation programs in every position within a program. They know what the effects of local conditions are on themselves. They are likely to have a good understanding of those effects on their peers with disabilities. They also know what impairment really means in the context of their family, community and nation. This knowledge enables them to be very effective members of a rehabilitation team. They can be more effective than nondisabled people as role models for and counsellors of other people with disabilities. People with disabilities have an important role in community education. As community educators, they serve as living examples of people with disabilities who make a significant contribution, provided that they are given the opportunity and the right type of assistance.
- ❖ **Families of people with disabilities:** Families have the primary responsibility for caring for all of their members. They are the first line of support and assistance for people with disabilities at the local level. As such, families must be included in rehabilitation program activities. Where the individual with a disability is not able, for whatever reason, to speak for himself or herself, a family member should represent him or her and should be considered a

legitimate member of disabled people's organizations. Members of families with experience in caring for people with disabilities are the people who most often initiate rehabilitation and are, or prove to be, the most effective contributors at all levels.

- **Communities:** Community members should be involved in rehabilitation programs at all levels because they already know the local environmental conditions, the local economy, the local political situation and how to work with them. They also know about the accessibility, availability and effectiveness of locally available rehabilitation services; who in the community cares enough about other people to become a program leader or worker; and, which community members have the knowledge and skills for training others in microeconomic activities. They are the people most likely to want to live, work and stay in the community. Community involvement usually requires the agreement and approval, both formal and informal, of the community leaders.
- **Governments (local, regional, national):** Governments have the most important role in the development and sustainability of rehabilitation programs. Their cooperation, support and involvement are essential if rehabilitation is to cover the total population and be sustainable. They should implement and coordinate the development of the entire program structure, including the development of the referral system, as well as the activities within the community. They also should provide resources for non-governmental organizations (NGOs) and community activities. Finally, they should ensure that discriminatory legislation is changed and that the rights of people with disabilities are guaranteed and protected.
- **Non-governmental organizations, local, regional, national and international organizations:** NGOs, including organizations of people with disabilities are often able to provide resources and skills to facilitate the development of new programs, especially in areas where none exist. They can develop new approaches to rehabilitation and provide training programs for government employees, rehabilitation workers, people with disabilities, families, and community members. NGOs are effective in facilitating the development of community members as rehabilitation program leaders. They are often best able to provide long-term care facilities for those people with extensive disabilities whose families cannot or will not look after them.
- **Medical professionals, allied health science professionals, educators, social scientists and other professionals:** Professionals are often in a position where they can, as trainers and educators, facilitate the development of new programs by making their knowledge and skills accessible to community members and rehabilitation program workers. They can also ensure that they support community efforts by making themselves available and accessible on a referral basis. When they are in government service, they can advocate and promote the development of rehabilitation programs as an effective way to provide local-level services quickly.
- **The private sector (business and industry):** The private sector has a social obligation to return some of the benefits of its operations to the communities that support it.

■ SUMMARY

Rehabilitation is the process of helping an individual to achieve the highest level of function, independence and quality of life possible. Rehabilitation does not reverse or undo the damage caused by disease or trauma, but rather helps to restore the individual to optimal health, functioning and well-being. The goals of rehabilitation program varies from person to person and these are self-care, mobility, functional independence, social participation, education and work. The main objectives in rehabilitation are prevention of disability or maximum reduction or elimination of disability and training the disabled person with residual abilities to achieve independent living. The team members involved in rehabilitation team are patient and family, physician, physical therapist, occupational therapist, psychologist, social worker, prosthetist and orthotist, recreational therapist, pharmacist, dietician, speech therapist and rehabilitation nurse. Rehabilitation can be divided into medical rehabilitation, vocational rehabilitation, social rehabilitation and psychosocial rehabilitation. The major strategies for carrying out rehabilitation programs are institutional-based rehabilitation, community-based rehabilitation.

■ REFERENCES

1. World Health Organization International classification of functioning, disability, and health. Geneva, World Health Organization; 2001.
2. Gender AR. Scope of rehabilitation and rehabilitation nursing. Rehabilitation nursing practice. New York: McGraw-Hills; 1996.
3. Mauk KL. Overview of rehabilitation. Rehabilitation nursing. A contemporary approach to practice; 2011.
4. World Health Organization. World Report on Disability 2011. Geneva: World Health Organization; 2011.
5. National Cancer Institute. Rehabilitation. 2002. Available at: https://www.cancer.gov.
6. Ona ED, Baeza P, Jardon H A, Balaguer C. Review of Automated systems for Upper Limb Functional Assessment in Neurorehabilitation. IEEE Access. 2019 Feb 26; pp 1-1.
7. Habel M. Rehabilitation: Philosophy, goals and process. In: McCourt AE (Ed); 1993.
8. Conti AA. Western Medical Rehabilitation through Time: A Historical and Epistemological Review. Sci World J [Internet]. 2014.
9. Gobelet C, Franchignoni F. Vocational Rehabilitation. Springer Science and Business Media; 2006. p. 404.
10. International Labour Organization. Vocational rehabilitation and employment of disabled persons. International Labour Conference, 86th Session. ILO: Geneva; 1998.
11. Delisa JA. DeLisas-Physical Medicine and Rehabilitation: Principles and Practice, 5th edition, Lippincott Publisher, Philadelphia; 1998.
12. Jackson H. Approaches to rehabilitation of people with disabilities: A review. Journal of Social Development in Africa. 1988;3(1):39-53.
13. Miller EJ, Gwynne GV. A Life Apart, Tavistock, London; 1974.
14. WHO. "Rehabilitation For All", in World Health Magazine, WHO, Geneva; 1984.
15. Sunder S. Textbook of Rehabilitation. New Delhi: Jaypee Brothers Medical Publishers; 2020.
16. Evans PJ, Zinkin P, Harpham T, Chaudury G. Evaluation of medical rehabilitation in community-based rehabilitation. Soc Sci Med. 2001;53:333-4.
17. Helander E, Mendis P, Nelson G. Training disabled people in the community: an experimental manual on rehabilitation for developing countries. WHO, Geneva; 1980.
18. Hartley S, Finkenflugel H, Kuipers P, Thomas M. Community-based rehabilitation: opportunity and challenge. The Lancet. 2009;374(9704):1803-4.
19. Khasnabis C, Heinicke Motsch K, Achu K, et al. Community-based Rehabilitation. CBR Guidelines. Geneva: World Health Organization; 2010.
20. ILO, UNESCO, and WHO. CBR A strategy for rehabilitation, equalization of opportunities, poverty reduction and social inclusion of people with disabilities. Joint Position Paper; 2004.
21. Velema JP, Cornielje H. Backbone principles of the CBR guidelines and their application in the field of leprosy. Asia Pacific Disability Rehabilitation Journal. Volume 21 (1).
22. Goel S. An Introduction to Community-based Rehabilitation Continuing Medical Education. Internet J Health. 2006;6(2).
23. Outreach_sessions_in_Urban _Areas. pdf
24. Helander E. Prejudice and Dignity. An Introduction to Community-based Rehabilitation. UNDP New York, 1992, 2nd edition; 1999.

CHAPTER 9

Evidence Based in Community Physiotherapy

Shrikant Bhimrao Darade

LEARNING OBJECTIVES

Through this chapter, the reader will be able to:
- What is evidence-based practice?
- Definitions of evidence-based medicine, evidence-based practice and evidence-based physiotherapy.
- Discuss the circumstances that have resulted in an increased emphasis on the employment of evidence in practice.
- Discuss the employment of evidence for physiotherapist decision-making
- Describe the different steps involved in evidence based in community physiotherapy
- Discuss the barriers to evidence based in community physiotherapy and possible strategies

■ INTRODUCTION

Evidence-based physiotherapy (EBP) is an emerging and increasing theme in rehabilitation and physiotherapy. Although it is increasingly used worldwide, a definite and appropriate definition has not been agreed on among clinicians and researchers. The World Confederation for Physical Therapy (WCPT) has defined EBP as "a commitment to use the foremost available evidence to inform decision-making about the care of individuals that involves integrating physiotherapist practitioners and individual professional judgement with evidence gained through systematic research."[1,2] Evidence-based practice (EBP), which originates from evidence-based medicine, has been described as 'the conscientious, explicit, and judicious use of current best evidence in making decisions about the care of individual patients. Evidence-based practice (EBP) includes integration of best available research, clinical expertise, and patient values and circumstances associated with patient and client management, practice management, and health policy decision-making.[3]

"Evidence-based practice" and "evidence-based health care" are labels that are created to link the behavior described by evidence-based medicine to other health care professionals. According Hicks point of view, he expanded definition—"care that 'takes place when decisions that affect the care of patients with due weight accorded to any or all valid, relevant information".[4] As per above said definitions, evidence does not replace clinical expertise rather, evidence is employed to tell more fully to call decision-making process within which expertise provides one perspective to the clinical problem.

Evidence-based practice in community physiotherapy is defined by Strauss et al., 2000 and Cimoli et al., 2012, the application and integration of the foremost available research evidence with clinical expertise and patient values by health care professionals delivering healthcare services **(Fig. 9.1)**.

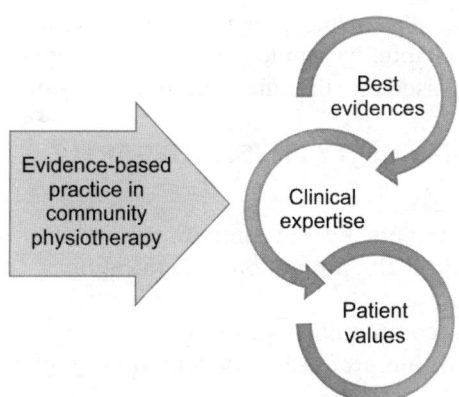

Figure 9.1: EBP in community physiotherapy.

EBP approach can result in enhanced quality of whole health care. That is important to professional development of physiotherapists. Within the due recent times, the Physiotherapy profession has been undergoing a period of change as a results of pressure from different health care provider groups. So as to fufill these challenges Physiotherapists (PTs) are encouraged to prove the effectiveness of their interventions through scientific evidence referred as evidence-based practice.[5,6]

The World Confederation for Physical Therapy (WCPT) believes that, Physiotherapist have a responsibility to make sure that the management of patients/clients, carers and communities is relied on the foremost available evidence. They even have a responsibility to not use techniques and technologies are shown to be ineffective or unsafe. Here EBP in community is an "open and thoughtful clinical decision-making" about physiotherapy management of patient at community level which integrates the "best available evidence with clinical judgments" and the patient preferences and values, and that further consider the larger social context in within which physiotherapy services are provided[7] **(Fig. 9.2)**.

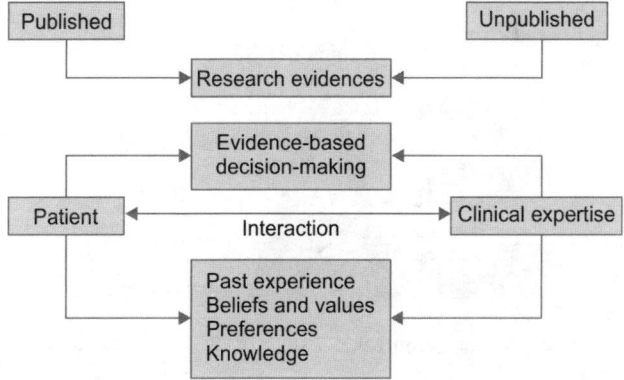

Figure 9.2: EBP in community physiotherapy in social context.
(*Source:* Bury T, Mead J. Evidence Based Healthcare: A practical guide for therapist; 1999).

Currently EBP dose not remain a component of the curriculum in many universities, but it is a part of few universities of Maharashtra and Gujarat in undergraduate and postgraduate courses. In accordance with Glasziou recommended that, EBP training should be introduced early, and embedded and applied throughout entry-level training.[8,9]

Hence the through this chapter we would like to define, increase emphasis, steps, barriers and strategies of evidence-based practice inn community physiotherapy.

■ GOALS OF EBP IN COMMUNITY PHYSIOTHERAPY[7,9]

- ❖ To create supportive ideas
- ❖ To build new principles and practices in community
- ❖ Help and assist to provide health promotion and education
- ❖ To provide health delivery service
- ❖ To build wellness among community population
- ❖ Promote collaboration within profession and with other profession at local, national and international levels
- ❖ Provide evidence-based data to practicing community physiotherapist
- ❖ Resolves the patient problems in the clinical settings and at community levels
- ❖ Assists with efficient and effective decision-making
- ❖ Reduces variation in physiotherapy care
- ❖ Using best evidence to implement the regulation of physiotherapist
- ❖ To introduce innovation
- ❖ Achieve the excellence in the field of community physiotherapy.

■ STEPS IN EVIDENCE-BASED COMMUNITY PHYSIOTHERAPY

According to Sackett et al.,[10] originally described the fundamental principles and the 5 steps of evidence-based practice follows **(Fig. 9.3)**:
1. **Ask:** Formulate a research question
2. **Acquire:** Knowledge related to search engines/databases, literature search
3. **Appraise:** Inclusion of levels/hierarchy of evidence and statistical methods, types of study designs, validity and reliability and tools of critical appraisal
4. **Apply:** Application of evidence in clinical decision making
5. **Assess:** How the previous four steps were performed?

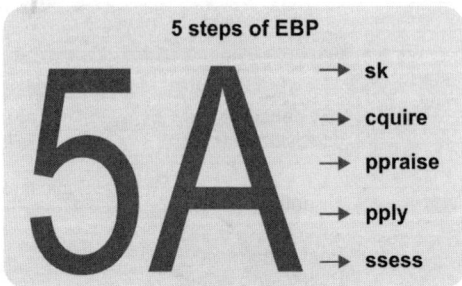

Figure 9.3: 7 steps of EBP.

Recently few research shows that evidence-based practice (EBP) provides higher quality care, improves patients outcome, reduced costs, and satisfaction among nurses than traditional approaches to care.[11-15]

According to Melnyk el al., (2010), explained the 7 steps of evidence-based practices **(Fig. 9.4)** as follows:

Step 0—Cultivate a spirit of inquiry
Start to ask question which lay the groundwork for EBP, e.g., in patients with head injuries, how does supine positioning compared with elevating the head of the bed 30 degrees affect intracranial pressure? Without this spirit of inquiry, the next step in EBP process are not likely happen.

Step 1 – Ask clinical Questions in PICOT format
P – Population of interest
I – Intervention or area of interest
C – Comparison of intervention or group
O – Outcome
T – Time
This format provides an efficient framework for searching data.

Step 2 – Search the best evidence
Search for evidence to inform clinical practice is tremendously streamlined when questions are in PICOT format.

The hierarchy of evidence may be useful:
1. Systemic reviews
2. Meta-analysis
3. RCTs
4. Cohort studies
5. Others

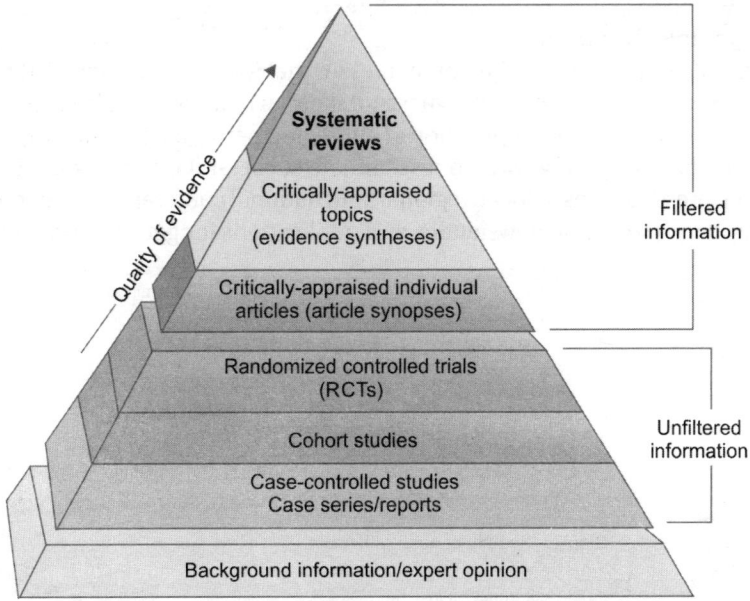

Figure 9.4: Pyramid for quality of evidence.

These are the evidences which acquire from internet, textbooks, journals, medline, Cochrane library, pubmed, PEDro, etc., are used in clinical practices or at community level to make decision.

Step 3 – Critically appraise the evidence

Once the articles selected for review, they must be rapidly appraised to determine which are most relevant, valid, reliable and applicable to clinical question.

There are three most important questions which evaluates the study,
1. Are the results of study valid?
2. What are the results and are they important?
3. Will the results are helpful to take care for my patient?

Step 4 – Integrate the evidence with clinical expertise and patient preferences and values

Research evidence alone is not sufficient to justify a change in practice. Clinical expertise, based on patient assessments, laboratory data, and data from outcomes management programs, as well as patients' preferences and values are important components of EBP. There is no magic formula for how to weigh each of these elements; implementation of EBP is highly influenced by institutional and clinical variables. For example, say there is a strong body of evidence showing reduced incidence of depression in burn patients where they received eight sessions of cognitive-behavioral therapy prior to hospital discharge. You want your patients also to have this therapy and so do they. But due to budget constraints at your hospital, it prevent to hiring a therapist to offer the treatment.

Step 5 - Evaluate the outcomes of practice decision or changes based on evidence

After implementing EBP in community, it is important to monitor and re-evaluate any changes in outcomes so that positive effects can be supported and negative ones remedied. Just because of an intervention was effective in a rigorously controlled trial does not mean that, it will work exactly the same way in the clinical setting. Monitoring the effect of an EBP change on health care quality and outcomes can help clinician's spot flaws in implementation and identify more precisely which patients are most likely to benefit.

Step 6 – Disseminate EBP results

Clinicians can get best results with their outcomes for their patients through EBP, but may often fail to share their experiences with colleagues and their own or other health care organizations or groups. This leads to needless duplication of effort, and perpetuates clinical approaches that are not evidence-based. Among ways to disseminate successful initiatives are EBP rounds in your institution, presentations at local, regional, and national conferences, and reports in peer-reviewed journals, professional newsletters, and publications for general audiences.

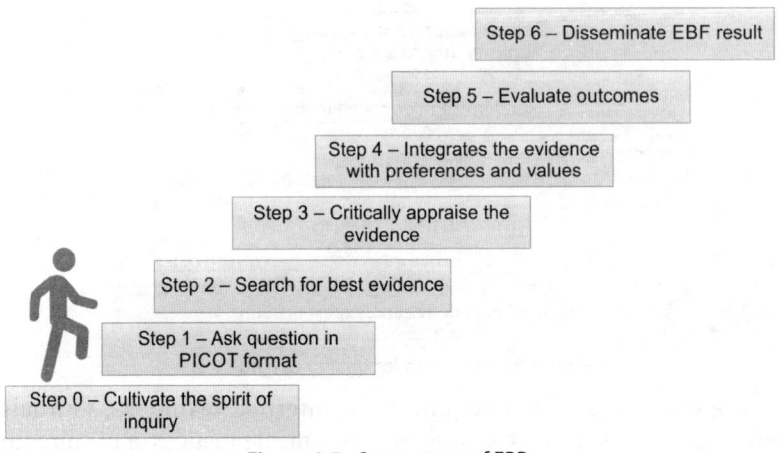

Figure 9.5: Seven steps of EBP.
(*Source:* Melnyk, 2010)

■ CHALLENGES TO IMPLEMENT EBP IN COMMUNITY PHYSIOTHERAPY[16]

Although the importance of research-based practice was identified decades ago and has gradually been adopted by the physiotherapy profession, there are a number of challenges for physiotherapy who are attempting to be use research to aid in clinical decision-making. Most challenges can be grouped under one of three areas:
1. Research methods
2. Clinician skills
3. Administrative factors

Challenge 1: Research methods

In accordance with the theory given by Sackett et al, the standard and solidity of research is classified according to a 5 hierarchy (5A), which sorts evidence in compliance to the thoroughness and potential for confounding variables to influence, the research outcomes. To give an instance, scientific proof generated by systemic reviews of RCTs is at the top peak of this hierarchy while case report and expert opinion are at the lowest point. Physiotherapists are motivated and uplifted to consider a study's "level of evidence" in the citation of making verification-based clinical resolution. EBP suggests that clinicians use the premier available finding, in accordance to this hierarchy, to escort clinical resolution, intervention, while making a decision regarding patient management.

Challenge 2: Clinician skills

With help of current experimentation writings, acknowledging research methodology and incorporating the best and foremost proofs into practice are some of the pre-requisites of a clinician in EBP. Whatsoever, a large number of healthcare providers have trouble to utilize client secured practice. Interpreting and implementing research proofs also needs objective skill, judgments and experience. It is not easy to determine, what constitutes the proof that gives grounds for a substitute in practice, and opportunity for bias exists at every stage of the activity. For instance, a bunch of people recommend that the base and nature of research-based inference leads to an inescapable subjectivity in interpreting and applying the substantiation, while others suggest that modifying or replacing the clinical practice to execute therapies that have not been tested is unprofessional.

Physical therapists must frequently question habituated and conventional practice and look for proofs to brace the clinical determination.

Challenge 3: Logical considerations

The clinicians who are trying to utilize proofs to guide clinical decision making face a bulk of challenges due to several factors. Practitioners who are not from teaching, mentoring or research centers usually get in contact with difficulties related to accessing the relevant practical proofs into practice.

EBP is not always economical, hence it modifies in practice as a cumulative outcome might face certain opposition.

■ STRATEGIES FOR EFFECTIVE EVIDENCE-BASED PRACTICE[16]

Regardless of certain challenges faced, physical therapists proved that they care and respect the integration of scientific and technological research into clinical practice.

In a latest survey, it is proved that physical therapists have a strong willingness and confidence for the betterment of skills related to EBP. Students who have just stepped into clinical practice did not have and thoughts and beliefs about the relevant sources of authority for treatment determination that were entrenched during entry-level education.

In spite of the prevalence of such factors, a number of strategies have been suggested and they are as follows:

Strategy 1: Develop, implement, and evaluate dissemination techniques specific to EBP
Unexpectedly, there is very less knowledge in deciding the foremost way to get the outcome of ideal physical therapy analysis into clinical practice. An essential aspect is to make a change in management culture and a modification in administrators and supervisors attitudes. The strategies that focus on a particular issue, include the collaboration among clinicians, enforce desirable practices and target obstructions to modify, like the organizational factors in the settlement of practice are prone to lead to enduring behavioral modifications. There is little evidence to support the utilization of passive circulatory techniques, like seminars, lectures, workshops and handouts etc., however a variety of strategies that are constricted to EBP in community and focus on a comprehensive implementation plan have been successful in creating behavioral modification in relation to EBP.

With the help of other evidences specifics strategies to effectively implement each of the component of EBP within a specific community. To minimize the barriers need to promote certain factors which improve implementation along with focus on ethics, incentives, motivation, social norms, patient problem and decision support system at community level. In the end several other strategies have emphasized on miscellaneous and interactive educational and academicals programming, utilization of small groups of staff to assess and evaluate research findings.

Strategy 2: Rethink traditional continuing education courses
One plan of action that continues to be employed by physiotherapist to be gain additional skills and to guide practice decision is attendance at continuing education and academically conferences. Shortly practitioners have been promoted to plead evidence from conference speaker's contemplation to essentially evaluate any assertion of effectiveness. Other have suggested that the time spends at progressive education and conferences might be better spent by people or in smaller groups of community retorting their own clinical queries through to EBP. Rather than focusing on conferences or seminars need to concentrate on structured and focused EBP in community area.

Strategy 3: Development, implementation and evaluation of "user friendly" knowledge transfer activities
Physiotherapist are conventionally trying to use proven and effective treatment along with presence of evidence of top most research. They may also benefit from hands on practical guidance from academician, practitioners and researchers with best clinical evidence.

Multi-dimensional interventions like interactive educational approach, journals, outreach visits, clinician and researchers should be employed.

Physiotherapist are promoted to follow specific guidelines when seeking and utilizing scientific and technological evidence to brace to aid clinicians to systematically evaluate the available evidence and decides its usefulness to clinical and community level practices. Many researchers have suggested that it might be more appropriate and suitable for clinician as well as community physiotherapist to utilize subordinate sources such as clinical guidelines and instructions, systemic reviews, published journals and research database.

Strategy 4: Highly visible role for professional associations
Professional associations need to play of prominent role in fostering EBP and aiding change in pessimistic attitude that prevails among the community physiotherapist. Professional associations must work to establish a framework for implementing EBP and work to create

increased consistency of the process. Postulate information about appropriate and suitable resources for scientific and technological proofs and access to computerized database for members are some of the methodology for professional organization to forester, support and promote EBP in community physiotherapist. Professional association should promote the development and execution of clinical as well as community physiotherapy practice norms. Norms must also be developed to aid and support clinical and community practitioner in evaluating non-standard therapies that may lack the support of scientific and research-based evidence.

Strategy 5: Start early
There is proof that off late graduates and therapists with additional educational background tend to have a more optimistic attitude and increased skills in accessing and utilizing scientific research to guide practice rather than there ore experience co-workers and colleagues. It is essential that academic program or educational program including both entry level and post professional, continue to foster the development of EBP skills and strategies. Educational activities and curricula utilized for entry level students, as well as progressing educational programing for practicing clinician's and health care providers are better and fruitful starting points.

Strategy 6: Increase clinician's involvement in research
All physiotherapist must participate in cycle of research and evidence-based publication, dissemination and implementation. It is of immense importance that there is increased collaboration in research in order to move the profession further. Joint in initiatives between academia, where students are learning, studying and inculcating research skills and developing research and technological competencies, and the clinicians, who provide working laboratories for inquiries, must be encourage and promoted. These initiatives should also consist of interactive educational and academic programs, research project development and implementation, and support in the form of access to databases and other library resources that lend themselves to EBP activities and workshops.

■ METHODOLOGY FOR EBP IN COMMUNITY PHYSIOTHERAPY[7 9,16]

With respect to challenges and strategies in EBP the overall methodology and preparation for community physiotherapist is given in **Figure 9.6**.

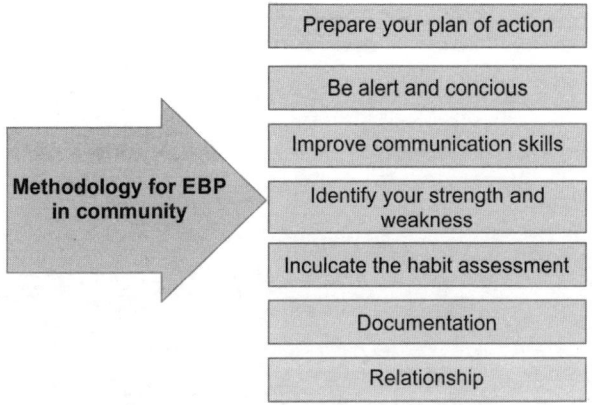

Figure 9.6: Methodology for EBP in community.

REFERENCES

1. World Confederation for Physical Therapy—European Region. Evidence based physiotherapy [Internet]. Brussels: The Confederation; 2015. [cited 2015 Mar 24]. Available from: http://www.erwcpt.eu/education/evidence_based_physiotherapy_evidence_and_research.
2. Sackett DL, Rosenberg WM, Gray JA, et al. Evidence-based medicine: what it is and what it isn't. BMJ. 1996;312(7023):71-2. http://dx.doi.org/10.1136/bmj.312.7023.71. Medline: 85559241.
3. Dawes M, Summerskill W, Glasziou P et al. Sicily statement on evidence-based practice. BMC Med Ed. 2005;5(1).
4. Hicks N. Evidence-based healthcare. Bandolier, 1997;4(39):8.
5. Taylor Pillae PE. Establishing Evidence-based practice. Issues and implication in critical care nursing. Intensive Care Nursing. 1998;14:30-37.
6. Herbert R, Jamtvedt G, Mead J, Hagen KB. Practical evidence-based physiotherapy. Butterworth Heinemann; 2005. pp. 170-97.
7. WCPT Guidelines [Internet]. Policy Statement: Evidence Based Practice. London: World confederation for physical therapy. 2012 [Updated: Mon 10 Apr 2017]. Available from: www.wcpt.org/policy/ps-EBP.
8. Glasziou P, Burls A, Gilbert R. Evidence-based medicine and the medical curriculum. The search engine is now as essential as the stethoscope. BMJ. 2008;337(a1253):a704-5.
9. Bhatt CJ, Sheth MS. Knowledge, attitude and practice towards evidence based practice in post-graduate physiotherapy students. Int J Health Sci Res. 2021;11(8):17-26. DOI: https://doi.org/10.52403/ijhsr.20210804
10. Sackett DL, Strauss SE, et al. Evidence-based medicine: how to practice and teach EBM. 2nd ed. Churchill Livingstone, New York; 2000.
11. Grimshaw J, et al. Toward evidence-based quality improvement. Evidence (and its limitations) of the effectiveness of guideline dissemination and implementation strategies 1966-1998. J Gen Intern Med. 2006;21(Suppl 2):S14-20.
12. McGinty J, Anderson G. Predictors of physician compliance with American Heart Association guidelines for acute myocardial infarction. Crit Care Nurs. 2008;31(2):161-72.
13. Shortell SM, et al. Improving patient care by linking evidence-based medicine and evidence-based management. JAMA. 2007;298(6):673-6.
14. Strout TD. Curiosity and reflective thinking: renewal of the spirit. Indianapolis, IN: Sigma Theta Tau International; 2005.
15. Williams DO. Treatment delayed is treatment denied. Circulation 2004;109(15):1806-8.
16. Schreiber J, Stern P. A review of the literature on evidence-based practice in physical therapy. The Internet Journal of Allied Health Sciences and Practices. 2005;3:4.

Section 3 Basic Concepts of National and International Legislation for Persons with Disability

CHAPTER 10

Role of National Institutes, District Rehabilitation Center and Primary Health Center

Deepali Nivrutti Hande

LEARNING OBJECTIVES

Through this chapter, the reader will be able to:
- Understand importance of National Rehabilitation Center, District Rehabilitation Center and Primary Health Center in rehabilitation of differently abled persons
- Understand burden of disabilities
- Gain knowledge of role of physiotherapy concern to primary healthcare level
- Acquire insights of primary healthcare centers in India

■ INTRODUCTION

Rehabilitation is defined as "a set of interventions designed to optimize functioning and reduce disability in individuals with health conditions in interaction with their environment". Alma Ata declaration (1978) stated that promotive, preventive, curative, and rehabilitative care should be incorporated in comprehensive primary health care. There are three approaches to rehabilitation namely Institution-based Rehabilitation (IBR), Outreach-based Rehabilitation, and Community-based Rehabilitation (CBR). The major goal of Community-based Rehabilitation is to make sure that people with disabilities (PwDs) are able to maximize their physical and mental abilities. Another goal is that PwDs should get access to resources and opportunities, and achieve full integration within their communities. CBR is a comprehensive approach at primary health care level where resources for rehabilitation are accessible from the community. Multi-sectoral coordination with involvement of community needed as it will transfer the knowledge pertaining to skill development in various types of rehabilitation methods. Community participation will be involved in planning, decision-making, and evaluation of the CBR program.

A number of International commitments and guidelines are focusing on the welfare of the disabled persons. India is associated with the 'Declaration on the Full Participation and Equality of People with Disabilities in the Asia Pacific Region' (2000) and 'Biwako Millennium Framework' (2002). India has signed the 'UN Convention on the Rights of Persons with Disabilities' (2008).

Population with disability is 10% of the world's population. From this 10% disabled population around 80% of these people live in socioeconomically vulnerable developing countries. According to the Census of India 2011, India has a about 26 million population suffering from various kinds of disability which accounts for 2.21% of the total population.

About 69% of the disabled population live in rural areas which itself is a challenge for equal distribution of provision of health care. PwDs face many hurdles in education and employment which is reflected in the low effective literacy rate of 59%, which is less than national level i.e., 74.04% as well as a low work participation rate at 36.3%. Hence the resource generation in the rural areas pertaining to rehabilitation of PwDs is utmost important for their social inclusion.

PRIMARY HEALTHCARE CENTERS

In the Declaration of Alma-Ata (1978) principles of PHC were outline. It was an important milestone in global health. Forty years later, it was ratified as the Declaration of Astana (Kazakhstan) at the Global Conference on Primary Health Care in October 2018. The rural public health system in India has a unique three-tiered pyramidal pattern which consist of primary, secondary and tertiary care. PHCs are considered as first-access points of patients to health care within the public system. These centers responsibly provide "preventive" services with primary-level clinical care.

The goals of PHC are to ensure the highest possible level of health and well-being of the people. It focuses to provide health promotion and disease prevention to treatment, rehabilitation and palliative care, and as close as feasible to people by equitable distribution. A vision for primary health care in the 21st century is to enhance Universal Health Coverage (UHC) and the Sustainable Development Goals (SDGs).

PHC ensures people receive quality comprehensive care including health promotion and prevention to treatment, rehabilitation and palliative care—as close as feasible. PHC plays utmost important role to enhance people's physical and mental health, as well as social well-being by delivering the most inclusive, equitable, cost-effective and efficient approach. In crisis such as the COVID-19 pandemic evidence shows that PHC has plays important role in catering health services to large number of populations.

Functions of PHC

At the PHC level 2 Multi Rehabilitation Workers (MRWs) for about 30,000 population will be responsible to provide services to the PwDs. They will provide information to community leaders, to the PwDs and their families about disability. MRWs will make sure that the services provided should be available from local resources. The MRW will work in coordination with PHC, education, Labour, NGOs and other persons, so that services will be available and open opportunities for PWDs. They will also make referral of cases to the District Rehabilitation Center (DRC) who require more advance healthcare services which are not possible at PHC level.

At the district level DRC will be headed by District Rehabilitation Officer (DRO) who will monitor and guide the work carried out at peripheral levels. Functionaries of the department of rural development, social welfare, labour and employment and women and child development will also provide specialist services at the district level.

At the national level, national center for disability rehabilitation under the national program of rehabilitation called National Institutes (NIs) for Rehabilitation.

Role of Primary Health Centers in Rehabilitation of PwDs

Due to inadequate resources only 1% of the total disabled population receives different support services. A PHC is the only existing infrastructure at primary ground level to provide various

CHAPTER 10: Role of National Institutes, District Rehabilitation Center and Primary Health Center

disability prevention and rehabilitation services. PHC has network with its subcenters in rural areas and health posts in urban areas. Health workers at subcenters get help from village health guides (VHGs), traditional birth attendants (TBAs) and Anganwadi workers for in identification of disabled along with CBR workers. WHO has developed a training package for community level functionaries of DRC.

Education and sensitization of medical officers and health teams in PHCs on important aspects of disability prevention, early identification, referral and rehabilitation, the valuable services is very essential. Training the Medical Officers in Disability Prevention and Rehabilitation can bring significant benefits to the PwDs. Most of the disable people live in the rural areas with very poor infrastructure for providing rehabilitation services. Rehabilitation Council of India has launched the National Programme on Orientation of Medical Officers working in Primary Health Centers for Disability Management on 15th July 1999, with a goal that the Medical Officers of PHCs could be trained in various disability issues. This program has been designed to provide health services for PwDs residing in rural areas.

Empowerment of PHC Medical Officers to help create better sensitization at the grass root level which will ultimately ensure better implementation of the Persons with Disabilities Act, 1995.

National Programs

Following are the few national programs run by government of India through PHCs for disability limitation and rehabilitation of PwDs
* National Leprosy Eradication Programme
* National Programme for Control of Blindness (NPCB)
* National Programme for Prevention and Control of Deafness (NPPCD)
* National Mental Health Programme (NMHP)
* National Programme for Prevention and Control of Cancer, Diabetes, CVD and Stroke (NPCDCS)
* National Programme for Health Care of Elderly

Health Promotion in Children Facilitated by PHCs

* Screening, health care and referral
* Screening of general health, assessment of anemia/nutritional status, visual acuity, hearing problems, dental checkup, common skin conditions, neonatal disorders, behavior problems, etc.
* Basic medicines for young school going children for common ailments.
* Referral cards for appropriate cases to higher center, e.g., district/subdistrict hospitals.

Immunization

* As per national schedule
* Fixed day activity
* Coupled with education about the issue.

Micronutrient (Vitamin A and IFA) Management

Distribution of iron-folate tablets coupled with education.

■ DE-WORMING

Role of Physiotherapy in Primary Health Care

* Physiotherapists can incorporate individualized exercise Programs
* Self-management and education for all musculoskeletal complaints
* Mobility aides assessment and assistance.

Table 10.1: Few examples of role of physiotherapy in different health problems at PHC level.

Non-communicable diseases	• To educate patient on the benefits of regular physical activity • Execute knowledge and training to prescribe individualized exercise plans • To coordinate comprehensive obesity management programs. • Lung health programs: teach patients skills to manage their acute periods and counseling for those with chronic cardiorespiratory conditions such as asthma, COPD • Referral to community-based treatment programs • Identification of need for additional diagnostics, specialist referral programs with obesity, pre-diabetes, diabetes, arthritis and other chronic diseases • Support and education for caregivers in chronic diseases of the vascular or peripheral neuropathy complications • Balance disorders and preventive strategies of fall. • Education on Type 1 diabetes of Type 1 diabetes children and caregivers to encourage the children in physical activity
	• Education self-management programs • Referral to community-based treatment programs Identification of need for additional diagnostics, specialist referral programs with obesity, pre-diabetes, diabetes, arthritis and other chronic diseases • Facilitate linkages with community programs • Support and education for caregivers in non-communicable diseases

Geriatric health	• **Incontinence**
	  – Patient education regarding urinary incontinence
	  – Evidence based management of pelvic floor muscle weakness and rehabilitation of same as a treatment approach for incontinence
	• **Falls prevention programs**
	  – Screening of intrinsic and extrinsic risk factors for fall
	  – Balance training
	  – Lower extremity strength training
	  – Appropriate specialist referral
	  – Lifestyle and behavioral modifications.
	  – Ergonomics advice for ADLs
	• **Arthritis**
	  – Patient education regarding arthritis
	  – Provide adequate information on exercise in arthritis
	  – Education to cope with arthritis pain and self-management of pain
	  – Rehabilitation of patients with RA and OA
	  – Lifestyle and behavioral modifications.
	  – Ergonomics advice for ADLs

Contd...

Contd...

Women's health	**Antenatal physiotherapy** • Prevention of musculoskeletal strains • Education and advice on physical discomforts • To increase and maintain physical fitness • Assessment and management of musculoskeletal disorder • Can teach coping skills for labor • Education on physiological changes during pregnancy and after childbirth • Ergonomic advice on ADLs and lifestyle **Postnatal physiotherapy** • Information and advice on physical discomforts • To increase and maintain physical fitness • Assessment and treatment of musculoskeletal disorder • Breathing exercise • Abdominal exercise • Pelvic tilting exercise • Pelvic floor muscles strengthening • Back care advice • Physiotherapy management of following postnatal problem • Painful perineum • Diastasis recti • Back pain • Symphysis pubis • Bladder and bowel problem • Circulatory problem • Afterpains • Breast engorgement and mastitis • Tiredness
Postmenopausal women's health	• Breathing exercises • Postural training • Weight reduction • Physical activity • Osteoporosis • Patient education regarding osteoporosis • Weight reduction • Aerobic training • Resistance training
Mental health	• Enhancement in physical activity • Breathing exercises • Yoga • Meditation

A holistic approach to health care should integrate all levels of health promotion and disease prevention.

■ DISTRICT DISABILITY REHABILITATION CENTER

Background

Disability limitation at early stage when they are amenable to preventive and rehabilitative measures, so that progression to severe disability can be minimized is a vital component in rehabilitation of disabled. There are many measures initiated by Ministry of Social Justice and Empowerment and Health and Family Welfare in India and initiative like District Disability Rehabilitation Center (DDRC) is one of them. DDRCs were established to facilitate comprehensive services to Persons with Disabilities in the rural areas. They have a group of rehabilitation professionals to cater experts services like identification of Persons with Disabilities, Awareness Generation, Early detection and Intervention, Provision/Fitment, Follow-up and repairing of Assistive Devices, Rehabilitative Services and Physiotherapy, Speech Therapy, etc. They also help the PwDs to obtain Disability Certificates, Buss Passes and other concessions/facilities for Persons with Disabilities.

DDRCs work in collaboration of both Central and State Governments wherein Central Government will establish, initiate, implement the center for three years involving funding for man power contingencies as well as required equipments and coordination. State Government will provide provision for rent-free, well-connected building, basic infrastructure, furniture, monitoring and coordination of activities through District Management Team (DMT) Chaired by the District Collector and also identification of implementing agency. During 1985-1990, District Disability Rehabilitation Center (DDRCs) started under the Scheme for implementation of Persons with Disabilities Act 1995 (SIPDA). Originally, DDRCs were started to provide comprehensive services to the persons with disabilities at the grass root level. Section 66 of PWD Act, 1995 was revised in 1999 and all schemes then existing for rehabilitation of persons with disabilities were amalgamated into a single scheme called the "Scheme to Promote Voluntary Action for Persons with Disabilities". On 1.04.2003 this scheme was renamed as the "Deendayal Disabled Rehabilitation Scheme (DDRS)". The DDRS funds District Disability Rehabilitation center.

Objectives of Setting up of DDRC

- ❖ To do survey and identification of persons with disabilities through screening camp; facilitation of disability certificate, bus passes and other concession/facilities for persons with disabilities; assisting in the issue of Unique Disability Identity Card (UDID) to divyangjan in the district
- ❖ Enhancing prevention of disabilities and awareness generation for encouraging and, early detection and intervention as well as maintaining data of organizations working for the empowerment of persons with disabilities in the district etc.
- ❖ To create awareness and facilitating Insurance Schemes launched by the National Trust/ Department for Divyangjan
- ❖ Assessment of disability and appropriate assistive devices, provision/fitment of assistive devices, follow up/repair of assistive devices, assisting the ADIP/ALMICO camps for distribution of aids and assistive devices in the district; Therapeutic Services, e.g., Physiotherapy, Occupational Therapy, Speech Therapy, etc.
- ❖ Referral and arrangement of surgical correction through Government and Charitable institutes
- ❖ Help to get loans for self-employment, through banks and other financial institutions
- ❖ To provide counselling services to PwDs, their parents and family members
- ❖ Enhance barrier free environment and to play an active role in the Accessible India campaign of the department

CHAPTER 10: Role of National Institutes, District Rehabilitation Center and Primary Health Center

- ❖ To deliver supportive and complimentary services to promote education, assisting students with disabilities for availing Scholarship Schemes of the Department, vocational training/ skill training of eligible Divyangjan and employment for persons with disabilities through:
  - To provide orientation training to teachers, community and families
  - To train PwDs for early motivation and early stimulation for education, vocational training and employment.
  - Identifying suitable vocations for persons with disabilities, keeping in view local resources and designing and providing vocational training and identifying suitable jobs, so as to make them economically independent.
  - Provide referral services for existing educational training, vocational institutions and to act as outreach center for the services provided by the National Institutes.

A Nodal Officer, i.e., District Disability Rehabilitation Officer is responsible for coordination, management and administration of DDRCs on a day-to-day basis. Red Cross Society or any such autonomous/semi-autonomous bodies of State Govt. or a reputed NGO are consider to run DDRC.

Staff for DDRC

Each DDRC may have a maximum of 10 staff members, having specified qualifications. The rehabilitation professionals should preferably be registered with Rehabilitation Council of India (RCI).

Table 10.2: Staff for DDRC.

Sr. No.	Post	Qualification
1.	Clinical Psychologist/Psychologist	MPhil in clinical Psychology/MA in Psychology preferably with 2 years experience in the field of disability rehabilitation
2.	Senior Physiotherapist/ Occupational Therapist	Postgraduate in related field with 5 years experience
3.	Orthopedically Handicapped Senior Prosthetist/Orthotist	Degree in Prosthetic and Orthotic preferably from National Institute with 5 years experience or a diploma in Prosthetic and Orthotic with 6 years experience
4.	Prosthetist/Orthotist Technician	ITI trained with 2/3 years experience
5.	Senior Speech Therapist/Audiologist	Postgraduate in related field/BSc (Speech and Hearing)
6.	Hearing Assistant/Junior Speech Therapist	Diploma in Speech and Hearing with knowledge of hearing aids repair/ear mold making
7.	Mobility Instructor	Matriculation + Certificate/Diploma in Mobility
8.	Multipurpose Rehabilitation Worker	10 + 2 with diploma in CBR/MRW course or one year diploma course in early childhood special education with two years of experience
9.	Accountant-cum-Clerk-cum-Storekeeper	B Com/SAS with 2 years experience
10.	Attendant-cum-Peon-cum-Messenger	VIII class pass

Role of State Government

State Governments are expected to play a more proactive role in the effective working of DDRCs by involving State/District Administration.

DDRCs in India

In the prerevised scheme 199 DDRCs were approved for setting up in various districts of the country, i.e., up to March, 2010. Out of which 185 are functional as per records available with this Department.

In all DDRCs have been approved for setting up in 310 districts and 263 DDRCs have been set up.

Equipment

The equipment for fabrication and fitment of assistive devices related to all kind of disabilities is to be purchased from this scheme. These equipments can also be procured from the ALIMCO (Artificial Limbs Manufacturing Corporation of India, Lucknow Road, Kanpur—an organization under the Department of Disability Affairs).

Training to Manpower of DDRCs in Coordination with State Government

The staff of the NGO and DDRCs are trained though National Institutes (NIs) for capacity building.

National Institutes undertake the following training programs in coordination with State Government are as follows:

- One day workshop of District Collectors and State Government Officials: Sensitization to disabilities issues, main provisions of PWD Act, DDRC scheme and effective delivery through them, sharing of best practices.
- Three days training for Nodal officers of Implementing agency and Social Welfare Officers: DDRC Scheme, processing of proposals under ADIP, DDRS, etc., maintenance of accounts and other records, facilities, concessions and Schemes for Persons with Disabilities and important referral addresses
- Up to 15 days in-service training for technical and professional manpower in DDRCs: Focus especially on early intervention and follow-up, new techniques of treatment and rehabilitation.
- Special courses for in-service training courses, which include bridge courses for under-qualified manpower of DDRCs—for 6 months to 1 year sandwich programs.
- Workshop on communication skills and preparation of educative material.
- Repairs and maintenance of aids and appliances for technical staff, multipurpose workers.
- Exposure visits to CRC/NIs and other DDRC.

Action plan of DDRCs should broadly be as follows:
- Survey of the Person with Disabilities and their needs in the districts—10–15 villages per month
- Assessment camps at headquarters—twice in a week
- At civil hospital—once every week
- Assessment cum distribution camps at villages—twice a month

CHAPTER 10: Role of National Institutes, District Rehabilitation Center and Primary Health Center

- Awareness generation activities like visits to school/awareness camp in villages for various target groups/training program of grass root level functionaries—4 times a month.
- Follow-up camps in villages—4 times a month
- Survey of persons with disabilities.

The data can be collected with the help of anganwadi workers/other grassroots level workers like ASHA about the disabled persons in each village.

Assessment/Fitment/Follow-up and repair of assistive devices

Actual fitment of assistive devices would be one of the major important activities of District Center.

The organization of the camps for this is done in collaboration with Anganwadi Workers (AWWs), Health Workers, Para teachers NREGA, Panchayati Raj Institutions, Local NGOs and other grass-root level functionaries.

The district center provides for repair services, adjustment and follow-up of assistive devices on nominal charges. They also provide training for effective and correct use of assistive devices to PwDs.

Promotion of Prevention

The district centers provides information about dissemination on prevention of different disabilities through various National Health Program to emphasize the linkage between Health Programs and Schemes and prevention of disability. This is implemented in the form of distribution and publicizing the information available with the implementing agencies on prevention and early intervention in local language with support of ICDS workers, Health Workers, CBRWs with a focus on identification, prevention and early detection.

Early Intervention

Early identification of disabilities and early intervention is very important for avoiding secondary disabilities and ensuring successful integration of children with disabilities with other children at all levels which is done by early intervention unit of each DDRC.

Barrier Free Environment

Provision of barrier free environment is as important as of appropriate assistive devices for providing accessibility to PwDs. This is another aspect of DDRC functioning which is implemented through construction of barrier free buildings, especially public sector and public utility, e.g., schools and hostels, Panchayat and other Government buildings, hospitals, markets, bus stands, parks, public toilets.

National Institutes

National Institutes (NIs) are autonomous bodies established under Society Registration Act focusing on specific types of disabilities. These institutes are primarily engaged in Human Resources Development in the field of disability by conducting various courses, providing rehabilitation services to persons with disabilities (PwDs) and promotes research. They also provide vocational skill training, placement and distribution of assistive aids and appliances to PwDs.

SECTION 3: Basic Concepts of National and International Legislation for Persons with Disability

Table 10.3: List of nine national institutes working for the welfare of PwDs in India.

Sr. No.	Name of the national institute	Place
1.	National Institute for the Empowerment of Persons with Visual Disabilities (NIEPVD)	Dehradun
2.	Ali Yavar Jung National Institute of Speech and Hearing Disabilities (AYJNISHD)	Mumbai
3.	National Institute for the Empowerment of Persons with Intellectual Disabilities (NIEPID)	Secunderabad, Telangana
4	National Institute for Empowerment of Persons with Multiple Disabilities (NIEPMD)	Chennai
5.	Pt. Deendayal Upadhyaya National Institute for Persons with Physical Disabilities (PDUNIPPD)	New Delhi
6.	Swami Vivekanand National Institute of the Rehabilitation Training and Research (SVNIRTAR)	Cuttack
7.	National Institute for Locomotor Disabilities (NILD)	Kolkata
8.	Indian Sign Language Research and Training Center (ISLRTC)	New Delhi
9.	National Institute of Mental Health and Rehabilitation (NIMHR)	Sehore, Madhya Pradesh

Main activities of these Institutes are as follows:

National Institute for the Empowerment of Persons with Visual Disabilities (NIEPVD), Dehradun

This is one of the major organizations launched by the Government of India for the People with Visual Disability (PVD).
- Residential school for the Visually Impaired up to the 12th standard.
- Central Braille press which is the largest press of Braille literature for school and college education
- Rehabilitative services for persons with visual disabilities
- Early intervention and assessment services
- Postgraduate, Undergraduate and Diploma courses in Special Education and Rehabilitation Psychology
- Undertakes Research and developmental activities
- This institute is instrumental in providing following skill development courses for PVD:
  - Nursery workers
  - Vermi Compost Producer
  - Grower with mushrooms
  - Cultivator of medicinal plants
  - Organic producers
  - Seed producers of consistency
  - Secretary of Government
  - Agarbatti Maker Hand Rolling
  - Delivery of items for disposable paper (Tumbler and Dona Paper Cups, Plates)
  - Stationery products produce
  - Manufacture of handmade paper and so on.

Ali Yavar Jung National Institute of Speech and Hearing Disabilities (AYJNISHD), Mumbai
- PhD, Post Graduate, Under Graduate and Diploma courses in Audiology, Speech Language

CHAPTER 10: Role of National Institutes, District Rehabilitation Center and Primary Health Center

Pathology, Special Education, etc.
- Nodal agency for Cochlear Implant Surgery and postoperative rehabilitation. At present 186 hospitals empanelled for the said surgery.
- Tertiary level care, evaluation and diagnosis of speech-language and audiology impairment.
- Diagnostic, therapeutic, educational and vocational services to persons with speech and/or hearing disabilities.
- Early intervention and assessment services.

National Institute for the Empowerment of Persons with Intellectual Disabilities (NIEPID), Secunderabad
- Rehabilitative services for persons with Intellectual disabilities with evidential and visible positive outcomes of cognitive recovery.
- M Phil, Postgraduate, Undergraduate and Diploma level Courses in Special Education and Rehabilitation Psychology.
- Special Education, Clinical Psychology, Cognitive Therapy and Vocational/skill training.
- Model Special Education Center located at Secunderabad/Noida/New Delhi up to Pre-Vocational Level (i.e., up to 18 years).

National Institute for Empowerment of Persons with Multiple Disabilities (NIEPMD), Chennai
- M Phil, Postgraduate, Undergraduate and Diploma courses in Clinical Psychology, Special Education, Physiotherapy, Occupational Therapy, P&O, Speech Language Pathology, etc.
- Renders rehabilitative services to persons with multiple disabilities.
- Early Intervention and assessment Services.
- Psychological Assessments and Interventions.
- Inclusive preparatory School and Vocational training.

Pt. Deendayal Upadhyaya National Institute for Persons with Physical Disabilities (PDUNIPPD), Delhi
- Comprehensive rehabilitative services to persons with Locomotor disabilities.
- Prosthetics and Orthotics, Physiotherapy, Occupational Therapy, Vocational and Psychological counseling services.
- Specialty Clinical services.
- Early Intervention and assessment services.
- Postgraduate, Undergraduate courses in Prosthetics and Orthotics, Physiotherapy, and Occupational Therapy.

Swami Vivekanand National Institute of the Rehabilitation Training and Research (SVNIRTAR), Cuttack
- Comprehensive rehabilitative services to Persons with Locomotor Disabilities.
- Prosthetics and Orthotics, Physiotherapy, Occupational Therapy, and Vocational counseling services.
- Providing Early Intervention and assessment services.
- Postgraduate, Undergraduate courses in Prosthetics and Orthotics, Physiotherapy, and Occupational Therapy. Also conducts DNB in Physical Medicine and Rehabilitation (PMR) of National Board of Examination (NBE), New Delhi.
- 100-bedded hospital and Cerebral Palsy Clinic.
- 2 well equipped operation theatres for corrective and reconstructive surgeries.
- Radiological and Pathological investigation Units.

National Institute for Locomotor Disabilities (NILD), Kolkata
- Comprehensive rehabilitation services to the Persons with Locomotor Disabilities.
- Prosthetics and Orthotics, Physiotherapy, Occupational Therapy, and Vocational counseling services.
- Early Intervention and assessment services.
- Postgraduate, Undergraduate courses in Prosthetics and Orthotics, Physiotherapy, and Occupational Therapy. Also conducts DNB (PMR).
- 50-bedded hospital and engaged in corrective surgery.
- Physical medicine and Rehabilitation.
- OPD and Radiology Services.

Indian Sign Language Research and Training Centre (ISLRTC), New Delhi
- They trained professional for using, teaching and conducting research in Indian Sign Language.
- They have Diploma course in Indian Sign Language Interpretation (DISLI) and Diploma in Teaching Indian Sign Language (DTISL).
- They have well researched dictionary of Indian sign language (10,000 words) developed.
- Have an MoU with NCERT to convert course books and materials for classes-I to XII into sign language.
- They promote accessible Indian Sign Language in audiovisual and social media.

National Institute of Mental Health and Rehabilitation (NIMHR), Sehore
The Institute has started functioning recently from 30.09.2019.
- They conduct Psychological Assessment and testing are services that help mental health professionals to identify mental health disorders through combination of interviews, self-report measures, psychological batteries and assessment tools.
- They do neuropsychological assessment is a performance-based method to assess cognitive functioning are available at institute for various neuropsychological disorders, developmental disabilities and severe mental illnesses.
- They provide Psycho-Education, Guidance and Counselling are provided in institute by trained clinical professionals.
- Motivational Enhancement Therapy (MET), Cognitive Behavior Therapy (CBT), Rational Emotive Therapy (RET), Behavior Therapy (BT), Exposure and Response Prevention Therapy (ERP), Family/couple Therapy, etc., are available here in the form of Psychotherapy treatment.
- Institute conducts awareness generation activities and screening programs on the different issues related to Mental Health and Mental Illnesses like awareness at grassroots level of aganwadi, schools and colleges etc.

Composite Regional Center for Skill Development, Rehabilitation and Empowerment of Persons with Disabilities (CRCs)
Composite Regional Centers (CRCs) as extended centers of National Institutes. Goal of CRCs are to provide rehabilitation services to all PwDs, training of rehabilitation professionals, workers. They also undertake programs of education and skill development for PwDs and to generate awareness among parents and the community regarding needs and rights of PwDs.

BIBLIOGRAPHY

1. Deendayal Disabled Rehabilitation Scheme: (As revised w.e.f. 01.04.2018) Department of Empowerment of Persons with Disabilities, Ministry of Social Justice and Empowerment Government of India, New Delhi: https://disabilityaffairs.gov.in/upload/uploadfiles/files/Revised%20DDRS%20Scheme.pdf
2. Department of empowerment of persons with disabilities: Ministry of social justice and empowerment: GOI http://disabilityaffairs.gov.in/content/page/national-institutes.php
3. disabledhelpline.org/ddrc-scheme/
4. Kumar SG, Gautam Roy, Kar SS. Disability and rehabilitation services in India: Issues and challenges. Journal of Family Medicine and Primary Care. 2012;1(1):69-73.
5. mospi.nic.in/sites/default/files/publication_reports/Disabled_persons_in_India_2016.pdf
6. niepid.nic.in
7. nimhr.ac.in
8. Rajamohan S, Saranya Devi E. Roles and responsibility of the National Institute for the Empowerment of Person with Visual Disabilities in India: A Study. International Journal of Management (IJM). 2000;11(9):408-17.
9. Ramani S, Sivakami M. Community perspectives on primary health centers in rural Maharashtra: What can we learn for policy? Journal of Family Medicine and Primary Care. 2019;8:2837-44.
10. Role of Physiotherapy in Primary Health Care: Opportunities and Challenge: Conference Paper University of Manitoba.https://researchgate.net/publication/262179007_Role_of_Physiotherapy_in_Primary_Health_Care_Opportunities_and_Challenge
11. Sharma AK, Vashist P. Continuing Medical Education—Community Based Rehabilitation in Primary Health Care: Indian Journal of Community Medicine. 2000;27(3):139-1.
12. Training Manual for NCD Programme Managers at State and District Level: Sep 2017. https://main.mohfw.gov.in/sites/default/files/Training%20Manual%20for%20NCD%20Programme%20Managers%20at%20State%20and%20Disctrict%20Level_0.pdf
13. www.censusindia.gov.in
14. www.nhfdc.nic.in/upload/nhfdc/Persons_Disabilities_31mar21.pdf
15. www.specialeducationnotes.co.in/paper1Unit5.htm?i=1
16. www.svnirtar.nic.in/
17. www.swavlambancard.gov.in
18. www.un.org/disabilities/documents/toolaction/pwdfs.pdf3.
19. www.who.int/
20. www.who.int/news-room/fact-sheets/detail/primary-health-care

CHAPTER

Appropriate Technology, Assistive Devices Used for Disabled

Shyam D Ganvir, Pratima Sarwadikar

LEARNING OBJECTIVES

Through this chapter, the reader will be able to:
- Learning the definition of appropriate technology
- Knowing the use of appropriate technology to the person with disability
- Learning the various assistive devices and use of the same to the person with disability

■ APPROPRIATE TECHNOLOGY

The term *appropriate technology* is more difficult to define. Should not all kinds of technology for people with disabilities be appropriate? Appropriate technology normally means that assistive devices should be produced locally by locally available material and tools. However, socioeconomic and cultural aspects also are involved.

❖ Appropriate technology is a system that provides proper fit and alignment based on sound biomechanical principles, which suit the needs of the individual and can be sustained by the country at the most economical and affordable price.
❖ An appropriate technology should meet the physical needs of people with disabilities within their environment and economic situation.
❖ Local production of components from locally available materials should be encouraged.
❖ Use of different methods, procedures, and materials should be investigated, tested, and evaluated.
❖ Experiences related to appropriate technologies and use of materials should be properly documented and made available to others.[1]

■ ASSISTIVE TECHNOLOGY

❖ Any assistive, adaptive, or rehabilitative device used by the elderly population or people with disabilities, including the procedure of selection, location, and usage comes under the broadly defined term "assistive technology."
❖ These devices can reduce the effects of disabilities of such people in performing activities of daily living (ADLs) and grant them superior independence in performing tasks which were previously in adequate to carry out and executed with difficulty.
❖ **Adaptive technology** is designed specifically for persons with disabilities and would seldom be used by nondisabled persons.

CHAPTER 11: Appropriate Technology, Assistive Devices Used for Disabled

❖ "**Assistive technology** is an object or system that maintains or increases the abilities of persons with disabilities," while **Adaptive technology** is "any object or system that is explicitly designed for increasing or maintaining the capabilities of people with disabilities."[1]

■ ASSISTIVE DEVICES

1. **Wheelchairs:** It is an electrically or manually propelling mobility device which includes a seating system. They are designed to allow people with impaired mobility to perform ADLs such as feeding, toileting, dressing, grooming, and bathing. They are a substitute for normal movement for such people, allowing them to perform mobility related activities. Wheelchairs or walkers are the devices often required by people with both sitting and walking disability.

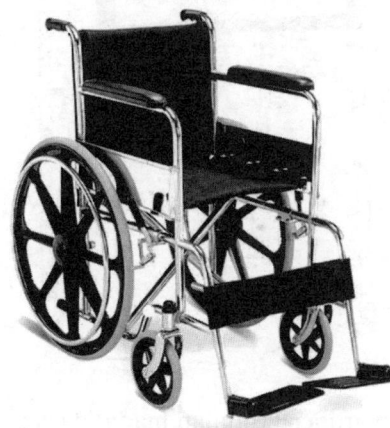

2. **Low-cost robotic wheelchair:** Semiautonomous mobile robots have conventionally been focused at executing surveillance, delivery, or similar tasks. Mobile robots can play a very different role as part of assistive technology. Power wheelchairs are customarily used by people who are compromised with upper body strength and do not have the ability to operate manual wheelchair.

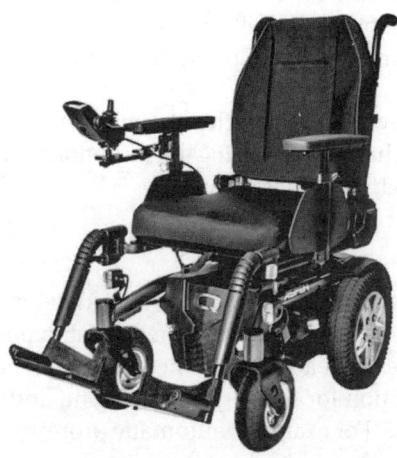

3. **Transfer devices:** These devices are mainly used by caregivers to move patients with mobility disability between beds, a bed to wheelchair or chair, transfer to commodes, toilets, shower benches, stretchers, and automobiles.
4. **Walkers:** Walking frame or rollator is a tool that provides additional support to patients for maintenance of balance or stability while standing in place or walking. It comprises a waisthigh frame, approximately 12 inch deep, and must be marginally more extensive than the user. Walkers may be height adjustable and available in different sizes for varied populations such as children or heavy individuals.

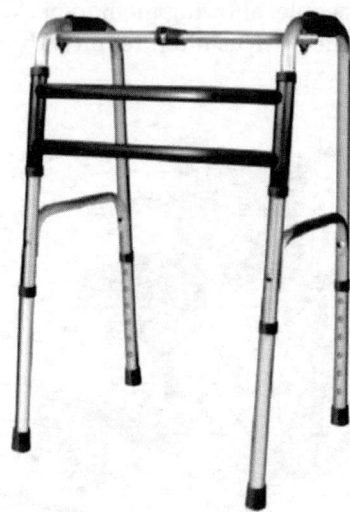

5. **Prosthesis:** Prosthesis is an artificial (human made) device to replace part. It is a device designed to substitute the function or appearance of a missing limb or body part as much as possible. In a broadest sense, prosthesis includes dentures, wigs, and plastic heart valves. However, we primarily concerned with limb prosthesis (i.e., artificial legs and arms). They are employed to replace missing body parts occurring as a result of congenital disabilities (congenital) or injury (traumatic).
6. **Desktop video magnifier:** Amplified versions of texts and pictures can be produced using this device for the benefit of individuals with poor vision. These magnifiers can be used as to read printed material, photographs, and illustrations; write checks; and complete forms. They come in various makes pertaining to size, portability, and features concerning magnification, lighting, contrasting, etc.
7. **Wearable technology:** They are smart electronic devices to be used as an accessory implant. An example of this is the technology exploring the reception of visual information by a visually impaired individual through wearable devices.[1]

■HOME AUTOMATION

Assistive domotics could be a style of home automation that enables the senior and disabled population to live independently. It slowly becomes a viable possibility for such people that opt to keep in their own homes instead of a healthcare center. The technology and equipment are almost like home automation for security, amusement, and energy conservation but are readymade for elderly people. "For example, automatic prompts and prompters operate using motion sensors and pre-recorded audio messages; an automatic prompt within the room might recall the resident to show off the kitchen appliance, and one by the outside door might keep in mind the resident to lock the door."[1]

With the advancement of medical technology, survival beyond critical illness and trauma is increasingly becoming possible. In intensive care unit patients who are with the critical illness and prolonged hospitalization, they develop muscle weakness. Maintaining the muscle strength and function becomes a secondary concern for stabilization of the patient. Complications related to prolonged bed rest are hypotension, skin breakdown, osteoporosis, contractures, and respiratory disease. The different assistive technology was used for early mobilization of the patient in the critical care unit.[1]

ASSISTIVE TECHNOLOGY IN DIABETIC FOOT

Diabetic foot is a syndrome characterized by a triad of conditions such as neuropathy, vascular compromise, and musculoskeletal deformities in the foot. Early detection and prevention strategies will be useful to prevent further complications such as ulcer formation and subsequent gangrene formation and amputation.[1]

Types of assistive devices used in diabetic foot:
- Offloading footwear
- Modified insoles
- Plantar pressure analysis using various software such as Win track and SIMI three-dimensional (3D) motion gait analysis to prevent gait deformities raised due to diabetic foot
- Pulse flow DF footwear which is used in diabetic foot ulcer which uses pneumatic compression technology to offload the affected area.

A variety of foot orthoses, custommade and prefabricated, inserted inappropriate footwear, which aims to compensate for the loss of function, to protect the feet from trauma and to redistribute high plantar pressures. Casting, foam boxes, and foot scanning are equipment's and techniques that are used to capture the shape and morphology of the feet. These impressions, manual or digital, are used in the production of custom-made foot orthoses. Based on the digital data, foot orthoses can be automatically produced by carving out the orthoses from a block or by 3D printing.[1]

REFERENCE

1. Maiya AG, Kumar AS, Anche P, Yadav H. Assistive technology in locomotor disability: Physiotherapy and rehabilitation perspectives. Indian Journal of Physical Therapy and Research. 2019;1;1(1):66.

CHAPTER 12

Schemes and Legislations for Person with Disabilities

Nitin Suhas Nikhade, Pradnya Dumore

LEARNING OBJECTIVES

Through this chapter, the reader will be able to:
- Understand schemes for person with disabilities
- Gain knowledge on legislations for person with disabilities
- Acquire insights on National policy for person with disabilities

■ INTRODUCTION

What is Disability?

Disability is complex, dynamic, multidimensional, and contested. Over recent decades, the disabled people's movement—have identified the role of social and physical barriers in disability. The transition from an individual, medical perspective to a structural, social perspective has been described as the shift from a "medical model" to a "social model" in which people are viewed as being disabled by society rather than by their bodies. According to The Rights of Persons with Disabilities Act, 2016 "Person with disability" means *a person with long-term physical, mental, intellectual or sensory impairment which, in interaction with barriers, hinders his full and effective participation in society equally with others.*[1]

According to Census 2011, there are 2.68 crore persons with disabilities in India who constitute 2.21% of the total population. This includes persons with visual, hearing, speech, locomotor and mental disabilities. Out of the total population of persons with disabilities (PWDs), about 1.50 crore are male and 1.18 crore, female. Further, 0.82 crore PWDs live in urban areas and 1.86 crore PWDs live in rural areas.[2]

Intersection of disability with gender, poverty, age and other factors compound the problem. The women and girls with disabilities remain hidden and silent, their concerns unknown and their rights unrecognized. In the urban and rural communities alike, they face triple discrimination because of their disabilities, gender and poverty. Studies on women with disabilities in rural areas of many countries in the Asian region have found that more than 80% of women with disabilities have no independent means of livelihood, and are thus totally dependent on others for their very existence. People with disabilities are discriminated against in matters of education and employment, and are therefore, at a disadvantage when it comes to earning incomes and contributing to the family economy.

People with disabilities are also very vulnerable to poverty, if they are not already poor, since disability often results in loss of income and demands additional expenditure. Consequently, more than two-thirds of the people with moderate and severe disabilities live in poverty. Disabled persons, their families and caregivers incur substantial additional expenditure for facilitating activities of daily living, medical care, purchase and maintenance of assistive devices, transportation to access rehabilitation and medical facilities, etc. In the absence of adequate societal support and government services, the family's resources are stretched to provide additional supports to a member with a disability. Therefore, there is a need to provide them comprehensive social security through various schemes by central government as well as the state governments.[3]

■ PROVISIONS FOR PERSONS WITH DISABILITIES IN CONSTITUTION OF INDIA

The Constitution of India ensures equality, freedom, justice and dignity of all individuals and implicitly mandates an inclusive society for all including persons with disabilities. In the recent years, there have been vast and positive changes in the perception of the society towards persons with disabilities. It has been realized that a majority of persons with disabilities can lead a better quality of life if they have equal opportunities and effective access to rehabilitation measures.[4]

Under the constitution the disabled have been guaranteed the following fundamental rights:

1. The constitution secures to the citizens including the disabled, a right of justice, liberty of thought, expression, belief, faith and worship, equality of status and of opportunity and for the promotion of fraternity.
2. Article 15(1) enjoins on the government not to discriminate against any citizen of India (including disabled) on the ground of religion, race, caste, sex or place of birth.
3. Article 15(2) states that no citizen (including the disabled) shall be subjected to any disability, liability, restriction or condition on any of the above grounds in the matter of their access to shops, public restaurants, hotels and places of public entertainment or in the use of wells, tanks, bathing ghats, roads and places of public resort maintained wholly or partly out of government funds or dedicated to the use of the general public. Women and children and those belonging to any socially and educationally backward classes or the scheduled castes and tribes can be given the benefit of special laws or special provisions made by the state.
4. There shall be equality of opportunity for all citizens (including the disabled) in matters relating to employment or appointment to any office under the state.
5. No person including the disabled irrespective of his belonging can be treated as an untouchable. It would be an offence punishable in accordance with law as provided by Article 17 of the constitution.
6. Every person including the disabled has his life and liberty guaranteed under Article 21 of the constitution.
7. There can be no traffic in human beings (including the disabled), and beggar and other forms of forced labor is prohibited and the same is made punishable in accordance with law (Article 23).
8. Article 25 guarantees to every citizen (including the disabled) the right to freedom of religion. Every disabled person (like the non-disabled) has the freedom of conscience to practice and propagate his religion subject to proper order, morality and health.
9. Every disabled person can move the Supreme Court of India to enforce his fundamental rights and the rights to move the Supreme Court is itself guaranteed by Article 32.

10. No disabled person owning property (like the non-disabled) can be deprived of his property except by authority of law though right to property is not a fundamental right. Any unauthorized deprivation of property can be challenged by suit and for relief by way of damages.
11. Every disabled person (like the non-disabled) on attainment of 18 years of age becomes eligible for inclusion of his name in the general electoral roll for the territorial constituency to which he belongs.[4]

■ NATIONAL POLICY FOR PERSONS WITH DISABILITIES

The National Policy for Persons with Disabilities (2006) recognizes that persons with disabilities are a valuable human resource for the country and seeks to create an environment that provides them equal opportunities, protection of their rights and full participation in society. The national policy also recognizes the fact that a majority of persons with disabilities can lead a better quality of life if they have equal opportunities and effective access to rehabilitation measures. The Department of Empowerment of Persons with Disabilities (Divyangjan) was carved out of the Ministry of Social Justice and Empowerment in May 2012 as Department of Disability Affairs to ensure greater focus on policy matters to effectively address disability issues and to act as a nodal department for greater coordination among stakeholders, organizations, state governments and related central ministries.[5]

The salient features of the national policy are:
 i. Physical rehabilitation, which includes early detection and intervention, counselling and medical interventions and provision of aids and appliances. It also includes the development of rehabilitation professionals.
 ii. Educational rehabilitation which includes vocational training.
 iii. Economic rehabilitation, for a dignified life in society.

Physical Rehabilitation Strategies

Early Detection and Intervention

Early detection of disability and intervention through drug or non-drug therapies helps in minimization of impact of disability. Therefore, there will be emphasis on early detection and early intervention, and necessary facilities will be created towards this end. Government will take measures to disseminate information regarding availability of such facilities to the people especially in rural areas.

Ministry of Health and Family Welfare implements various programs for prevention and control of disabilities, which are:
- Universal Immunisation Programme
- National Programme for Control of Blindness
- Pulse-polio Programme
- National Iodine Deficiency Disorder Control Programme
- National Leprosy Eradication Programme
- National Programme for Prevention and Control of Deafness
- National Programme for Prevention and Control of Fluorosis.

Counseling and Medical Rehabilitation

Physical rehabilitation measures including counseling, strengthening capacities of persons with disabilities and their families, physiotherapy, occupational therapy, psychotherapy, surgical correction and intervention, vision assessment, vision stimulation, speech therapy, audiological rehabilitation and special education shall be extended to cover all the districts in the country by active involvement and participation of state governments, local level institutions, NGOs including associations of parents and persons with disabilities.

Currently, rehabilitation services are largely available in and around urban areas. Since 75% persons with disabilities live in rural areas, the services run by professionals will be extended to cover uncovered and unserved areas. Privately owned rehabilitation service centers shall be regulated for maintenance of minimum standards which shall be laid down.

To expand coverage in rural and unserved areas, new District Disability Rehabilitation Centres (DDRCs) will be set up with support from the State Government.

The National Rural Health Mission through Accredited Social Health Activist (ASHA) addresses the health needs of rural population, especially the vulnerable sections of society. The ASHA inter-alia will take care of the comprehensive services to the persons with disabilities at the grass root level.

Assistive Devices

The Government of India has been assisting persons with disabilities in procuring durable and scientifically manufactured, modern aids and appliances of ISI standard that can promote their physical, social and psychological independence by reducing the effect of disabilities.

Every year through national institutes, state governments, DDRCs and NGOs, persons with disabilities are provided with devices such as prostheses and orthoses, tricycles, wheel chair, surgical footwear and devices for activities of daily living, learning equipment (Braille writing equipment, Dictaphone, CD player/tape recorder), low vision aids, special mobility aids like canes for blind, hearing aids, educational kits, communication aids, assistive and alerting devices and devices suitable for the persons with mental disabilities. The availability of devices will be expanded to cover uncovered and under-serviced areas. Private, public and joint sector enterprises involved in the manufacture of high-tech assistive devices for persons with disabilities will be provided financial support by the public sector banks.

Development of Rehabilitation Professionals

Human resource requirements for rehabilitation of persons with disabilities will be assessed and development plan will be prepared so that the rehabilitation strategies do not suffer from lack of manpower.

Education for Persons with Disabilities

Education is the most effective vehicle of social and economic empowerment. In keeping with the spirit of the Article 21A of the constitution guaranteeing education as a fundamental right and Section 26 of the Persons with Disabilities Act, 1995, free and compulsory education has to be provided to all children with disabilities up to the minimum age of 18 years.

Sarva Shiksha Abhiyan (SSA) launched by the government has the goal of 8 years of elementary schooling for all children including children with disabilities in the age group of 6–14 years. Children with disabilities in the age group of 15–18 years are provided free education under Integrated Education for Disabled Children (IEDC) scheme.

Facilities for technical and vocational education designed to inculcate and bolster skill development suited to various types of productive activities by adaptation of the existing institutes or accelerated setting up of institutes in un-served/underserved areas will be encouraged. NGOs will also be encouraged to provide vocational training.

Persons with disabilities will be provided access to the universities, technical institutions and other institutions of higher learning to pursue higher and professional courses[5].

Economic Rehabilitation of Persons with Disabilities

Economic rehabilitation of Persons with disabilities comprise of both wage employment in organized sector and self-employment. Supporting structure of services by way of vocational rehabilitation centers and vocational training centers will be developed to ensure that disabled persons in both urban and rural areas have increased opportunities for productive and gainful employment. Strategies for economic empowerment of persons with disabilities would be the following.

Employment in Government Establishments

The PWD Act, 1995 provides for 3% reservation in employment in the establishments of Government of India and public sector undertakings (PSUs) against identified posts. The status of reservation for government in various ministries/departments against identified posts in Group A, B, C and D is 3.07%, 4.41%, 3.76% and 3.18% respectively. In PSUs, the reservation status in Group A, B, C and D is 2.78%, 8.54%, 5.04% and 6.75%, respectively. Government will ensure reservation in identified posts in the government sector including public sector undertakings in accordance with the provisions of the PwD Act, 1995.

Wage Employment in Private Sector

Development of appropriate skills in persons with disabilities will be encouraged for their employability in private sector. Vocational rehabilitation and training centers engaged in developing appropriate skills amongst persons with disabilities keeping in view their potential and abilities will be encouraged to expand their services. Considering rapid growth of employment opportunities in service sector, persons with disabilities will be encouraged to undertake skill training suitable to the market requirement. Proactive measures like incentives, awards, tax exemptions, etc., will be taken to encourage the employment of persons with disabilities in the private sector.

Self-employment

Considering slow pace of growth in employment opportunities in the organized sector, self- employment of persons with disabilities will be promoted. This will be done through vocational education and management training. The government vocational training centers for persons with disabilities operating in the country are part of the vocational and skilling network for providing skill training. Efforts are taken to develop capacity in training of trainers in association with National Skill Development Corporation and Sector Skill Council for Persons with Disabilities.

National Handicapped Finance Development Corporation implements schemes for financial assistance for skill and entrepreneur development program for persons with disabilities in the age group of 18–59 years. It also provides loans at concessional rate of interest to persons with disabilities for promoting self-employment. Priority in financial support will be given to self-help groups formed by the persons with disabilities.

The Small Industries Development Bank of India (SIDBI) is the nodal public central bank for providing subsidized loan facility for startups. SIDBI Startup Mitra is a digital initiative of SIDBI to address the gaps in the Startup eco system. It acts as a virtual platform to bring together all stakeholders, startup entrepreneurs, incubators, investors, industry bodies, banks to meet the financing and developmental needs of early age startup enterprises.[5]

Women with Disabilities

Women with disabilities require protection against exploitation and abuse. Special programs will be developed for education, employment and providing of other rehabilitation services to women with disabilities keeping in view their special needs. Special educational and vocation training facilities will be setup. Programs will be undertaken to rehabilitate abandoned disabled women/girls by encouraging their adoption in families, support to house them and impart them training for gainful employment skills. The government will encourage the projects where representation of women with disabilities is ensured at least to the extent of 25% of total beneficiaries.

Steps shall be taken to provide short duration stay homes for women with disabilities, hostels for working disabled women, and homes for aged disabled women. It has been noted that women with disabilities have serious difficulty in looking after their children. The government will take up a program to provide financial support to women with disabilities so that they may hire services to look after their children. Such support will be limited to two children for a period not exceeding two years.

Children with Disabilities

Children with disabilities are the most vulnerable group and need special attention. The government would strive to: (a) Ensure right to care, protection and security for children with disabilities. (b) Ensure the right to development with dignity and equality creating an enabling environment where children can exercise their rights, enjoy equal opportunities and full participation in accordance with various statutes. (c) Ensure inclusion and effective access to education, health, vocational training along with specialized rehabilitation services to children with disabilities. (d) Ensure the right to development as well as recognition of special needs and of care, and protection of children with severe disabilities.

Barrier-free Environment

Barrier-free environment enables people with disabilities to move about safely and freely, and use the facilities within the built environment. The goal of barrier-free design is to provide an environment that supports the independent functioning of individuals so that they can participate without assistance, in everyday activities. Therefore, to the maximum extent possible, buildings/places/transportation systems for public use will be made barrier-free.

Issue of Disability Certificates

The Government of India has notified guidelines for evaluation of the disabilities and procedure for certification. These guidelines provide composition of medical authorities for assessment and certification process. For disability certification, various experts such as Ophthalmologist, ENT Specialist, Audiologist, Speech and Language Pathologist, Orthopedic/PMR Specialist, Clinical Psychologist/Rehabilitation Psychologist, Neurologist, Psychiatrist, Special Educator, Physiotherapist, Occupational Therapist, etc., are required at the district level. The central government has launched the Unique Disability Identity (UDID) project which provides an online platform for application and certification of disability. Online certification through UDID portal is now made mandatory from 1st June 2021. The government will ensure that the persons with disabilities obtain the disability certificates without any difficulty in the shortest possible time by adoption of simple, transparent and client-friendly procedures.

Social Security

Disabled persons, their families and caregivers incur substantial additional expenditure for facilitating activities of daily living, medical care, transportation, assistive devices, etc. Therefore, there is a need to provide them social security by various means. Central government has been providing tax relief to persons with disabilities and their guardians. The state governments/UT administrations have been providing unemployment allowance or disability pension. The state governments will be encouraged to develop a comprehensive social security policy for persons with disabilities.

Parents of severely disabled persons with autism, cerebral palsy, mental retardation and multiple disabilities feel a sense of insecurity regarding the welfare of their wards after their death. National trust for persons with autism, cerebral palsy, mental retardation and multiple disabilities has been providing legal guardians through local level committee. They are also implementing the Supported Guardianship Scheme to provide financial security to persons with the above-mentioned severe disabilities who are destitute and abandoned by supporting the cost of guardianship. This scheme, which is presently implemented in a few districts, shall be expanded to cover other areas in a phased manner.

Promotion of Non-governmental Organizations (NGOs)

The national policy recognizes the NGO sector as a very important institutional mechanism to provide affordable services to complement the endeavors of the government. The NGO sector is a vibrant and growing one. It has played a significant role in the provisions of services for persons with disabilities. Some of the NGOs are also undertaking human resource development and research activities. Government has also been actively involving them in policy formulation, planning, implementation, monitoring and has been seeking their advice on various issues relating to persons with disabilities. Interaction with NGOs will be enhanced on various disability issues regarding planning, policy formulation and implementation. Networking, exchange of information and sharing of good practices amongst NGOs will be encouraged and facilitated. The following programs will be undertaken:

- A directory of NGOs working in the field of disability will be prepared properly mapping them by geographic regions along with their major activities. For NGOs supported by the central/state governments, their resource position, both financial and manpower will also be reported. Disabled persons organizations, family associations and advocacy groups of parents of disabled persons shall also be covered in the directory identifying them separately.
- There are regional/state imbalances in the development of the NGO movement. Steps will be taken to encourage and accord preference to NGOs working in the underserved and inaccessible areas. Reputed NGOs shall also be encouraged to take up projects in such areas.
- NGOs will be provided opportunities for orientation and training of their human resource. Training in management skill which is already being provided, will be strengthened. Transparency, accountability, procedural simplification, etc., will be guiding factors for improvement in the NGO–government partnership.
- The NGOs shall be encouraged to mobilize their own resources to reduce the dependence on grants-in-aid from the government and also to improve the availability of funds in the sector. Tapering of assistance in a schematic manner will also be considered so that the number of NGOs to be helped within the available resources could be maximized.[5]

Collection of Regular Information on Persons with Disabilities

There is a need for regular collection, compilation and analysis of data relating to socioeconomic conditions of persons with disabilities. The National Sample Survey Organization has been collecting information on socioeconomic conditions of persons with disabilities on regular basis once in 10 years since 1981. The census has also started collection of information on persons with disabilities from the census 2001. The National Sample Survey Organization will have to collect the information on persons with disabilities at least once in 5 years. The differences in the definitions adopted by the two agencies will be reconciled.

A comprehensive website for persons with disability will be created under the Ministry of Social Justice and Empowerment. Organizations both in public and private sector will be encouraged to make their websites accessible to the persons with disabilities.

Research

For improving the quality of life of persons with disabilities, research will be supported on their socioeconomic and cultural context, cause of disabilities, early childhood education methodologies, development of user-friendly aids and appliances and all matters connected with disabilities which will significantly alter the quality of their life and civil society's ability to respond to their concerns. Wherever persons with disabilities are subjected to research interventions, their or their family member or caregiver's consent is mandatory.

Sports, Recreation and Cultural Life

The contribution of sports for its therapeutic and community spirit is undeniable. Persons with disabilities have right to access sports, recreation and cultural facilities. For promoting sports, the government is committed to providing quality infrastructure in terms of training facilities for sportspersons with disabilities. In this regard, the government is setting up a Center for Disability Sports at Gwalior with a view to provide world class infrastructure for Divyang sportspersons so that they can compete effectively and win medals for the country in various international events like Paralympics and special olympics.

The earlier emphasis on medical rehabilitation has now been replaced by an emphasis on social rehabilitation. There has been an increasing recognition of abilities of persons with disabilities and emphasis on mainstreaming them in the society based on their capabilities.

The Government of India has enacted three legislations for persons with disabilities viz.
 i. Persons with Disability (Equal Opportunities, Protection of Rights and Full Participation) Act, 1995, which provides for education, employment, creation of barrier free environment, social security, etc.
 ii. National Trust for Welfare of Persons with Autism, Cerebral Palsy, Mental Retardation and Multiple Disability Act, 1999 has provisions for legal guardianship of the four categories and creation of enabling environment for as much independent living as possible.
 iii. Rehabilitation Council of India Act, 1992 deals with the development of manpower for providing rehabilitation services.

I. The Persons with Disabilities (PWD) Act, 1995

"The Persons with Disabilities (Equal Opportunities, Protection of Rights and Full Participation) Act, 1995" had come into enforcement on February 7, 1996. It is a significant step which ensures equal opportunities for the people with disabilities and their full participation in the nation building.[6] The Act provides for both the preventive and promotional aspects of rehabilitation like education, employment and vocational training, reservation, research and manpower development, creation of barrier-free environment, rehabilitation of persons with disability, unemployment allowance for the disabled, special insurance scheme for the disabled employees and establishment of homes for persons with severe disability, etc.

Main provisions of the Act[6] are:
- **Prevention and early detection of disabilities:**
  - Surveys, investigations and research shall be conducted to ascertain the cause of occurrence of disabilities.
  - Various measures shall be taken to prevent disabilities. Staff at the primary health center shall be trained to assist in this work.
  - Measures shall be taken for prenatal, perinatal, and postnatal care of the mother and child.
  - All the children shall be screened once in a year for identifying 'at-risk' cases.
  - Awareness campaigns shall be launched and sponsored to disseminate information.
- **Education:**
  - Every child with disability shall have the rights to free education till the age of 18 years in integrated schools or special schools.
  - Appropriate transportation, removal of architectural barriers and restructuring of modifications in the examination system shall be ensured for the benefit of children with disabilities.
  - Children with disabilities shall have the right to free books, scholarships, uniform and other learning material.
  - Special schools for children with disabilities shall be equipped with vocational training facilities.
  - Nonformal education shall be promoted for children with disabilities.
  - Teachers' training institutions shall be established to develop requisite manpower.
- **Skill development and employment**
  - 3% of vacancies in government employment shall be reserved for people with disabilities, 1% each for the persons suffering from: Blindness or low vision, hearing impairment, locomotor disabilities and cerebral palsy.
  - Suitable scheme shall be formulated for the training and welfare of persons with disabilities.
  - The relaxation of upper age limit in the employment.
  - Health and safety measures and creation of a non-handicapping, environment in places where persons with disabilities are employed.
  - Government educational institutes and other educational institutes receiving grant from government shall reserve at least 3% seats for people with disabilities.
  - No employee can be sacked or demoted if they become disabled during service, although they can be moved to another post with the same pay and condition. No promotion can be denied because of impairment.
- **Affirmative action**
  - Aids and appliances shall be made available to the people with disabilities.
  - Allotment of land shall be made at concessional rates to the people with disabilities for: House, business, special recreational centers, special schools, research schools, factories by entrepreneurs with disability, etc.

- **Non-discrimination**
  - Public building, rail compartments, buses, ships and air-crafts will be designed to give easy access to the disabled people.
  - In all public places and in waiting rooms, the toilets shall be wheelchair accessible. Braille and sound symbols are also to be provided in all elevators (lifts).
  - All the places of public utility shall be made barrier-free by providing the ramps.

- ❖ **Research and manpower development**
  - Research shall be sponsored and promoted for prevention of disability, community-based rehabilitation, development of assistive devices.
  - Job identification and on-site modifications of offices and factories.
  - Financial assistance shall be made available to the universities, other institutions of higher learning, professional bodies and non-government research-units or institutions, for undertaking research for special education, rehabilitation and manpower development.
- ❖ **Social security**
  - Financial assistance to non-government organizations for the rehabilitation of persons with disabilities.
  - Insurance coverage for the benefit of the government employees with disabilities.
  - Unemployment allowance to the people with disabilities who are registered with the special employment exchange for more than a year and could not find any gainful occupation.
- ❖ **Grievance redressal**
  - In case of violation of the rights as prescribed in this act, people with disabilities may move an application to the chief commissioner for persons with disabilities in the center, or commissioner for persons with disabilities in the state.

II. The Rights of Persons with Disabilities (RPwD) Act, 2016

An Act to give effect to the United Nations Convention on the rights of persons with disabilities and for matters connected therewith or incidental thereto. The RPwD Act, 2016 was enacted on 28.12.2016 which came into force from 19.04.2017. The salient features of the Act[1] are:
- ❖ Responsibility has been cast upon the appropriate governments to take effective measures to ensure that the persons with disabilities enjoy their rights equally with others.
- ❖ Disability has been defined based on an evolving and dynamic concept.

The Act covers the following specified disabilities:[1]
- ❖ **Physical disability**
  - Locomotor disability
    - Leprosy cured person
    - Cerebral palsy
    - Dwarfism
    - Muscular dystrophy
    - Acid attack victims
  - Visual impairment
    - Blindness
    - Low vision
  - Hearing impairment
    - Deaf
    - Hard of hearing
  - Speech and language disability
- ❖ **Intellectual disability**
  - Specific learning disabilities
  - Autism spectrum disorder
- ❖ **Mental behavior (mental illness)**
- ❖ **Disability caused due to:**
  - Chronic neurological conditions such as:

- Multiple sclerosis
- Parkinson's disease
- Blood disorder:
  - Hemophilia
  - Thalassemia
  - Sickle cell disease

❖ **Multiple disabilities**
- Additional benefits have been provided for persons with benchmark disabilities and those with high support needs.
- Every child with benchmark disability between the age group of 6 and 18 years shall have the right to free education.
- 5% reservation in seats in government and government-aided higher educational institutions for persons with benchmark disabilities.
- Stress has been given to ensure accessibility in public buildings (both government and private) in a prescribed time-frame.
- 4% reservation in government jobs for certain persons or class of persons with benchmark disability.
- The Act provides for grant of guardianship by District Court or any authority designated by the state government under which there will be joint decision-making between the guardian and the persons with disabilities.
- Broad based central and state advisory boards on disability to be set up as policy making bodies.
- The Act provides for strengthening of the office of chief commissioner of persons with disabilities and state commissioners of disabilities which will act as regulatory bodies and Grievance Redressal agencies and also monitor implementation of the Act. These offices will be assisted by an advisory committee comprising of experts in various disabilities.
- Creation of national and state fund to provide financial support to the persons with disabilities.
- The Act provides for penalties for offences committed against persons with disabilities.
- Designated special courts to handle cases concerning violation of rights of PwDs.

III. National Trust for the Welfare of Persons with Autism, Cerebral Palsy, Mental

Retardation and Multiple Disability Act, 1999

The national trust is a statutory body set up in 2000 under the National Trust for the Welfare of Persons with Autism, Cerebral Palsy, Mental Retardation and Multiple Disabilities Act, 1999. The national trust has been set up to discharge two basic duties—legal and welfare. Legal duties are discharged through local level committee and providing legal guardianship. Welfare duty is discharged through the schemes.

National trust runs a bouquet of schemes and programs ranging from early intervention for children up to 6 years to residential centers for adults with severe disabilities. The activities of the national trust interalia include training, awareness and capacity building programs and shelter, care giving and empowerment. The national trust offers registration to voluntary organization, association of person with disabilities and association of parents of persons with disabilities. There are around 425 registered organizations of the national trust in the country.[7]

CHAPTER 12: Schemes and Legislations for Person with Disabilities

Major Activities under different schemes and programs of the national trust:[7]

- **DISHA (Early Intervention and School Readiness Scheme):** This is an early intervention and school readiness scheme for children in the age group of 0–10 years with the four disabilities covered under the National Trust Act and aims at setting up DISHA centers for early intervention for persons with disabilities (PWDs) through therapies, trainings and providing support to family members. Registered organizations should provide day-care facilities to PWDs for at least 4 hours in a day (between 8 am to 6 pm) along with age specific activities. There should be a Special Educator or Early Intervention Therapist, Physiotherapist or Occupational Therapist and Counsellor for PWDs along with caregiver and Ayas in the center. The revised Early Intervention Scheme will have provision to cover 0–10 years age group of children in place of 0–6 years age group as envisaged in the earlier scheme. The set up cost has been increased from ₹ 50,000 to ₹ 1.55 lakh.

- **VIKAAS (Day Care):** This is a day-care scheme, primarily to expand the range of opportunities available to persons with disabilities for enhancing interpersonal and vocational skills as they are on a transition to higher age groups. The center will also offer care-giving support to persons with disabilities (PWDs) when they are in the Vikaas center. In addition it also helps in supporting family members of the persons with disabilities covered under the National Trust Act to fulfill other responsibilities. Registered organizations should provide day-care facilities to PWDs for at least 6 hours in a day (between 8 am to 6 pm) along with age specific activities. Day-care should be open for at least 21 days in a month.

- **SAMARTH (Respite Care):** The objective of Samarth scheme is to provide respite home for orphans or abandoned, families in crisis and also for persons with disabilities (PWDs) from BPL and LIG families including destitute with at least one of the four disabilities covered under the National Trust Act. It also aims at creating opportunities for family members to get respite time in order to fulfill other responsibilities. This scheme aims at setting up Samarth centers for providing group home facility for all age groups with adequate and quality care service with acceptable living standards including provision of basic medical care from professional doctors.

- **GHARAUNDA (Group Home for Adults):** The objective of Gharaunda scheme is to provide an assured home and minimum quality of care services throughout the life for the persons with autism, cerebral palsy, mental retardation and multiple disabilities. This scheme aims to provide adequate and quality care service with acceptable living standards including provision of basic medical care from professional doctors. Gharaunda centers should provide vocational activities, pre-vocational activities and assistance for further training.

- **'NIRAMAYA' Health Insurance Scheme:** The scheme is to provide affordable health insurance to persons with autism, cerebral palsy, mental retardation and multiple disabilities. The enrolled beneficiaries get a health insurance cover up to ₹ 1.0 lakh, by paying a nominal fee. This scheme gives facility for OPD treatment including the medicines, pathology, diagnostic tests, etc. Regular medical checkup for non-ailing disabled, dental preventive dentistry, surgery to prevent further aggravation of disability, non-surgical/hospitalization, corrective surgeries for existing disability including congenital disability, ongoing therapies to reduce impact of disability and disability-related complications, and alternative medicine.

- **SAHYOGI (Caregiver Training Scheme):** This scheme aims at setting up caregiver cells (CGCs) to provide training and create a skilled workforce of caregivers to provide adequate and nurturing care for persons with disabilities (Divyangjan) and their families who require it. It also seeks to provide parents an opportunity to get trained in care giving, if they so desire.

This scheme will provide a choice of training through two levels of courses primary and advanced to allow it to create caregivers suited to work both with persons with disabilities (Divyangjan) families and other institutions catering to the needs of the Divyangjan (NGOs, work centers, etc.).

There is a provision of training cost of Rs.4,200 per trainee, for primary course and Rs.8,000 for advanced course. Also, stipend for trainee @ Rs.5,000 for primary and Rs.10,000 for advanced course has been introduced in the scheme.

- **GYAN PRABHA (Educational Support):** Gyan Prabha scheme aims to encourage people with autism, cerebral palsy, mental retardation and multiple disabilities for pursuing educational courses like graduation courses, professional courses and vocational training leading to employment or self-employment. The national trust is providing a specific amount per course to a Divyangjan which covers fees, transportation, books, out of pocket expenses (OPEs), etc. Wide range of courses covered in the revised scheme in place of only vocational training/ skill development courses.
- **PRERNA (Marketing Assistance):** This is the marketing assistance scheme of the national trust with an objective to create viable and widespread channels for sale of products and services produced by persons with disabilities (PWDs) covered under the National Trust Act. This scheme aims at providing funds to participate in events such as exhibitions, melas, fairs, etc. for marketing and selling products and services prepared by PWDs. The scheme also provides an incentive to the registered organizations (ROs) based on the sales turnover of the products made by PWDs. However, at least 51% of employees of these work centers should be persons with disabilities covered under the National Trust Act.
- **SAMBHAV (Aids and Assisted Devices):** This is a scheme to setup additional resource centers, one each in each city of the country with population greater than 5 million (As per 2011 census), to collate and collect the aids, software and other form of assistive devices developed with a provision of display and demonstration of the devices. The scheme also includes maintaining information, pertaining to aids and assistive devices present at Sambhav center, on the national trust website. These centers aim to provide information and easy access to devices, appliances, aids, software, etc., for betterment and empowerment of PWDs.
- **BADHTE KADAM (Awareness and Community Interaction):** This scheme shall support registered organizations (ROs) of the national trust to carry out activities that focus on increasing the awareness of the disabilities. Aim of scheme is to create community awareness, sensitization, social integration and mainstreaming of persons with disabilities. The national trust shall sponsor a maximum of 4 events for each RO per year. Each RO should conduct at least 1 event (either for community, educational institutes or medical institutes) in a year. Badhte Kadam was earlier an initiative of the national trust which is now converted into a scheme.

IV. Rehabilitation Council of India Act, 1992

The Rehabilitation Council of India (RCI) is the apex government body, constituted under the Rehabilitation Council of India Act, 1992 to regulate and monitor the training programs and courses targeted at disabled, and special education requirement communities; promotes research in rehabilitation and special education. It is the only statutory council in India that maintains the central rehabilitation register (CRR) which mainly documents details of all qualified professionals who operate and deliver training and educational programs for the disabled. In the year 2000, the Rehabilitation Council of India (Amendment) Act, 2000 was introduced to make it more broad-based. The mandate given to RCI for regulating and monitoring services given to persons with disability, standardizing syllabi and maintaining a central rehabilitation register of all qualified professionals and personnel working in the field of rehabilitation and special education. The Act also prescribes punitive action against unqualified persons delivering services to persons with disability.[5]

Central Government Schemes for Disabled Persons

- **Assistance to disabled persons for purchase/fitting of aids and appliances (ADIP scheme):** The main objective of the scheme is to assist needy person with disabilities in procuring durable sophisticated and scientifically manufactured, modern, standard aids and appliances that can promote their physical, social and psychological rehabilitation by reducing the effects of disabilities and enhance their economic potential.

  The scheme is implemented through implementing agencies such as the NGO's, national institutes under administrative control of the Ministry of Social Justice and Empowerment and ALIMCO (a PSU). The agencies should preferably possess professional/technical expertise in the form of professionally qualified staff (from recognized courses) for the identification, prescription of the required artificial aids/appliance; fitment and post-fitment care of the beneficiaries as well as the aid/appliance. The agency should also preferably possess infrastructure in the form of machinery/equipment for the fabrication, fitment and maintenance of artificial aid/appliance to be given to a disabled person under ADIP scheme. Aids and appliances which do not cost more than ₹ 10,000 are covered under the scheme for single disability. In the case of multiple disabilities, the limit will apply to individual items separately in case more than one aid/appliance is required.

  Quantum of assistance and income limit under the ADIP scheme:

Total income	Amount of assistance
Up to ₹ 15,000 per month	Full cost of aid/appliance
15,001 to ₹ 20,000 per month	50% of the cost of aid/appliance

  In case of dependents, the income of parents/guardians should not exceed ₹ 20,000 per month.

  Motorized tricycles and wheelchairs for severely disabled and for quadriplegic (SCI), muscular dystrophy, stroke, cerebral palsy, hemiplegic and any other person with similar conditions, where either three/four limbs or one half of the body are severely impaired. The extent of subsidy provided is ₹ 25,000. The minimum age for availing motorized tricycle and wheelchairs is 16 years. The assistance will be provided once in 10 years.

  Travelling cost would be admissible separately to the person with disabilities and one escort limited to bus fare or railway, subject to a limit of ₹ 250 each person, irrespective of number of visits to the centre. Further, boarding and lodging expenses at the rate of ₹ 100 per day for maximum duration of 15 days would be admissible, only for those patients whose total income is up to Rs.15, 000 per month and the same will be allowed to attendant/escort.[8]

- **Scheme for Implementation of Persons with Disabilities Act (SIPDA):** This scheme provides grant-in-aid to state governments, organizations of central/state governments, including autonomous bodies and universities, for creating barrier free access to their buildings; making websites accessible; early intervention; awareness generation, skill development, etc.[8]

- **Deendayal Disabled Rehabilitation Scheme (DDRS):** The umbrella Central Sector Scheme of the Ministry of Social Justice and Empowerment called the "Scheme to Promote Voluntary Action for Persons with Disabilities" was revised and renamed as the "Deendayal Disabled

Rehabilitation Scheme (DDRS)" on 01.04.2003. The DDRS scheme facilitates delivery of various services to persons with disabilities by voluntary organizations. The objectives of the scheme are: (1) To create an enabling environment to ensure equal opportunities, equity, social justice and empowerment of persons with disabilities. (2) To encourage voluntary action for ensuring effective implementation of the People with Disabilities (Equal Opportunities and Protection of Rights) Act of 1995.

The approach of this scheme is to provide financial assistance to NGOs to make available all the services necessary for rehabilitation of persons with disabilities including early intervention, development of daily living skills, education, skill-development oriented towards employability, training and awareness generation. With a view to inclusion of persons with disabilities in the mainstream of society and actualizing their potential, the thrust would be on education and training programs. Under this scheme grants-in-aid is provided through NGOs for various projects such as vocational training centers, sheltered workshops, special schools for the persons with disabilities, project for cerebral palsied children, home based rehabilitation program, project for rehabilitation of leprosy cured persons (LCPs), project relating to survey, identification, awareness and sensitization, project for community based rehabilitation, environment friendly and eco-promotive projects for the handicapped, district disability rehabilitation centers (DDRCs), seminars/ workshops/rural camps, etc. The maximum level of support could be up to 90% of the eligible amount of grant for the project.[8]

- **Indira Gandhi National Disability Pension Scheme (IGNDPS):** This scheme was launched as a component of the National Social Assistance Program on 17th February 2009 by the ministry of rural development. The objective of scheme is to provide financial assistance to disabled persons belonging to below poverty line household. Person who are within the age group of 18–79 years and having 80% and above/multiple disabilities and belonging to a household below poverty line are eligible to get the pension.

  Under IGNDPS, a sum of Rs. 300 is paid as pension for disabled people whose age ranges between 18 and 79 years and a sum of ₹ 500 is provided for people ≥80 years age. Central government is providing financial assistance of Rs. 300 per month per beneficiary. In addition to this state government is providing ₹ 200 per month to each beneficiaries. Dwarfs are also an eligible category for this pension. To get this pension the beneficiaries has to apply in the prescribed form to the concerned Block Development Officer (BDO) or executive officer of the municipality. The sub-collector sanctions pension in favor of the beneficiaries on the recommendation of the BDOs. The eligible applications are being sanctioned on first come first serve basis from the waiting list.[9]

- **Inclusive Education for Disabled (IED) Under Sarva Shiksha Abhiyan (SSA):** The main focus of Sarva Shiksha Abhiyan (SSA) is on increasing access, enrollment and retention of all children with special needs (CWSN) as well as improvising the quality of education for them. The Ministry of Human Resource Development, Government of India issued guidelines for inclusive education for disabled as follows:
  - A zero rejection policy for education: It ensures that every child with special needs, irrespective of the kind, category and degree of disability, is provided meaningful and quality education.
  - Education to child with special needs should be provided in an environment most suited to his/her learning needs.
  - The education to child with special needs should be need based and district centric for effective utilization of resources.

- Education to CWSN should be given in an appropriate environment till 18 years. CWSN need to be taught by a trained teacher.
  Under SSA, a continuum of educational options, learning aids and tools, mobility assistance, support services, etc., are being made available to students with disabilities. This includes education through an open learning system and open schools, alternative schooling, distance education, special schools, wherever necessary home-based education, itinerant teacher model, remedial teaching, part time classes, community-based rehabilitation (CBR) and vocational education.[5]
- **Inclusive Education of the Disabled at Secondary Stage Scheme:** The Scheme of Inclusive Education for Disabled at Secondary Stage (IEDSS) has been launched from the year 2009–2010. This scheme replaces the earlier scheme of Integrated Education for Disabled Children (IEDC) and provides assistance for the inclusive education of the disabled children in classes IX-XII. This scheme now subsumed under Rashtriya Madhyamik Shiksha Abhiyan (RMSA) from 2013.
  The aim of the scheme is to enable all students with disabilities, to pursue further four years of secondary schooling after completing eight years of elementary schooling in an inclusive and enabling environment. The scheme covers all children studying at the secondary stage in government, local body and government-aided schools, with one or more disabilities as defined under the Persons with Disabilities Act (1995) in the class IX to XII, namely blindness, low vision, leprosy cured, hearing impairment, locomotor disabilities, mental retardation, mental illness, autism, and cerebral palsy, etc. Girls with the disabilities receive special focus to help them gain access to secondary schools, as also to information and guidance for developing their potential. Under the scheme, student-oriented facilities such as medical and educational assessment, books and stationery, uniforms, transport allowance, reader allowance, stipend for girls, support services, assistive devices, boarding the lodging facility, therapeutic services, teaching learning materials, etc., are provided. Other facilities include appointment of special education teachers, allowances for general teachers for teaching such children, teacher training, orientation of school administrators, establishment of resource room, providing barrier free environment, etc. Financial assistance is provided by the central government for all items covered in the scheme. The state governments are only required to make provisions for scholarship of ₹ 600 per disabled child per annum.[5]
- **Accessible India Campaign/Sugamya Bharat Abhiyan:** The Ministry of Social Justice and Empowerment has launched the Accessible India Campaign (Sugamya Bharat Abhiyan) on 3rd December, 2015 on the occasion of International Day for Persons with Disabilities. This nationwide campaign focuses on three verticals, i.e., built environment; public transportation and information and communication technologies for achieving universal accessibility for persons with disabilities. The government is creating an enabling and barrier free environment in which equal opportunities and access is provided for the growth and development of persons with disabilities to lead productive, safe and dignified lives. This includes creation of disabled friendly barrier free environment in buildings, public toilets, buses, bus-stands, railway stations, airports and other public places.[10]

❖ **National Institutes (NIs) and Composite Regional Centre (CRC):** The Ministry of Social Justice and Empowerment, Government of India, has set up national institutes (NIs) and composite regional centre for skill development, rehabilitation and empowerment of persons with disabilities (Divyangjan) in various states to provide both preventive and promotional aspects of rehabilitation like education, health, employment and vocational training, research and manpower development, rehabilitation for persons with disabilities, etc. There are eight national institutes (NIs) and sixteen composite regional center (CRCs) functioning in the country.[11]

The following eight national institutes are working for development of manpower in different areas, namely:
- Pt. Deendayal Upadhyaya National Institute for Person with Physical Disabilities, New Delhi.
- Indian Sign Language Research and Training Center (ISLRTC), New Delhi.
- National Institute for the Empowerment of Persons with Visual Disabilities, Dehradun.
- Ali Yavar Jung National Institute of Speech and Hearing Disabilities, Mumbai.
- National Institute for Locomotor Disabilities (NILD), Kolkata.
- National Institute for Empowerment of Persons with Multiple Disabilities, Chennai.
- National Institute for the Empowerment of Persons with Intellectual Disabilities (NIEPID), Secunderabad.
- Swami Vivekanand National Institute of Rehabilitation Training and Research (SVNIRTAR), Cuttack.

❖ **District Disability Rehabilitation Centers (DDRCs):** The scheme was launched by the Ministry of Social Justice and Empowerment, Government of India in January 2000. Initially, establishment of DDRCs started as an outreach activity for providing comprehensive services to the persons with disabilities at the grass root level and for facilitating creation of the infrastructure and capacity building at the district level for awareness generation, rehabilitation and training of rehabilitation professionals. The District Disability Rehabilitation Centers are set up under the plan scheme—"Scheme for implementation of Persons with Disabilities (Equal Opportunities, Protection of Rights and Full Participation) Act, 1995 (SIPDA)." 310 districts have been identified and 263 DDRCs have been set up. The major objectives of these centers are:
- Awareness generation for encouraging and enhancing prevention of disabilities, early detection and intervention, etc.
- Assessment of need of assistive devices, provision/fitment of assistive devices, follow up/repair of assistive devices.
- Therapeutic services, e.g., physiotherapy, occupational therapy, speech therapy, etc., for person with disabilities through rehabilitation professionals.
- To provide supportive and complimentary services to promote education, vocational training and employment for persons with disabilities.

The state governments are expected to play a more proactive role in the effective working of DDRCs. In order to ensure greater involvement of state/district administration, the state government may suitably supplement the honorarium and other requirements of the DDRCs for undertaking their various activities in an effective manner. The state governments may authorize district collectors in their capacity as chairperson of district management team (DMT), to make minor modifications for effective functioning of DDRCs, considering the ground realities within the broad stipulation of the DDRC scheme.[11]

❖ **Vocational Rehabilitation Centers (VRCs):** The Department of Empowerment of Persons with Disabilities (Divyangjan) is running 03 vocational rehabilitation centers at Ludhiana, Bathinda and Hoshiarpur and a workshop for handicapped at Shimlapuri in Ludhiana district to impart training to persons with disabilities in the age group of 18–40 years in different types of trades like tailoring, cutting, embroidery, typing/stenography, etc. The trainees are given a stipend of ₹ 2,000 per month through their bank accounts. Training to physically

CHAPTER 12: Schemes and Legislations for Person with Disabilities

handicapped persons is provided in various trades like weaving, hosiery, tailoring, canning, candle making, etc., so as to make them economically self-reliant. All applicants should have 40% and above disability certificate and the age should be between 18–40 years.

In order to facilitate speedy rehabilitation of the handicapped, seven skill training workshops (STWs) have also been attached to seven VRCs at Ahmedabad, Bengaluru, Chennai, Hyderabad, Kanpur, Mumbai and Thiruvananthapuram for imparting non-formal training in the trades best suited to an individual disabled person. Rehabilitation services of the VRCs have also been extended to the disabled persons at their door steps living in rural areas through the mobile camps and rural rehabilitation extension centers (RRECs). These RRECs have been set up in eleven blocks under five VRCs namely, Chennai, Kanpur, Kolkata, Ludhiana and Mumbai.

Services Rendered to the Handicapped Persons by the VRCs

- Evaluation of persons with disabilities to assess their physical efficiencies, functional capacities, psychological strengths and weaknesses in respect of their intelligence, aptitude, and areas of interest.
- Testing of the handicapped persons on the job capabilities in different trades sanctioned under VRC's programs such as electronics, automobile, tailoring, computer applications, wood work and chair canning, arts and crafts, screen printing, photography, Painting, etc.
- Imparting workshop training to develop vocational adjustment best suited to their strengths and weaknesses.
- Imparting non formal in-plant training and tailor made module based vocational training to persons with disabilities for enhancing their levels of knowledge and skills suited to local job market needs and also assisting, guiding and motivating them for channelizing them towards self-employment.
- Sponsoring the handicapped persons to the employers against vacancies notified to the VRCs and taking follow-up action.
- Recommending the handicapped persons for grant of loans by the concerned financial institutions under differential rate of interest or setting up of different ventures under various self-employment schemes.[11]

Central Public Sector Enterprises (CPSEs) Schemes

- **National Handicapped Finance and Development Corporation (NHFDC):** This corporation has been set up by the Ministry of Social Justice and Empowerment, Government of India on 24th January 1997. It is registered as a company not for profit. The NHFDC functions as an apex institution for providing financial assistance to the persons with disabilities (Divyangjan) for their economic rehabilitation and provides number of skill development programs to empower them to grow and sustain their enterprises. The schemes include following loans facilities:[8]
  - **Divyangjan Swavalamban Yojna:** The main objective of the scheme is to assist the needy disabled persons by providing concessional loan for economic and overall empowerment. Any Indian citizen with 40% or more disability and age above 18 years can apply for loan. However, in case of persons with mental retardation, the eligible age would be above 14 years. The upper limit of concessional loan under various NHFDC schemes would be ₹ 50 lakhs per beneficiary/unit. The actual loan amount shall be determined by implementing agencies based on the needs of the project being funded as well as repaying capacity of

the borrower within the repayment period. The rate of interest varies from 5 to 9 % based on the quantum of loan amount.
- **Vishesh Microfinance Yojana:** The objective of the scheme is to provide need-based finance for the disabled persons at reasonable rate of interest through state level organizations to pursue small/micro business and developmental activities.

   Under this scheme, the unit cost of the project shall not exceed ₹ 60,000. The NHFDC's shares 90% of the project cost and 10% is contributed by the implementing agencies and/or beneficiaries. The rate of interest would be 12% pa. The loan amount shall be repaid in quarterly installments within a maximum period of 3 years from the date of each disbursement.
- **Educational loan:** Any Indian citizen with 40% or more disability is eligible to apply for education loan under NHFDC schemes through the implementing agencies. Loan up to Rs.10 lakh for study in India and Rs.20 lakh for study at abroad is provided. The rate of interest for education loan is 4% for a loan of up to ₹ 20 lakh. A rebate of 0.5% on interest is allowed to female students with disabilities in education loan scheme. The repayment period for educational loan is maximum of 7 years.

❖ **Artificial Limbs Manufacturing Corporation (ALIMCO):** Artificial Limbs Manufacturing Corporation of India (ALIMCO) is a central public sector enterprise, registered under Section 8 (not for profit motive) of the Companies Act, 1956. It is functioning under the aegis of the Ministry of Social Justice and Empowerment, Department of Empowerment of Persons with Disabilities. ALIMCO has been engaged in manufacturing, supply and distribution of artificial limbs, assistive devices and other rehabilitation aids for persons with disabilities since 1976. The corporation is equipped with sophisticated machines and is backed by its own research and development for constantly updating designs and quality of products. The corporation conducts camps in association with various state government/district authorities for fitting and distribution of aids and appliances in rural and semi urban areas of the country.[8]

National Awards for the Empowerment of Persons with Disabilities

❖ **Scheme of National Awards for the Empowerment of Persons with Disabilities:** The scheme was launched by ministry of social justice and empowerment. The scheme is dedicated to the outstanding employers of persons with disabilities as well as the most outstanding employees. In order to recognize their effort and encourage others to strive to achieve excellence in this field, every year on the occasion of the international day for the disabled persons, i.e., 3rd December, the national awards are conferred on individuals, institutions, states, districts, etc., for outstanding work done by them in the field of empowerment of persons with disabilities. The scheme is funded by the central government. Awards are given under following 14 categories—best employees/self-employed with disabilities, best employers and best placement officer or agency, best individual and best institution working for the cause of persons with disabilities, role model, best braille press, outstanding creative adult persons with disabilities, best creative child with disabilities, best applied research or outstanding innovation or product development aimed at improving the life of persons with disabilities, outstanding work in the creation of barrier-free environment for the persons with disabilities, best district in providing rehabilitation services, best state channelizing agency of National Handicapped Finance and Development Corporation (NHFDC), best "accessible" website, best state in promoting empowerment of persons with disabilities; and best sports person with disability.[12]

Government Concessions for the Disabled

- **Income Tax Relief for Handicapped: Section 80 DD:** Section 80 DD provides for a deduction in respect of the expenditure incurred by an individual or Hindu undivided family resident in India on the medical treatment (including nursing) training and rehabilitation, etc., of handicapped dependents. For officiating the increased cost of such maintenance, or amount paid to Life Insurance Company (LIC) or any other insurer in respect of a scheme for the maintenance of a disabled dependent, the limit of the deduction under section 80 DD is ₹ 75,000 for disabled individuals with a 40–80% disability (non-severe disability) and ₹ 1,25,000 for disabled individuals with 80% or more disability (severe disability). The disabilities covered under Section 80 DD are blindness, low vision, leprosy-cured, hearing impairment, locomotor disability, autism, cerebral palsy, mental retardation and mental illness.[8]
- **Travel Concessions for the Disabled: By Rail:** As per the Order of Ministry of Railways, Government of India, the following concessions are available for the disabled persons.[8]

	Element of concession		
		Season tickets	
Category of persons	Single journey tickets	I Class	II Class
1. Completely blind persons traveling alone or with an escort	• 75% in second, sleeper, first classes and AC 3-tire • 50% in AC 2-tire and AC first classes	50%	50%
2. Orthopedically handicapped/paraplegic persons who cannot travel without an escort		50%	50%
3. Mentally retarded persons who cannot travel without an escort		50%	50%
4. Totally deaf and dumb persons travelling alone or with an escort	50% in second, sleeper, first classes	50%	50%

■ INTERNATIONAL LEGISLATIONS FOR PEOPLE WITH DISABILITY

The Role of Disability Legislation

Persons with disabilities often are excluded from the mainstream of the society and denied their human rights. Discrimination against persons with disabilities takes various forms, ranging from invidious discrimination, such as the denial of educational opportunities, to more subtle forms of discrimination, such as segregation and isolation because of the imposition of physical and social barriers. Effects of disability-based discrimination have been particularly severe in fields such as education, employment, housing, transport, cultural life and access to public places and services. Most disability legislation and policies are based on the assumption that persons with disabilities simply are not able to exercise the same rights as nondisabled persons.

A need exists for more comprehensive legislation to ensure the rights of disabled persons in all aspects political, civil, economic, social and cultural rights on an equal basis with persons without disabilities. Appropriate measures are required to address existing discrimination and to promote thereby opportunities for persons with disabilities to participate on the basis of equality in social life and development. Discriminatory practices against persons with disabilities thus may be the result of social and cultural norms that have been institutionalized by law. Though legislation is not the only means of social progress, it represents one of the most powerful vehicles of change, progress and development in society. Legislation at country level is fundamental in promoting the rights of persons with disabilities. While the importance and increasing role of international law in promoting the rights of persons with disabilities is recognized by the international community, domestic legislation remains one of the most effective means of facilitating social change and improving the status of disabled persons. International norms concerning disability are useful for setting common standards for disability legislation.[13]

International Legal Framework

- ❖ **International treaties that are binding on states and create legal obligations to the states parties:**

  All international human rights instruments protect the human rights of persons with disabilities, as they apply to all persons. This principle of universality is reinforced by the principles of equality and nondiscrimination, which are included in human rights instruments.

  Some international and regional human rights conventions protect the rights of persons with disabilities specifically, or have provisions concerning persons with disabilities. These include:
  - ILO Convention concerning Vocational Rehabilitation and Employment (Disabled Persons)
  - Inter-American Convention on the Elimination of All Forms of Discrimination Against Persons with Disabilities Convention on the Rights of the Child (Article 23)
  - African Charter of Human and People's Rights [Article 18(4)]
  - The African Charter on the Rights and Welfare of the Child (Article 13)
  - European Social Charter (Article 15)
  - Protocol of San Salvador (Additional Protocol to the American Convention on Human Rights in the Area of Economic, Social and Cultural Rights) (Article 6 and 9).

  International human rights treaties are binding on states parties that have ratified the instruments. Some universal instruments, such as the Universal Declaration of Human Rights, and some specific provisions, such as the principle of nondiscrimination, have become part of customary international law and are considered binding on all states, even those that have not ratified a human rights treaty that embodies norms of customary law.[14]

- ❖ **International instruments that are nonbinding, such as declarations and rules, and are useful in interpreting international standards and implementing them in national legislation:**

  General policy instruments, such as the outcome documents of world summits and conferences, are applicable to persons with disabilities which include, for example, the Copenhagen Declaration and Programme of Action adopted at the World Summit for Social Development (6–12 March 1995), and the Millennium Declaration and the Millennium Development Goals adopted at the United Nations Millennium Summit in September 2000.

  Several disability-specific nonbinding international instruments have been adopted at the international level.[14] The instruments include:

- ❖ Declaration of the Rights of Mentally Retarded Persons, Declaration on the Rights of Disabled Persons
- ❖ World Programme of Action Concerning Disabled Persons
- ❖ Tallinn Guidelines for Action on Human Resources Development in the Field of Disability
- ❖ Principles for the Protection of Persons with Mental Illness and the Improvement of Mental Health Care

- Standard Rules on the Equalization of Opportunities for Persons with Disabilities
- ILO Recommendation concerning Vocational Rehabilitation of the Disabled
- ILO Recommendation concerning Vocational Rehabilitation and Employment (Disabled Persons)
- Sundberg Declaration on Actions and Strategies for Education
- Prevention and Integration, adopted by the UNESCO World Conference on Actions and Strategies for Education
- Prevention and Integration, Malaga (Spain), 2–7 November 1981
- Salamanca Statement and Framework for Action on Special Needs Education, adopted by the UNESCO World Conference on Special Needs Education: Access and Quality, Salamanca (Spain), 7–10 June 1994.

Application of International Conventions, Standards and Norms to Domestic Law

Application of international law:

Translation from an international convention, standard or norm to national law and then to local implementation is slow and complex but fundamental.

Three main methods are available to implement international legal instruments in domestic law:

- Direct incorporation of rights recognized in the international instrument into what may be termed a **"bill of rights"** in the national legal order.
- Enactment of different legislative measures in the civil, criminal and administrative laws to give effect to the rights recognized in international legal instruments.
- Self-executing operation of international legal instruments in the national legal order.

Role of domestic courts incorporation of international norms and standards by domestic courts:

- Direct application of international law by domestic courts also can play an important role in implementing international human rights norms applicable to persons with disabilities by means of compliance with relevant international standards and citing precedents in other jurisdictions.
- Furthermore, judicial initiatives may propel executive and legislative branches of governments to act with regard to drafting, enforcing and evaluating disability legislation.
- The greater the extent to which international norms on disability is widely known, the greater the possibility of domestic courts complying with these norms.[14]

■ REFERENCES

1. The Rights of Persons with Disabilities Act, 2016 (PDF). www.disabilityaffairs.gov.in
2. Disabled population by type of disability, type of households and sex (India and States/UTs), 2011. Census Commissioner, Ministry of Home Affairs, Government of India. Website: http://www.censusindia.gov.in
3. Booklet Rights of the Disabled by National Human Rights Commission. Website: https://nhrc.nic.in
4. Bhattacharyya R. Disability Laws in India: A Study. Intern Jr of Research. 2014;1(4):99-115.
5. National Policy for Persons with Disabilities. Ministry of Social Justice and Empowerment, Government of India. Website: www.socialjustice.nic.in
6. The Persons with Disabilities (Equal Opportunities, Protection of Rights and Full Participation) Act, 1995. Website: www.legislative.gov.in
7. The National Trust for the welfare of persons with autism, cerebral palsy, mental retardation and multiple disabilities. Ministry of Social Justice and Empowerment, Government of India. Website: https://thenationaltrust.gov.in

8. Policies and Schemes of Central and State Governments for People with Disabilities. Published by Sightsavers. Ministry of Social Justice and Empowerment, Government of India. Website: www.ccdisabilities.nic.in
9. National Social Assistance Programme Guidelines. Ministry of Rural Development, Government of India. Website: https://nsap.nic.in/Guidelines
10. Accessible India Campaign—An Inclusive Society Creates a Sashakt Bharat. Ministry of Social Justice and Empowerment, Government of India. Website: www.disabilityaffairs.gov.in
11. Compendium of Schemes for the Welfare of Persons with Disability. Department of Empowerment of Persons with Disabilities (Divyangjan), Ministry of Social Justice and Empowerment, Government of India. Website: www.disabilityaffairs.gov.in
12. Scheme of National Award for the Welfare of Persons with Disability. Department of Empowerment of Persons with Disabilities (Divyangjan), Ministry of Social Justice and Empowerment, Government of India. Website: www.disabilityaffairs.gov.in
13. Hurst R. The International Disability Rights Movement and the ICF. Disabil Rehabil. 2003;25(11-12):572-6. doi: 10.1080/0963828031000137072. PMID: 12959330.
14. United Nations General Assembly Session 61 Resolution 106. Convention on the Rights of Persons with Disabilities A/RES/61/106 13 December 2006.

CHAPTER 13

Accessibility for Persons with Disability

Shyam D Ganvir, Deepak B Anap

LEARNING OBJECTIVES

Through this chapter, the reader will be able to:
- Learning the definition of appropriate technology
- Knowing the use of appropriate technology to the person with disability
- Learning the various assistive devices and use of the same to the person with disability

■ INTRODUCTION

Persons with Disabilities use several devices to overcome the specific conditions. Therefore, anthropometrics is used to ensure that dimensions in a building such as doors, doorways, passenger areas, reception desks, rest areas, relationship between desk and wheelchair, toilets are designed appropriately. Adequate space should be allocated for persons using mobility devices, e.g., wheelchairs, crutches and walkers, white cane, etc., as well as those walking with the assistance of other persons. These dimensions are required to suit and meet the Mobility Devices.

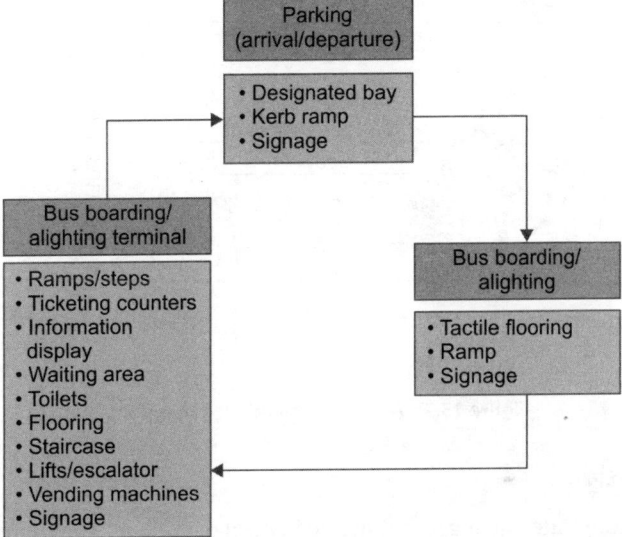

Figure 13.1: Schematic diagram shows steps from parking to bus boarding/alighting.

Wheelchair User

Dimensions of a standard wheelchair are extremely important and helps to get standards for space allowance, reach range, etc., of a wheelchair user. Electric wheelchairs may be of a larger dimension, much heavier and do not have the same manoeuvrability/capability as manual wheelchairs.

Manual Wheelchairs

Dimensions for consideration as per harmonized guidelines CPWD:

Dimensions for consideration as per harmonized guidelines CPWD	
Description	Dimension
Wheelchair Open	
Length	1000–1200 mm
Width	650–720 mm
Height	910–950 mm
Wheelchair footrest	350 mm (deep)
Wheelchair castor width	12 mm
Seat height	480 mm
Arm rest height	760 mm
Lap height	675 mm
Wheelchair Folded	
Width	300 mm
Height of armrest	760 mm

Structure of wheelchair and name of each part (standard type):[1]

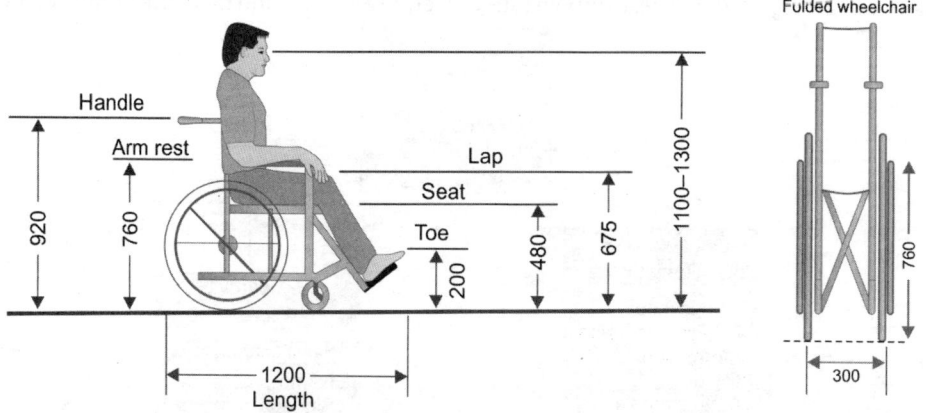

Figure 13.2: Wheelchair standard dimensions.

Accessibility of Wheelchair

A wheelchair has a footplate and leg rest attached in front of the seat. The footplate extends about 350 mm in front of the knee. The footplate may prevent a wheelchair user from getting close enough to an object. Hence, at least 350 mm deep and 700 mm high space under a counter, stand/stanmd, etc., should be given. The access to the wheelchair will be by handrail in the continuity.

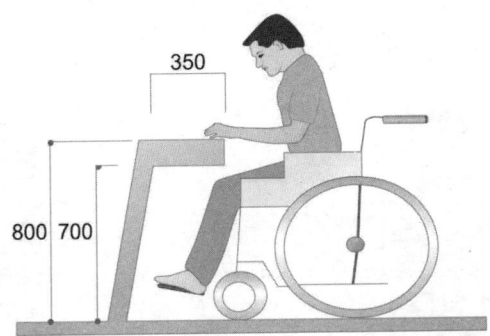

Figure 13.3: Knee clearance.

Wheelchair User Area

The minimum clear floor or ground area required accommodating a single, stationary wheel chair and occupant is:

Description	Dimension
Wheelchair User Area	
Length	1200 mm
Width	900 mm

Circulation Dimensions

The minimum clear floor ground area for a wheelchair to turn is 1500 mm whereas it may be ideal to provide 2000 mm.

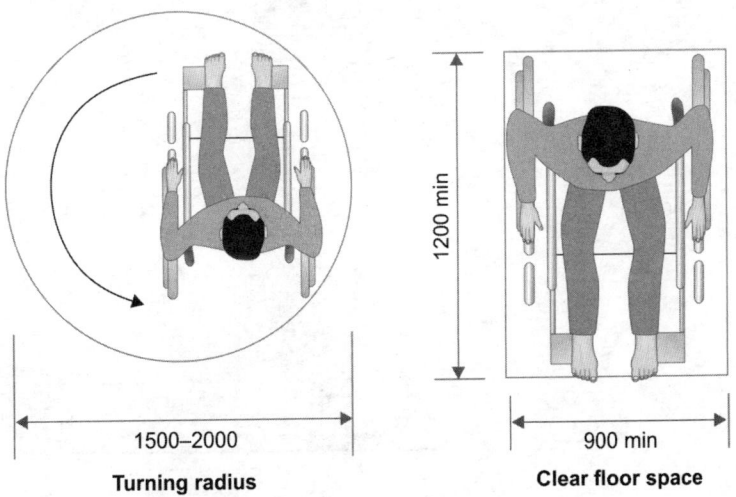

Figure 13.4: Turning radius and clear floor space.

Reach Range

A wheelchair user's movement pivots around his or her shoulders. The range of reach (forward and side; with or without obstruction) of a wheelchair user should be taken into consideration.

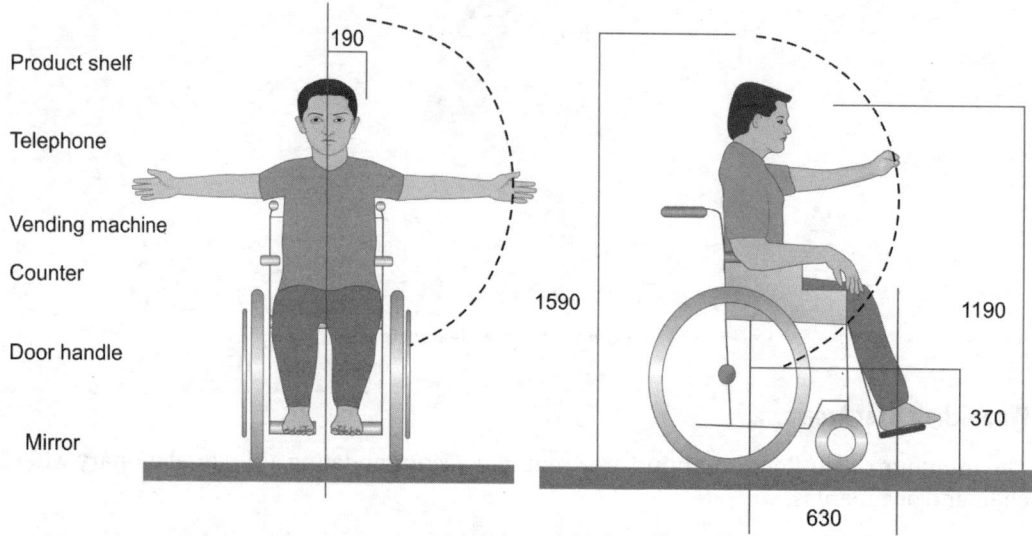

Figure 13.5: Range of reach of wheel chair user.

Reach Without Obstruction

Reach	Without obstructions	
Type	**Forward**	
Highest	1200 mm	
Lowest	380 mm	

CHAPTER 13: Accessibility for Persons with Disability

Common (most appropriate)	800–1200 mm	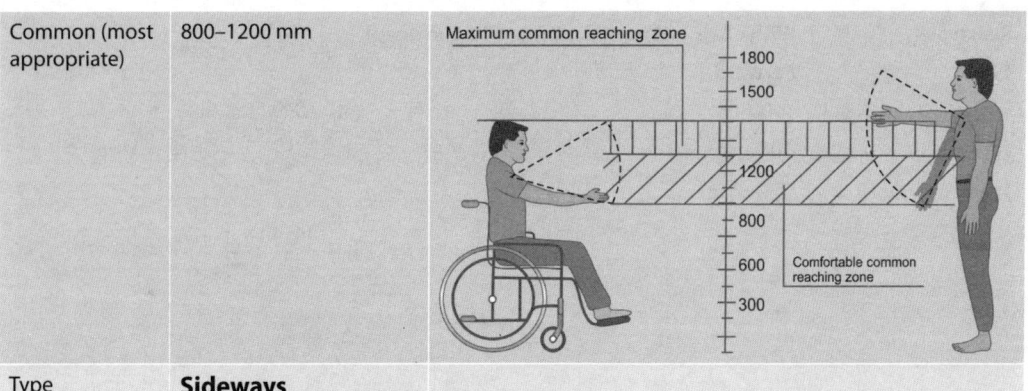
Type	**Sideways**	
Reach	**With obstructions**	
Highest	1300 mm	
Lowest	250 mm	

Reach Type	With obstructions (maximum 500 mm deep)
	Forward
Highest	1000 mm
Touch	600 mm
Grasp	500 mm
Type	Sideways
Highest	1200 mm
Lowest	860 mm
Touch	600 mm
Grasp	500 mm

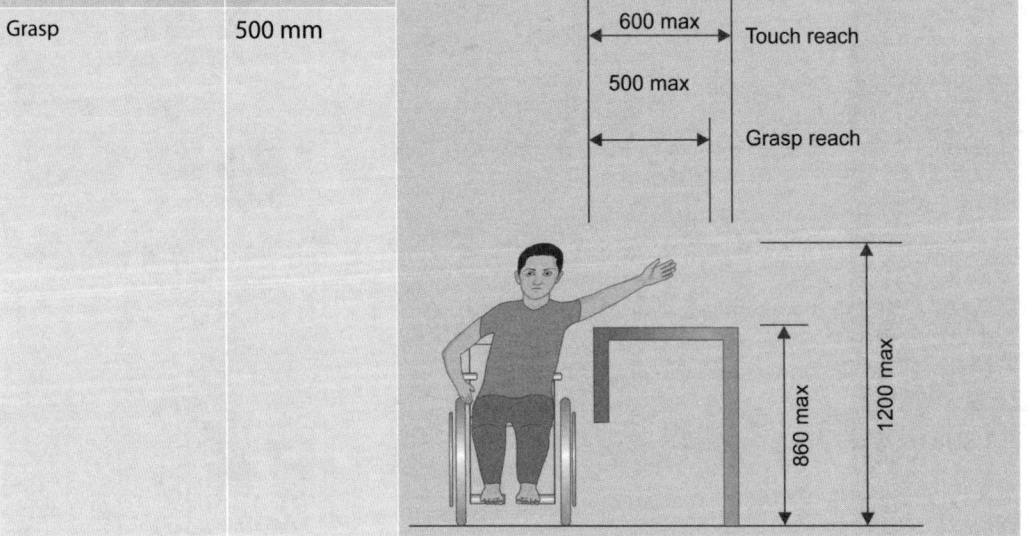

Vision Zone

Vision zone is 900–1800 mm and all signage should be designed based upon these dimensions. The smallest letter should not be less than 15 mm. Map and information panels along pathways should be placed at a height between 900 mm and 1800 mm. vi No obstruction should be there in the vision zone.

CHAPTER 13: Accessibility for Persons with Disability

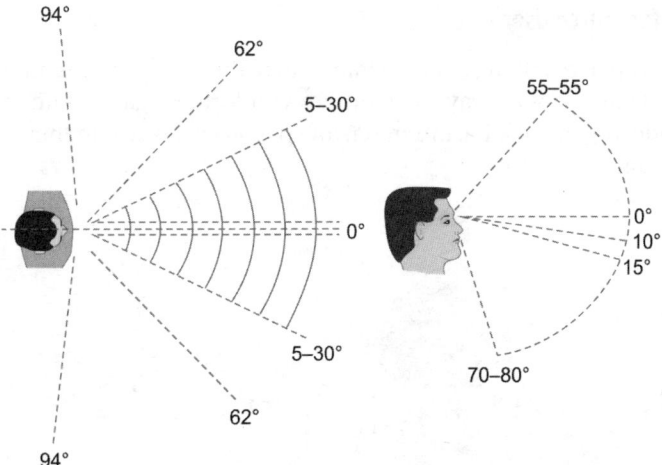

Figure 13.6: Field of vision.

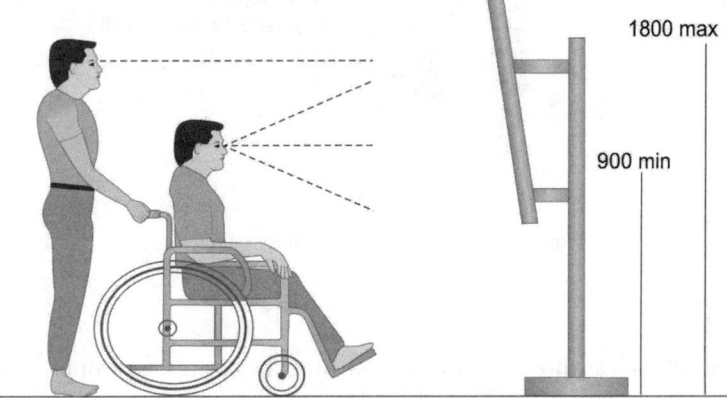

Figure 13.7: Vision zone.

Heights and Widths

Height of Controls: Electrical	
Switches (Light)	800–1100 mm
Switches (Power)	400–500 mm
Doors/Windows	
Handles	
Doors	900–1000 mm (900 mm minimum clear width)
Windows (Controls)	750–900 mm
Space required under the counter	350 mm deep for wheelchair footrest
Entrance/Exit Door	
Minimum width of Entrance/Exit door	900 mm
Minimum front approach doorways space	1200 mm
Minimum Latch approach doorways space	1250 mm

Space Allowance for Crutch User

Although people who use walking aids can manoeuvre through door openings of 900 mm clear width, they need wider passageways 920 mm for comfortable gait. Crutch tips, often extend down out at a wide angle, are a hazard in narrow passageways where they might not be seen by other pedestrians.

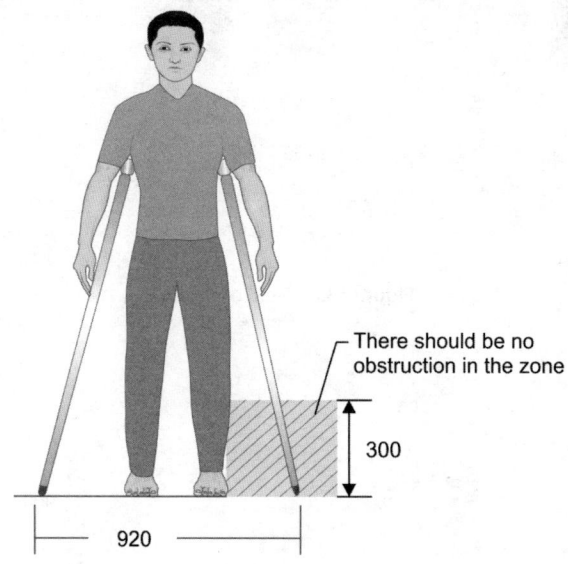

Figure 13.8: Space requirement for crutch user.

White Cane User

Protruding objects, such as directional signs, tree branches, wires, guy ropes, public telephone booths, benches and ornamental fixtures should be installed with consideration of the range of a person with vision impairment white cane. A barrier or sounding object to warn blind or visually

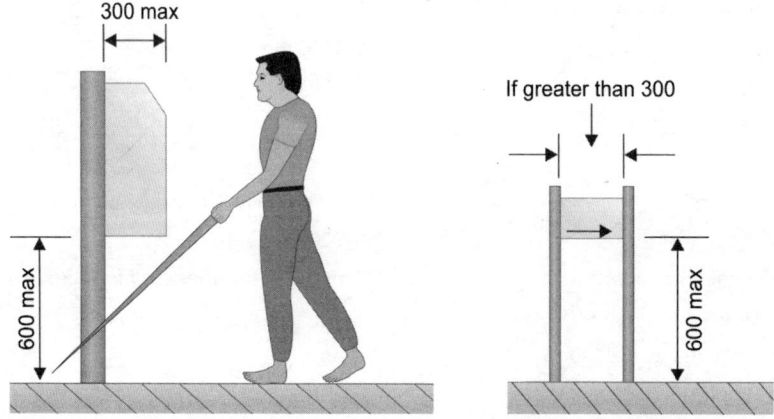

Figure 13.9: Radial range and object detection by the visually impaired.

impaired persons should be provided under stairways or escalators. Walkways, halls, corridors, passageways, aisles, or other circulation spaces should have clear headroom to minimize the risk of accidents. The radial range of the white cane is a band 1200 mm wide. Any obstacle above 600 mm cannot be detected by the white cane. If there are projections above this height, then the projections have to be reflected at the floor level in terms of level or textural differences.

■HANDRAILS

General

Handrails/grab bars are extremely important features and must be designed to be easy to grasp and to provide a firm and comfortable grip so that the hand can slide along the rail without obstruction. Many Persons with Disabilities and elderly rely upon handrails/grab bars to maintain balance or prevent serious falls. Handrails may be provided with Braille/tactile markings at the beginning and the end to give information to people with visual impairment.

Handrail with Braille Information Panel Handrail should:
* Be slip-resistant with round ends.
* Have a circular section of 38–45 mm in diameter.
* Have a minimum clear space of 50 mm from the walls.
* Be free of any sharp or abrasive elements.
* Have continuous gripping surfaces, without interruptions or obstructions that can break a hand hold

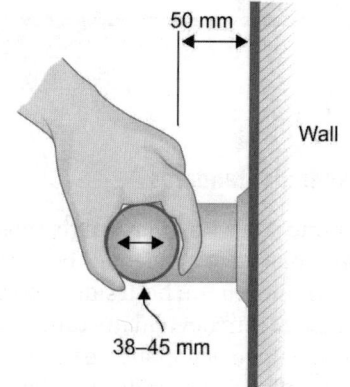

Figure 13.10: Grab bar details.

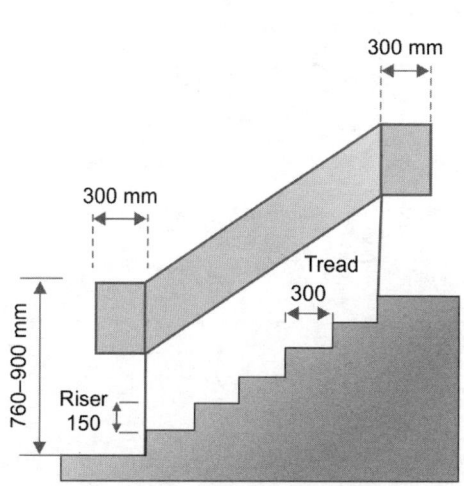

Figure 13.11: Handrails for steps.

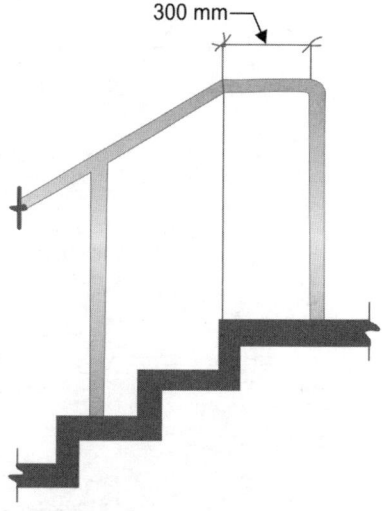

Figure 13.12: Handrails for extension.

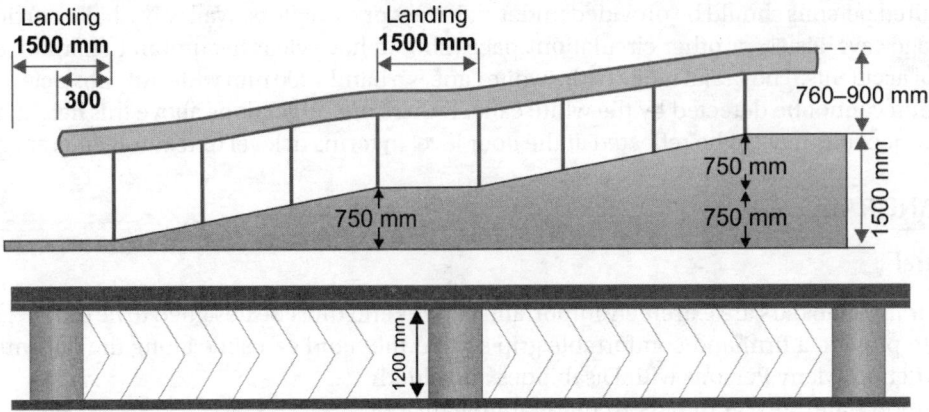

Figure 13.13: Handrails for ramps.

Handrails Standards

A ramp run with a vertical rise greater than 150 mm should have handrails that are on both the sides placed at a height of between 760 mm and 900 mm above the floor level handrails must be continuous on both sides and even at landings. Extend horizontally for a distance of not less than 300 mm beyond the top and bottom of the ramp to provide support for persons who may need help to negotiate the ramp not project into another path of travel. Provision of continuous handrail along corridor can be provided. This can be installed where staircases, ramps and corridors are provided. Handrails to have braille engravings.

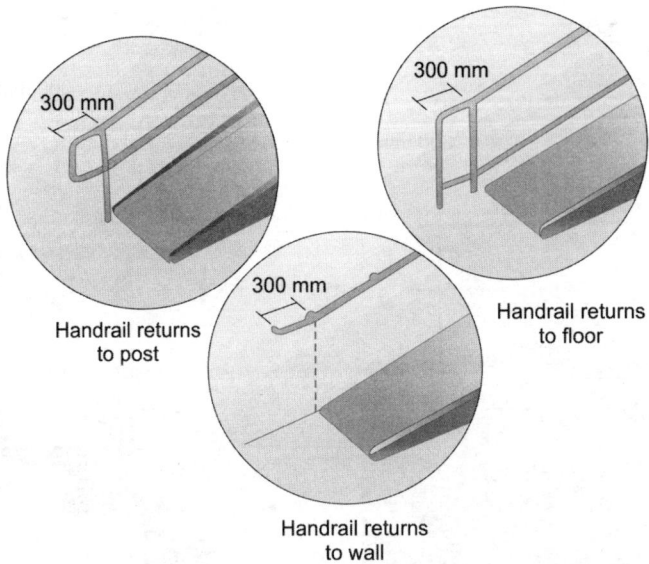

Figure 13.14: Typical handrail extensions.

CHAPTER 13: Accessibility for Persons with Disability

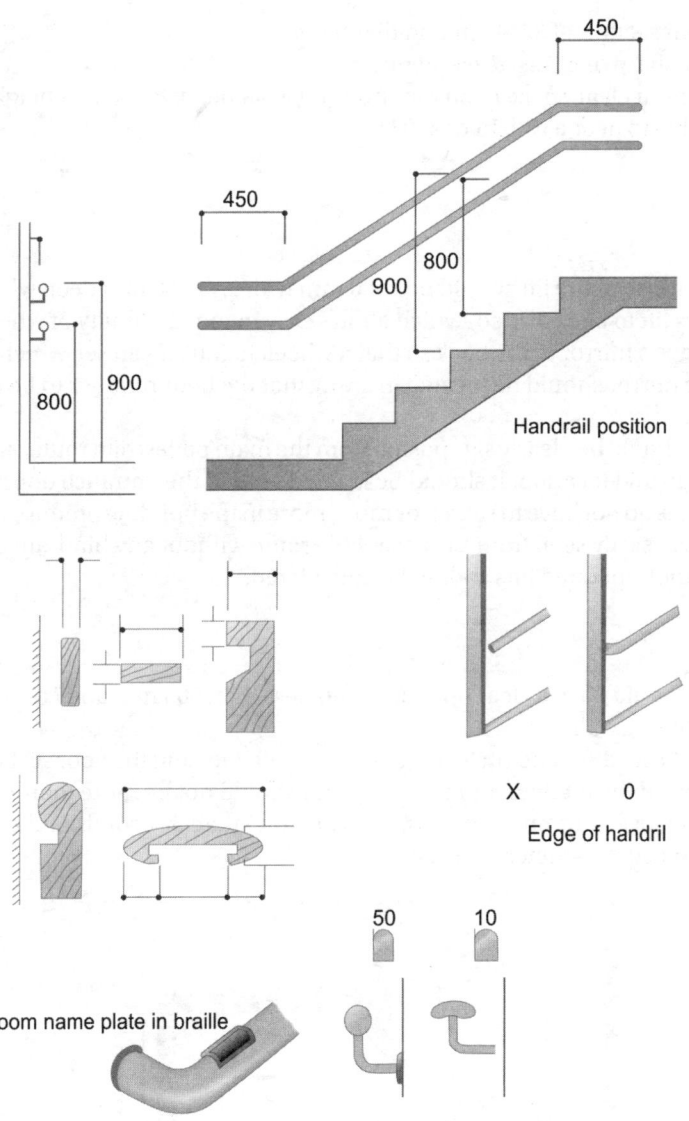

Handrail shape and clearance from wall surface

Figure 13.15: Handrail detail.

Grab Bar

Grab bars/rails should be manufactured from a material which contrasts with the wall finish (or use dark tiles behind light-colored rails), be not too warm/cold to the touch and provide good grip. It is essential that all grab rails are adequately fixed, since considerable pressure will be placed on the rail during manoeuvring. In rural areas, indigenous materials such as bamboo/wood/other can be used for making grab bars in toilets.

Grab bars should:
* Be slip-resistant with round ends.
* Preferably have knurled surfaces.

- Have a circular section of 38–45 mm in diameter.
- Be free of any sharp or abrasive elements.
- Have a minimum clear space of 50 mm from the wall be installed at a height of 760 mm to 900 mm be able to bear a weight of 250 kg.

Lift

Size

- The minimum size of the lift should be 1500 mm wide by 1500 mm deep wherever possible, 13 passengers lift to be provided, which allows easy manoeuvrability of wheelchair user.
- Each lift to have a mirror at the back so that a wheelchair user can see which floor they have reached. The mirror should be located in a way that the floor number to be easily indicated in the mirror.
- Lift locations should be clearly signposted from the main pedestrian route, and recognizable through design and location. It should be located near to the entrance door so that persons with disabilities do not have to search or move more in the building premises to search them. They should be easily seen from the accessible route without any hindrances in the route.
- Provision of foot-operated lifts should be considered.

Door

- The lift door should have a clear opening of not less than 900 mm and contrasting in colour from the adjoining wall.
- There should be no difference in level between the lift door and the floor surface at each level. The gap between the lift door and building floor should not be more than 12 mm.
- Time of closing of an automatic door should be more than 5 seconds and the closing speed should not exceed 0.25 meters per second.

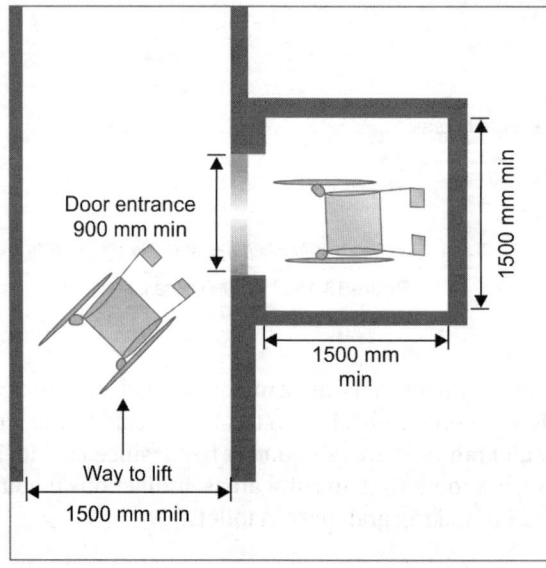

Figure 13.16: Placement of lift accessories.

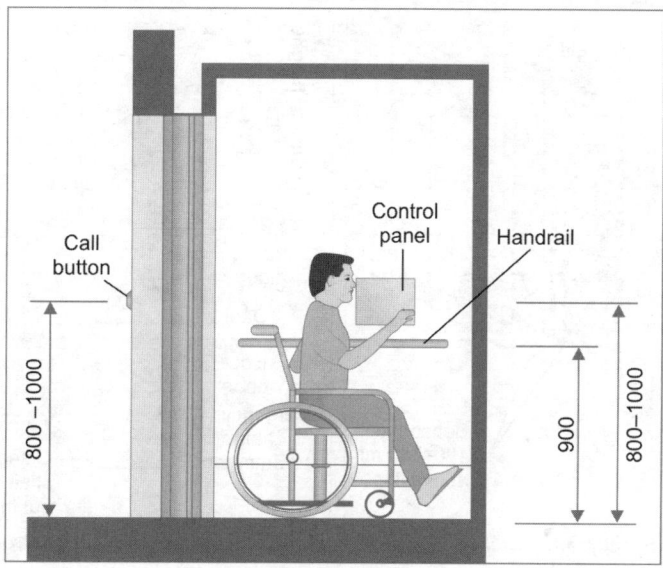

Figure 13.17: Size of lift.

Call Button

The call button located outside the lift should:
* Have a clear floor space of at least 900 mm × 1200 mm with no obstruction placed to prevent a wheelchair user from reaching the call button; and
* Be installed at a height between 800 mm and 1000 mm.
* The call to be connected to the guard, which handles the lifts mobility at the ground surface, and also to the help desk for persons with disabilities.
* Provision of call button at foot level in addition to hand operated level should be provided.

Control Panel

The control panel should:
* Have a clear floor space of at least 900 mm × 1200 mm with no obstruction placed to prevent a wheelchair user from reaching it; be placed at a height of between 800 mm and 1000 mm from the floor level
* Have buttons with Braille/raised letters and in sharp contrast from the background to aid people with visual impairments.
* The control panels to be regularly maintained and the buttons with braille/raised letters to be clean by dry materials on regular basis to avoid any dirt or damage.
* Provision of horizontal control panel should be given.

SECTION 3: Basic Concepts of National and International Legislation for Persons with Disability

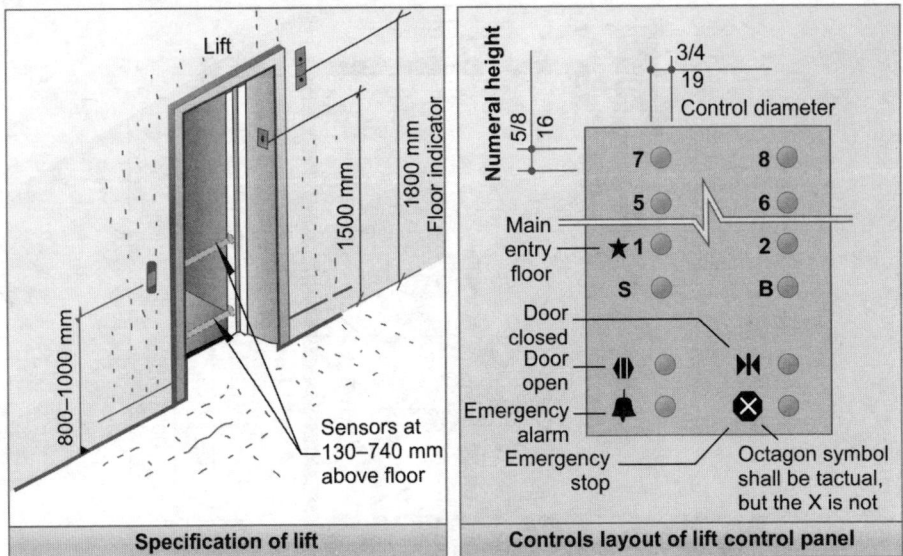

Figure 13.18: Specifications of lift; controls layout of lift control panel.

Audio and Visual Indicators

- The lift should have a voice announcement system along with a visual display to indicate the floor level and also the information that the door of the cage is open or closed for entrance or exit
- The announcement system should be clearly audible, i.e., the announcement should be 50 decibel.
- The visual indicators can be digital and can be hung from ceiling or wall hung signage.

Other Facilities

- The use of visually and acoustically reflective wall surfaces should be minimized within the lift car as visual reflections can cause discomfort and affect the visual acuity of people with visual impairments.
- The floor of the lift car should be slip resistant and have similar frictional qualities to the floor of the lift landing to decrease the risk of stumbling.
- The provision of a mirror on the wall of the lift car opposite the lift door is a positive aid to navigation for wheelchair users. It allows the wheelchair user to see if anyone is behind them and also to see the floor indicator panel. The mirror should not extend below 900 mm from the lift floor to avoid confusing people with impaired sight.
- The emergency communication system should be coupled with an induction loop system installed all around the lift. Telephone units, where provided, should have an inbuilt inductive coupler to assist persons using hearing aids.

■ REFERENCE

1. Accessibility guidelines for bus terminals and bus stops. Govt of India Ministry of Road Transport and Highways, November 2021.

CHAPTER 14

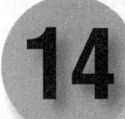

The UN Convention on the Rights of Person with Disabilities

Shyam D Ganvir, Sonyabapu Shewale

LEARNING OBJECTIVES

Through this chapter, the reader will be able to:
- Understand the rights of person with disabilities
- Gain knowledge about different articles for person with disabilities

ARTICLE 1

Purpose

The purpose of the present convention is to promote, protect and ensure the full and equal enjoyment of all human rights and fundamental freedoms by all persons with disabilities, and to promote respect for their inherent dignity.

Persons with disabilities include those who have long-term physical, mental, intellectual or sensory impairments which in interaction with various barriers may hinder their full and effective participation in society on an equal basis with others.

ARTICLE 2

Definitions

For the purposes of the present convention:
- "Communication" includes languages, display of text, Braille, tactile communication, large print, accessible multimedia as well as written, audio, plain-language, human-reader and augmentative and alternative modes, means and formats of communication, including accessible information and communication technology.
- "Language" includes spoken and signed languages and other forms of non spoken languages.
- "Discrimination on the basis of disability" means any distinction, exclusion or restriction on the basis of disability which has the purpose or effect of impairing or nullifying the recognition, enjoyment or exercise, on an equal basis with others, of all human rights and fundamental freedoms in the political, economic, social, cultural, civil or any other field. It includes all forms of discrimination, including denial of reasonable accommodation.
- "Reasonable accommodation" means necessary and appropriate modification and adjustments not imposing a disproportionate or undue burden, where needed in a particular

case, to ensure to persons with disabilities the enjoyment or exercise on an equal basis with others of all human rights and fundamental freedoms.
- ❖ "Universal design" means the design of products, environments, programmes and services to be usable by all people, to the greatest extent possible, without the need for adaptation or specialized design. "Universal design" shall not exclude assistive devices for particular groups of persons with disabilities where this is needed.

■ ARTICLE 3

General Principles

The principles of the present convention shall be:
a. Respect for inherent dignity, individual autonomy including the freedom to make one's own choices, and independence of persons;
b. Non-discrimination;
c. Full and effective participation and inclusion in society;
d. Respect for difference and acceptance of persons with disabilities as part of human diversity and humanity;
e. Equality of opportunity;
f. Accessibility;
g. Equality between men and women;
h. Respect for the evolving capacities of children with disabilities and respect for the right of children with disabilities to preserve their identities.

■ ARTICLE 4

General Obligations

1. States Parties undertake to ensure and promote the full realization of all human rights and fundamental freedoms for all persons with disabilities without discrimination of any kind on the basis of disability. To this end, States Parties undertake:
   a. To adopt all appropriate legislative, administrative and other measures for the implementation of the rights recognized in the present Convention
   b. To take all appropriate measures, including legislation, to modify or abolish existing laws, regulations, customs and practices that constitute discrimination against persons with disabilities
   c. To take into account the protection and promotion of the human rights of persons with disabilities in all policies and programmes
   d. To refrain from engaging in any act or practice that is inconsistent with the present Convention and to ensure that public authorities and institutions act in conformity with the present Convention
   e. To take all appropriate measures to eliminate discrimination on the basis of disability by any person, organization or private enterprise
   f. To undertake or promote research and development of universally designed goods, services, equipment and facilities, as defined in Article 2 of the present Convention, which should require the minimum possible adaptation and the least cost to meet the specific

needs of a person with disabilities, to promote their availability and use, and to promote universal design in the development of standards and guidelines
   g. To undertake or promote research and development of, and to promote the availability and use of new technologies, including information and communications technologies, mobility aids, devices and assistive technologies, suitable for persons with disabilities, giving priority to technologies at an affordable cost
   h. To provide accessible information to persons with disabilities about mobility aids, devices and assistive technologies, including new technologies, as well as other forms of assistance, support services and facilities
   i. To promote the training of professionals and staff working with persons with disabilities in the rights recognized in the present Convention so as to better provide the assistance and services guaranteed by those rights.
2. With regard to economic, social and cultural rights, each State Party undertakes to take measures to the maximum of its available resources and, where needed, within the framework of international cooperation, with a view to achieving progressively the full realization of these rights, without prejudice to those obligations contained in the present Convention that are immediately applicable according to international law.
3. In the development and implementation of legislation and policies to implement the present Convention, and in other decision-making processes concerning issues relating to persons with disabilities, States Parties shall closely consult with and actively involve persons with disabilities, including children with disabilities, through their representative organizations.
4. Nothing in the present Convention shall affect any provisions which are more conducive to the realization of the rights of persons with disabilities and which may be contained in the law of a State Party or international law in force for that State. There shall be no restriction upon or derogation from any of the human rights and fundamental freedoms recognized or existing in any State Party to the present Convention pursuant to law, conventions, regulation or custom on the pretext that the present Convention does not recognize such rights or freedoms or that it recognizes them to a lesser extent.
5. The provisions of the present Convention shall extend to all parts of federal States without any limitations or exceptions.

■ ARTICLE 5

Equality and Non-discrimination

1. States Parties recognize that all persons are equal before and under the law and are entitled without any discrimination to the equal protection and equal benefit of the law.
2. States Parties shall prohibit all discrimination on the basis of disability and guarantee to persons with disabilities equal and effective legal protection against discrimination on all grounds.
3. In order to promote equality and eliminate discrimination, States Parties shall take all appropriate steps to ensure that reasonable accommodation is provided.
4. Specific measures which are necessary to accelerate or achieve de facto equality of persons with disabilities shall not be considered discrimination under the terms of the present Convention.

ARTICLE 6

Women with Disabilities

1. States Parties recognize that women and girls with disabilities are subject to multiple discrimination, and in this regard shall take measures to ensure the full and equal enjoyment by them of all human rights and fundamental freedoms.
2. States Parties shall take all appropriate measures to ensure the full development, advancement and empowerment of women, for the purpose of guaranteeing them the exercise and enjoyment of the human rights and fundamental freedoms set out in the present Convention.

ARTICLE 7

Children with Disabilities

1. States Parties shall take all necessary measures to ensure the full enjoyment by children with disabilities of all human rights and fundamental freedoms on an equal basis with other children.
2. In all actions concerning children with disabilities, the best interests of the child shall be a primary consideration.
3. States Parties shall ensure that children with disabilities have the right to express their views freely on all matters affecting them, their views being given due weight in accordance with their age and maturity, on an equal basis with other children, and to be provided with disability and age-appropriate assistance to realize that right.

ARTICLE 8

Awareness-raising

1. States Parties undertake to adopt immediate, effective and appropriate measures:
    a. To raise awareness throughout society, including at the family level, regarding persons with disabilities, and to foster respect for the rights and dignity of persons with disabilities;
    b. To combat stereotypes, prejudices and harmful practices relating to persons with disabilities, including those based on sex and age, in all areas of life;
    c. To promote awareness of the capabilities and contributions of persons with disabilities.
2. Measures to this end include:
    a. Initiating and maintaining effective public awareness campaigns designed:
        i. To nurture receptiveness to the rights of persons with disabilities;
        ii. To promote positive perceptions and greater social awareness towards persons with disabilities;
        iii. To promote recognition of the skills, merits and abilities of persons with disabilities, and of their contributions to the workplace and the labour market;
    b. Fostering at all levels of the education system, including in all children from an early age, an attitude of respect for the rights of persons with disabilities;
    c. Encouraging all organs of the media to portray persons with disabilities in a manner consistent with the purpose of the present Convention;
    d. Promoting awareness-training programmes regarding persons with disabilities and the rights of persons with disabilities.

ARTICLE 9

Accessibility

1. To enable persons with disabilities to live independently and participate fully in all aspects of life, States Parties shall take appropriate measures to ensure to persons with disabilities access, on an equal basis with others, to the physical environment, to transportation, to information and communications, including information and communications technologies and systems, and to other facilities and services open or provided to the public, both in urban and in rural areas. These measures, which shall include the identification and elimination of obstacles and barriers to accessibility, shall apply to, inter alia:
   a. Buildings, roads, transportation and other indoor and outdoor facilities, including schools, housing, medical facilities and workplaces;
   b. Information, communications and other services, including electronic services and emergency services.
2. States Parties shall also take appropriate measures:
   a. To develop, promulgate and monitor the implementation of minimum standards and guidelines for the accessibility of facilities and services open or provided to the public;
   b. To ensure that private entities that offer facilities and services which are open or provided to the public take into account all aspects of accessibility for persons with disabilities;
   c. To provide training for stakeholders on accessibility issues facing persons with disabilities;
   d. To provide in buildings and other facilities open to the public signage in Braille and in easy to read and understand forms;
   e. To provide forms of live assistance and intermediaries, including guides, readers and professional sign language interpreters, to facilitate accessibility to buildings and other facilities open to the public;
   f. To promote other appropriate forms of assistance and support to persons with disabilities to ensure their access to information;
   g. To promote access for persons with disabilities to new information and communications technologies and systems, including the Internet;
   h. To promote the design, development, production and distribution of accessible information and communications technologies and systems at an early stage, so that these technologies and systems become accessible at minimum cost.

ARTICLE 10

Right to Life

States Parties reaffirm that every human being has the inherent right to life and shall take all necessary measures to ensure its effective enjoyment by persons with disabilities on an equal basis with others.

ARTICLE 11

Situations of Risk and Humanitarian Emergencies

States Parties shall take, in accordance with their obligations under international law, including international humanitarian law and international human rights law, all necessary measures to ensure the protection and safety of persons with disabilities in situations of risk, including situations of armed conflict, humanitarian emergencies and the occurrence of natural disasters.

ARTICLE 12

Equal Recognition before the Law

1. States Parties reaffirm that persons with disabilities have the right to recognition everywhere as persons before the law.
2. States Parties shall recognize that persons with disabilities enjoy legal capacity on an equal basis with others in all aspects of life.
3. States Parties shall take appropriate measures to provide access by persons with disabilities to the support they may require in exercising their legal capacity.
4. States Parties shall ensure that all measures that relate to the exercise of legal capacity provide for appropriate and effective safeguards to prevent abuse in accordance with international human rights law. Such safeguards shall ensure that measures relating to the exercise of legal capacity respect the rights, will and preferences of the person, are free of conflict of interest and undue influence, are proportional and tailored to the person's circumstances, apply for the shortest time possible and are subject to regular review by a competent, independent and impartial authority or judicial body. The safeguards shall be proportional to the degree to which such measures affect the person's rights and interests.
5. Subject to the provisions of this article, States Parties shall take all appropriate and effective measures to ensure the equal right of persons with disabilities to own or inherit property, to control their own financial affairs and to have equal access to bank loans, mortgages and other forms of financial credit, and shall ensure that persons with disabilities are not arbitrarily deprived of their property.

ARTICLE 13

Access to Justice

1. States Parties shall ensure effective access to justice for persons with disabilities on an equal basis with others, including through the provision of procedural and age-appropriate accommodations, in order to facilitate their effective role as direct and indirect participants, including as witnesses, in all legal proceedings, including at investigative and other preliminary stages.
2. In order to help to ensure effective access to justice for persons with disabilities, States Parties shall promote appropriate training for those working in the field of administration of justice, including police and prison staff.

ARTICLE 14

Liberty and Security of Person

1. States Parties shall ensure that persons with disabilities, on an equal basis with others:
   a. Enjoy the right to liberty and security of person;
   b. Are not deprived of their liberty unlawfully or arbitrarily, and that any deprivation of liberty is in conformity with the law, and that the existence of a disability shall in no case justify a deprivation of liberty.
2. States Parties shall ensure that if persons with disabilities are deprived of their liberty through any process, they are, on an equal basis with others, entitled to guarantees in accordance with

international human rights law and shall be treated in compliance with the objectives and principles of the present Convention, including by provision of reasonable accommodation.

■ ARTICLE 15

Freedom from Torture or Cruel, Inhuman or Degrading Treatment or Punishment

1. No one shall be subjected to torture or to cruel, inhuman or degrading treatment or punishment. In particular, no one shall be subjected without his or her free consent to medical or scientific experimentation.
2. States Parties shall take all effective legislative, administrative, judicial or other measures to prevent persons with disabilities, on an equal basis with others, from being subjected to torture or cruel, inhuman or degrading treatment or punishment.

■ ARTICLE 16

Freedom from Exploitation, Violence and Abuse

1. States Parties shall take all appropriate legislative, administrative, social, educational and other measures to protect persons with disabilities, both within and outside the home, from all forms of exploitation, violence and abuse, including their gender-based aspects.
2. States Parties shall also take all appropriate measures to prevent all forms of exploitation, violence and abuse by ensuring, inter alia, appropriate forms of gender- and age-sensitive assistance and support for persons with disabilities and their families and caregivers, including through the provision of information and education on how to avoid, recognize and report instances of exploitation, violence and abuse. States Parties shall ensure that protection services are age-, gender- and disability-sensitive.
3. In order to prevent the occurrence of all forms of exploitation, violence and abuse, States Parties shall ensure that all facilities and programmes designed to serve persons with disabilities are effectively monitored by independent authorities.
4. States Parties shall take all appropriate measures to promote the physical, cognitive and psychological recovery, rehabilitation and social reintegration of persons with disabilities who become victims of any form of exploitation, violence or abuse, including through the provision of protection services. Such recovery and reintegration shall take place in an environment that fosters the health, welfare, self-respect, dignity and autonomy of the person and takes into account gender- and age-specific needs.
5. States Parties shall put in place effective legislation and policies, including women- and child-focused legislation and policies, to ensure that instances of exploitation, violence and abuse against persons with disabilities are identified, investigated and, where appropriate, prosecuted.

■ ARTICLE 17

Protecting the Integrity of the Person

Every person with disabilities has a right to respect for his or her physical and mental integrity on an equal basis with others.

ARTICLE 18

Liberty of Movement and Nationality

1. States Parties shall recognize the rights of persons with disabilities to liberty of movement, to freedom to choose their residence and to a nationality, on an equal basis with others, including by ensuring that persons with disabilities:
   a. Have the right to acquire and change a nationality and are not deprived of their nationality arbitrarily or on the basis of disability;
   b. Are not deprived, on the basis of disability, of their ability to obtain, possess and utilize documentation of their nationality or other documentation of identification, or to utilize relevant processes such as immigration proceedings, that may be needed to facilitate exercise of the right to liberty of movement;
   c. Are free to leave any country, including their own;
   d. Are not deprived, arbitrarily or on the basis of disability, of the right to enter their own country.
2. Children with disabilities shall be registered immediately after birth and shall have the right from birth to a name, the right to acquire a nationality and, as far as possible, the right to know and be cared for by their parents.

ARTICLE 19

Living Independently and Being Included in the Community

States Parties to the present Convention recognize the equal right of all persons with disabilities to live in the community, with choices equal to others, and shall take effective and appropriate measures to facilitate full enjoyment by persons with disabilities of this right and their full inclusion and participation in the community, including by ensuring that:
a. Persons with disabilities have the opportunity to choose their place of residence and where and with whom they live on an equal basis with others and are not obliged to live in a particular living arrangement
b. Persons with disabilities have access to a range of in-home, residential and other community support services, including personal assistance necessary to support living and inclusion in the community, and to prevent isolation or segregation from the community
c. Community services and facilities for the general population are available on an equal basis to persons with disabilities and are responsive to their needs.

ARTICLE 20

Personal Mobility

States Parties shall take effective measures to ensure personal mobility with the greatest possible independence for persons with disabilities, including by:
a. Facilitating the personal mobility of persons with disabilities in the manner and at the time of their choice, and at affordable cost
b. Facilitating access by persons with disabilities to quality mobility aids, devices, assistive technologies and forms of live assistance and intermediaries, including by making them available at affordable cost
c. Providing training in mobility skills to persons with disabilities and to specialist staff working with persons with disabilities

d. Encouraging entities that produce mobility aids, devices and assistive technologies to take into account all aspects of mobility for persons with disabilities.

ARTICLE 21

Freedom of Expression and Opinion, and Access to Information

States Parties shall take all appropriate measures to ensure that persons with disabilities can exercise the right to freedom of expression and opinion, including the freedom to seek, receive and impart information and ideas on an equal basis with others and through all forms of communication of their choice, as defined in Article 2 of the present Convention, including by:
a. Providing information intended for the general public to persons with disabilities in accessible formats and technologies appropriate to different kinds of disabilities in a timely manner and without additional cost
b. Accepting and facilitating the use of sign languages, Braille, augmentative and alternative communication, and all other accessible means, modes and formats of communication of their choice by persons with disabilities in official interactions
c. Urging private entities that provide services to the general public, including through the Internet, to provide information and services in accessible and usable formats for persons with disabilities
d. Encouraging the mass media, including providers of information through the Internet, to make their services accessible to persons with disabilities
e. Recognizing and promoting the use of sign languages.

ARTICLE 22

Respect for Privacy

1. No person with disabilities, regardless of place of residence or living arrangements, shall be subjected to arbitrary or unlawful interference with his or her privacy, family, home or correspondence or other types of communication or to unlawful attacks on his or her honour and reputation. Persons with disabilities have the right to the protection of the law against such interference or attacks.
2. States Parties shall protect the privacy of personal, health and rehabilitation information of persons with disabilities on an equal basis with others.

ARTICLE 23

Respect for Home and the Family

1. States Parties shall take effective and appropriate measures to eliminate discrimination against persons with disabilities in all matters relating to marriage, family, parenthood and relationships, on an equal basis with others, so as to ensure that:
    a. The right of all persons with disabilities who are of marriageable age to marry and to found a family on the basis of free and full consent of the intending spouses is recognized
    b. The rights of persons with disabilities to decide freely and responsibly on the number and spacing of their children and to have access to age-appropriate information, reproductive and family planning education are recognized, and the means necessary to enable them to exercise these rights are provided

c. Persons with disabilities, including children, retain their fertility on an equal basis with others.
2. States Parties shall ensure the rights and responsibilities of persons with disabilities, with regard to guardianship, wardship, trusteeship, adoption of children or similar institutions, where these concepts exist in national legislation; in all cases the best interests of the child shall be paramount. States Parties shall render appropriate assistance to persons with disabilities in the performance of their child-rearing responsibilities.
3. States Parties shall ensure that children with disabilities have equal rights with respect to family life. With a view to realizing these rights, and to prevent concealment, abandonment, neglect and segregation of children with disabilities, States Parties shall undertake to provide early and comprehensive information, services and support to children with disabilities and their families.
4. States Parties shall ensure that a child shall not be separated from his or her parents against their will, except when competent authorities subject to judicial review determine, in accordance with applicable law and procedures, that such separation is necessary for the best interests of the child. In no case shall a child be separated from parents on the basis of a disability of either the child or one or both of the parents.
5. States Parties shall, where the immediate family is unable to care for a child with disabilities, undertake every effort to provide alternative care within the wider family, and failing that, within the community in a family setting.

■ARTICLE 24

Education

1. States Parties recognize the right of persons with disabilities to education. With a view to realizing this right without discrimination and on the basis of equal opportunity, States Parties shall ensure an inclusive education system at all levels and lifelong learning directed to:
    a. The full development of human potential and sense of dignity and self-worth, and the strengthening of respect for human rights, fundamental freedoms and human diversity
    b. The development by persons with disabilities of their personality, talents and creativity, as well as their mental and physical abilities, to their fullest potential
    c. Enabling persons with disabilities to participate effectively in a free society.
2. In realizing this right, States Parties shall ensure that:
    a. Persons with disabilities are not excluded from the general education system on the basis of disability, and that children with disabilities are not excluded from free and compulsory primary education, or from secondary education, on the basis of disability
    b. Persons with disabilities can access an inclusive, quality and free primary education and secondary education on an equal basis with others in the communities in which they live
    c. Reasonable accommodation of the individual's requirements is provided
    d. Persons with disabilities receive the support required, within the general education system, to facilitate their effective education
    e. Effective individualized support measures are provided in environments that maximize academic and social development, consistent with the goal of full inclusion.
3. States Parties shall enable persons with disabilities to learn life and social development skills to facilitate their full and equal participation in education and as members of the community. To this end, States Parties shall take appropriate measures, including:

a. Facilitating the learning of Braille, alternative script, augmentative and alternative modes, means and formats of communication and orientation and mobility skills, and facilitating peer support and mentoring
b. Facilitating the learning of sign language and the promotion of the linguistic identity of the deaf community
c. Ensuring that the education of persons, and in particular children, who are blind, deaf or deafblind, is delivered in the most appropriate languages and modes and means of communication for the individual, and in environments which maximize academic and social development.

4. In order to help ensure the realization of this right, States Parties shall take appropriate measures to employ teachers, including teachers with disabilities, who are qualified in sign language and/or Braille, and to train professionals and staff who work at all levels of education. Such training shall incorporate disability awareness and the use of appropriate augmentative and alternative modes, means and formats of communication, educational techniques and materials to support persons with disabilities.
5. States Parties shall ensure that persons with disabilities are able to access general tertiary education, vocational training, adult education and lifelong learning without discrimination and on an equal basis with others. To this end, States Parties shall ensure that reasonable accommodation is provided to persons with disabilities.

ARTICLE 25

Health

States Parties recognize that persons with disabilities have the right to the enjoyment of the highest attainable standard of health without discrimination on the basis of disability. States Parties shall take all appropriate measures to ensure access for persons with disabilities to health services that are gender-sensitive, including health-related rehabilitation. In particular, States Parties shall:

a. Provide persons with disabilities with the same range, quality and standard of free or affordable health care and programmes as provided to other persons, including in the area of sexual and reproductive health and population-based public health programmes
b. Provide those health services needed by persons with disabilities specifically because of their disabilities, including early identification and intervention as appropriate, and services designed to minimize and prevent further disabilities, including among children and older persons
c. Provide these health services as close as possible to people's own communities, including in rural areas
d. Require health professionals to provide care of the same quality to persons with disabilities as to others, including on the basis of free and informed consent by, inter alia, raising awareness of the human rights, dignity, autonomy and needs of persons with disabilities through training and the promulgation of ethical standards for public and private health care
e. Prohibit discrimination against persons with disabilities in the provision of health insurance, and life insurance where such insurance is permitted by national law, which shall be provided in a fair and reasonable manner
f. Prevent discriminatory denial of health care or health services or food and fluids on the basis of disability.

ARTICLE 26

Habilitation and Rehabilitation

1. States Parties shall take effective and appropriate measures, including through peer support, to enable persons with disabilities to attain and maintain maximum independence, full physical, mental, social and vocational ability, and full inclusion and participation in all aspects of life. To that end, States Parties shall organize, strengthen and extend comprehensive habilitation and rehabilitation services and programmes, particularly in the areas of health, employment, education and social services, in such a way that these services and programmes:
   a. Begin at the earliest possible stage, and are based on the multidisciplinary assessment of individual needs and strengths
   b. Support participation and inclusion in the community and all aspects of society, are voluntary, and are available to persons with disabilities as close as possible to their own communities, including in rural areas.
2. States Parties shall promote the development of initial and continuing training for professionals and staff working in habilitation and rehabilitation services.
3. States Parties shall promote the availability, knowledge and use of assistive devices and technologies, designed for persons with disabilities, as they relate to habilitation and rehabilitation.

ARTICLE 27

Work and Employment

1. States Parties recognize the right of persons with disabilities to work, on an equal basis with others; this includes the right to the opportunity to gain a living by work freely chosen or accepted in a labour market and work environment that is open, inclusive and accessible to persons with disabilities. States Parties shall safeguard and promote the realization of the right to work, including for those who acquire a disability during the course of employment, by taking appropriate steps, including through legislation, to, inter alia:
   a. Prohibit discrimination on the basis of disability with regard to all matters concerning all forms of employment, including conditions of recruitment, hiring and employment, continuance of employment, career advancement and safe and healthy working conditions
   b. Protect the rights of persons with disabilities, on an equal basis with others, to just and favourable conditions of work, including equal opportunities and equal remuneration for work of equal value, safe and healthy working conditions, including protection from harassment, and the redress of grievances
   c. Ensure that persons with disabilities are able to exercise their labour and trade union rights on an equal basis with others
   d. Enable persons with disabilities to have effective access to general technical and vocational guidance programmes, placement services and vocational and continuing training
   e. Promote employment opportunities and career advancement for persons with disabilities in the labour market, as well as assistance in finding, obtaining, maintaining and returning to employment
   f. Promote opportunities for self-employment, entrepreneurship, the development of cooperatives and starting one's own business
   g. Employ persons with disabilities in the public sector

h. Promote the employment of persons with disabilities in the private sector through appropriate policies and measures, which may include affirmative action programs, incentives and other measures
i. Ensure that reasonable accommodation is provided to persons with disabilities in the workplace
j. Promote the acquisition by persons with disabilities of work experience in the open labour market
k. Promote vocational and professional rehabilitation, job retention and return-to-work programmes for persons with disabilities.
2. States Parties shall ensure that persons with disabilities are not held in slavery or in servitude, and are protected, on an equal basis with others, from forced or compulsory labour.

ARTICLE 28

Adequate Standard of Living and Social Protection

1. States Parties recognize the right of persons with disabilities to an adequate standard of living for themselves and their families, including adequate food, clothing and housing, and to the continuous improvement of living conditions, and shall take appropriate steps to safeguard and promote the realization of this right without discrimination on the basis of disability.
2. States Parties recognize the right of persons with disabilities to social protection and to the enjoyment of that right without discrimination on the basis of disability, and shall take appropriate steps to safeguard and promote the realization of this right, including measures:
    a. To ensure equal access by persons with disabilities to clean water services, and to ensure access to appropriate and affordable services, devices and other assistance for disability-related needs
    b. To ensure access by persons with disabilities, in particular women and girls with disabilities and older persons with disabilities, to social protection programmes and poverty reduction programmes
    c. To ensure access by persons with disabilities and their families living in situations of poverty to assistance from the State with disability related expenses, including adequate training, counselling, financial assistance and respite care
    d. To ensure access by persons with disabilities to public housing programmes
    e. To ensure equal access by persons with disabilities to retirement benefits and programmes.

ARTICLE 29

Participation in Political and Public Life

States Parties shall guarantee to persons with disabilities political rights and the opportunity to enjoy them on an equal basis with others, and shall undertake:
a. To ensure that persons with disabilities can effectively and fully participate in political and public life on an equal basis with others, directly or through freely chosen representatives, including the right and opportunity for persons with disabilities to vote and be elected, inter alia, by:
    i. Ensuring that voting procedures, facilities and materials are appropriate, accessible and easy to understand and use
    ii. Protecting the right of persons with disabilities to vote by secret ballot in elections and public referendums without intimidation, and to stand for elections, to effectively hold

office and perform all public functions at all levels of government, facilitating the use of assistive and new technologies where appropriate

iii. Guaranteeing the free expression of the will of persons with disabilities as electors and to this end, where necessary, at their request, allowing assistance in voting by a person of their own choice

b. To promote actively an environment in which persons with disabilities can effectively and fully participate in the conduct of public affairs, without discrimination and on an equal basis with others, and encourage their participation in public affairs, including:

i. Participation in non-governmental organizations and associations concerned with the public and political life of the country, and in the activities and administration of political parties

ii. Forming and joining organizations of persons with disabilities to represent persons with disabilities at international, national, regional and local levels.

ARTICLE 30

Participation in Cultural Life, Recreation, Leisure and Sport

1. States Parties recognize the right of persons with disabilities to take part on an equal basis with others in cultural life, and shall take all appropriate measures to ensure that persons with disabilities:
   a. Enjoy access to cultural materials in accessible formats
   b. Enjoy access to television programmes, films, theatre and other cultural activities, in accessible formats
   c. Enjoy access to places for cultural performances or services, such as theatres, museums, cinemas, libraries and tourism services, and, as far as possible, enjoy access to monuments and sites of national cultural importance.
2. States Parties shall take appropriate measures to enable persons with disabilities to have the opportunity to develop and utilize their creative, artistic and intellectual potential, not only for their own benefit, but also for the enrichment of society.
3. States Parties shall take all appropriate steps, in accordance with international law, to ensure that laws protecting intellectual property rights do not constitute an unreasonable or discriminatory barrier to access by persons with disabilities to cultural materials.
4. Persons with disabilities shall be entitled, on an equal basis with others, to recognition and support of their specific cultural and linguistic identity, including sign languages and deaf culture.
5. With a view to enabling persons with disabilities to participate on an equal basis with others in recreational, leisure and sporting activities, States Parties shall take appropriate measures:
   a. To encourage and promote the participation, to the fullest extent possible, of persons with disabilities in mainstream sporting activities at all levels
   b. To ensure that persons with disabilities have an opportunity to organize, develop and participate in disability-specific sporting and recreational activities and, to this end, encourage the provision, on an equal basis with others, of appropriate instruction, training and resources
   c. To ensure that persons with disabilities have access to sporting, recreational and tourism venues
   d. To ensure that children with disabilities have equal access with other children to participation in play, recreation and leisure and sporting activities, including those activities in the school system

e. To ensure that persons with disabilities have access to services from those involved in the organization of recreational, tourism, leisure and sporting activities.

▪ ARTICLE 31

Statistics and Data Collection

1. States Parties undertake to collect appropriate information, including statistical and research data, to enable them to formulate and implement policies to give effect to the present Convention. The process of collecting and maintaining this information shall:
   a. Comply with legally established safeguards, including legislation on data protection, to ensure confidentiality and respect for the privacy of persons with disabilities
   b. Comply with internationally accepted norms to protect human rights and fundamental freedoms and ethical principles in the collection and use of statistics.
2. The information collected in accordance with this article shall be disaggregated, as appropriate, and used to help assess the implementation of States Parties' obligations under the present Convention and to identify and address the barriers faced by persons with disabilities in exercising their rights.
3. States Parties shall assume responsibility for the dissemination of these statistics and ensure their accessibility to persons with disabilities and others.

▪ ARTICLE 32

International Cooperation

1. States Parties recognize the importance of international cooperation and its promotion, in support of national efforts for the realization of the purpose and objectives of the present Convention, and will undertake appropriate and effective measures in this regard, between and among States and, as appropriate, in partnership with relevant international and regional organizations and civil society, in particular organizations of persons with disabilities. Such measures could include, inter alia:
   a. Ensuring that international cooperation, including international development programmes, is inclusive of and accessible to persons with disabilities
   b. Facilitating and supporting capacity-building, including through the exchange and sharing of information, experiences, training programmes and best practices
   c. Facilitating cooperation in research and access to scientific and technical knowledge
   d. Providing, as appropriate, technical and economic assistance, including by facilitating access to and sharing of accessible and assistive technologies, and through the transfer of technologies.
2. The provisions of this article are without prejudice to the obligations of each State Party to fulfil its obligations under the present Convention.

▪ ARTICLE 33

National Implementation and Monitoring

1. States Parties, in accordance with their system of organization, shall designate one or more focal points within government for matters relating to the implementation of the present Convention, and shall give due consideration to the establishment or designation of a

coordination mechanism within government to facilitate related action in different sectors and at different levels.
2. States Parties shall, in accordance with their legal and administrative systems, maintain, strengthen, designate or establish within the State Party, a framework, including one or more independent mechanisms, as appropriate, to promote, protect and monitor implementation of the present Convention. When designating or establishing such a mechanism, States Parties shall take into account the principles relating to the status and functioning of national institutions for protection and promotion of human rights.
3. Civil society, in particular persons with disabilities and their representative organizations, shall be involved and participate fully in the monitoring process.

■ARTICLE 34

Committee on the Rights of Persons with Disabilities

1. There shall be established a Committee on the Rights of Persons with Disabilities (hereafter referred to as "the Committee"), which shall carry out the functions hereinafter provided.
2. The Committee shall consist, at the time of entry into force of the present Convention, of twelve experts. After an additional sixty ratifications or accessions to the Convention, the membership of the Committee shall increase by six members, attaining a maximum number of eighteen members.
3. The members of the Committee shall serve in their personal capacity and shall be of high moral standing and recognized competence and experience in the field covered by the present Convention. When nominating their candidates, States Parties are invited to give due consideration to the provision set out in Article 4, Paragraph 3, of the present Convention.
4. The members of the Committee shall be elected by States Parties, consideration being given to equitable geographical distribution, representation of the different forms of civilization and of the principal legal systems, balanced gender representation and participation of experts with disabilities.
5. The members of the Committee shall be elected by secret ballot from a list of persons nominated by the States Parties from among their nationals at meetings of the Conference of States Parties. At those meetings, for which two thirds of States Parties shall constitute a quorum, the persons elected to the Committee shall be those who obtain the largest number of votes and an absolute majority of the votes of the representatives of States Parties present and voting.
6. The initial election shall be held no later than six months after the date of entry into force of the present Convention. At least four months before the date of each election, the Secretary-General of the United Nations shall address a letter to the States Parties inviting them to submit the nominations within two months. The Secretary-General shall subsequently prepare a list in alphabetical order of all persons thus nominated, indicating the State Parties which have nominated them, and shall submit it to the States Parties to the present Convention.
7. The members of the Committee shall be elected for a term of four years. They shall be eligible for re-election once. However, the term of six of the members elected at the first election shall expire at the end of two years; immediately after the first election, the names of these six members shall be chosen by lot by the chairperson of the meeting referred to in Paragraph 5 of this article.

8. The election of the six additional members of the Committee shall be held on the occasion of regular elections, in accordance with the relevant provisions of this article.
9. If a member of the Committee dies or resigns or declares that for any other cause she or he can no longer perform her or his duties, the State Party which nominated the member shall appoint another expert possessing the qualifications and meeting the requirements set out in the relevant provisions of this article, to serve for the remainder of the term.
10. The Committee shall establish its own rules of procedure.
11. The Secretary-General of the United Nations shall provide the necessary staff and facilities for the effective performance of the functions of the Committee under the present Convention, and shall convene its initial meeting.
12. With the approval of the General Assembly of the United Nations, the members of the Committee established under the present Convention shall receive emoluments from United Nations resources on such terms and conditions as the Assembly may decide, having regard to the importance of the Committee's responsibilities.
13. The members of the Committee shall be entitled to the facilities, privileges and immunities of experts on mission for the United Nations as laid down in the relevant sections of the Convention on the Privileges and Immunities of the United Nations.

ARTICLE 35

Reports by States Parties

1. Each State Party shall submit to the Committee, through the Secretary General of the United Nations, a comprehensive report on measures taken to give effect to its obligations under the present Convention and on the progress made in that regard, within two years after the entry into force of the present Convention for the State Party concerned.
2. Thereafter, States Parties shall submit subsequent reports at least every four years and further whenever the Committee so requests.
3. The Committee shall decide any guidelines applicable to the content of the reports.
4. A State Party which has submitted a comprehensive initial report to the Committee need not, in its subsequent reports, repeat information previously provided. When preparing reports to the Committee, States Parties are invited to consider doing so in an open and transparent process and to give due consideration to the provision set out in Article 4, Paragraph 3, of the present Convention.
5. Reports may indicate factors and difficulties affecting the degree of fulfilment of obligations under the present Convention.

ARTICLE 36

Consideration of Reports

1. Each report shall be considered by the Committee, which shall make such suggestions and general recommendations on the report as it may consider appropriate and shall forward these to the State Party concerned. The State Party may respond with any information it chooses to the Committee. The Committee may request further information from States Parties relevant to the implementation of the present Convention.
2. If a State Party is significantly overdue in the submission of a report, the Committee may notify the State Party concerned of the need to examine the implementation of the present Convention in that State Party, on the basis of reliable information available to the Committee,

if the relevant report is not submitted within three months following the notification. The Committee shall invite the State Party concerned to participate in such examination. Should the State Party respond by submitting the relevant report, the provisions of Paragraph 1 of this article will apply.
3. The Secretary-General of the United Nations shall make available the reports to all States Parties.
4. States Parties shall make their reports widely available to the public in their own countries and facilitate access to the suggestions and general recommendations relating to these reports.
5. The Committee shall transmit, as it may consider appropriate, to the specialized agencies, funds and programmes of the United Nations, and other competent bodies, reports from States Parties in order to address a request or indication of a need for technical advice or assistance contained therein, along with the Committee's observations and recommendations, if any, on these requests or indications.

ARTICLE 37

Cooperation between States Parties and the Committee

1. Each State Party shall cooperate with the Committee and assist its members in the fulfilment of their mandate.
2. In its relationship with States Parties, the Committee shall give due consideration to ways and means of enhancing national capacities for the implementation of the present Convention, including through international cooperation.

ARTICLE 38

Relationship of the Committee with other Bodies

In order to foster the effective implementation of the present Convention and to encourage international cooperation in the field covered by the present Convention:
a. The specialized agencies and other United Nations organs shall be entitled to be represented at the consideration of the implementation of such provisions of the present Convention as fall within the scope of their mandate. The Committee may invite the specialized agencies and other competent bodies as it may consider appropriate to provide expert advice on the implementation of the Convention in areas falling within the scope of their respective mandates. The Committee may invite specialized agencies and other United Nations organs to submit reports on the implementation of the Convention in areas falling within the scope of their activities
b. The Committee, as it discharges its mandate, shall consult, as appropriate, other relevant bodies instituted by international human rights treaties, with a view to ensuring the consistency of their respective reporting guidelines, suggestions and general recommendations, and avoiding duplication and overlap in the performance of their functions.

ARTICLE 39

Report of the Committee

The Committee shall report every two years to the General Assembly and to the Economic and Social Council on its activities, and may make suggestions and general recommendations based on the examination of reports and information received from the States Parties. Such suggestions and general recommendations shall be included in the report of the Committee together with comments, if any, from States Parties.

ARTICLE 40

Conference of States Parties

1. The States Parties shall meet regularly in a Conference of States Parties in order to consider any matter with regard to the implementation of the present Convention.
2. No later than six months after the entry into force of the present Convention, the Conference of States Parties shall be convened by the Secretary-General of the United Nations. The subsequent meetings shall be convened by the Secretary-General biennially or upon the decision of the Conference of States Parties.

ARTICLE 41

Depositary

The Secretary-General of the United Nations shall be the depositary of the present Convention.

ARTICLE 42

Signature

The present Convention shall be open for signature by all States and by regional integration organizations at United Nations Headquarters in New York as of 30 March 2007.

ARTICLE 43

Consent to be Bound

The present Convention shall be subject to ratification by signatory States and to formal confirmation by signatory regional integration organizations. It shall be open for accession by any State or regional integration organization which has not signed the Convention.

ARTICLE 44

Regional Integration Organizations

1. "Regional integration organization" shall mean an organization constituted by sovereign States of a given region, to which its member States have transferred competence in respect of matters governed by the present Convention. Such organizations shall declare, in their instruments of formal confirmation or accession, the extent of their competence with respect to matters governed by the present Convention. Subsequently, they shall inform the depositary of any substantial modification in the extent of their competence.
2. References to "States Parties" in the present Convention shall apply to such organizations within the limits of their competence.
3. For the purposes of Article 45, Paragraph 1, and Article 47, Paragraphs 2 and 3, of the present Convention, any instrument deposited by a regional integration organization shall not be counted.

4. Regional integration organizations, in matters within their competence, may exercise their right to vote in the Conference of States Parties, with a number of votes equal to the number of their member States that are Parties to the present Convention. Such an organization shall not exercise its right to vote if any of its member States exercises its right, and vice versa.

ARTICLE 45

Entry Into Force

1. The present Convention shall enter into force on the thirtieth day after the deposit of the twentieth instrument of ratification or accession.
2. For each State or regional integration organization ratifying, formally confirming or acceding to the present Convention after the deposit of the twentieth such instrument, the Convention shall enter into force on the thirtieth day after the deposit of its own such instrument.

ARTICLE 46

Reservations

1. Reservations incompatible with the object and purpose of the present Convention shall not be permitted.
2. Reservations may be withdrawn at any time.

ARTICLE 47

Amendments

1. Any State Party may propose an amendment to the present Convention and submit it to the Secretary-General of the United Nations. The Secretary General shall communicate any proposed amendments to States Parties, with a request to be notified whether they favour a conference of States Parties for the purpose of considering and deciding upon the proposals. In the event that, within four months from the date of such communication, at least one third of the States Parties favour such a conference, the Secretary-General shall convene the conference under the auspices of the United Nations. Any amendment adopted by a majority of two thirds of the States Parties present and voting shall be submitted by the Secretary-General to the General Assembly of the United Nations for approval and thereafter to all States Parties for acceptance.
2. An amendment adopted and approved in accordance with Paragraph 1 of this article shall enter into force on the thirtieth day after the number of instruments of acceptance deposited reaches two thirds of the number of States Parties at the date of adoption of the amendment. Thereafter, the amendment shall enter into force for any State Party on the thirtieth day following the deposit of its own instrument of acceptance. An amendment shall be binding only on those States Parties which have accepted it.
3. If so decided by the Conference of States Parties by consensus, an amendment adopted and approved in accordance with Paragraph 1 of this article which relates exclusively to Articles 34, 38, 39 and 40 shall enter into force for all States Parties on the thirtieth day after the number of instruments of acceptance deposited reaches two thirds of the number of States Parties at the date of adoption of the amendment.

ARTICLE 48

Denunciation

A State Party may denounce the present Convention by written notification to the Secretary-General of the United Nations. The denunciation shall become effective one year after the date of receipt of the notification by the Secretary-General.

ARTICLE 49

Accessible Format

The text of the present Convention shall be made available in accessible formats.

ARTICLE 50

Authentic Texts

The Arabic, Chinese, English, French, Russian and Spanish texts of the present Convention shall be equally authentic. IN WITNESS THEREOF the undersigned plenipotentiaries, being duly authorized thereto by their respective Governments, have signed the present Convention.

BIBLIOGRAPHY

1. https://www.un.org/disabilities/documents/convention/convoptprot-e.pdf

CHAPTER 15

Early Identification and Intervention for Detection of Disability

Suvarna S Ganvir, Maheshwari Harishchandre

LEARNING OBJECTIVES

Through this chapter, the reader will be able to:
- Define disability
- Gain knowledge about types of disability
- Understand about evaluation of disability
- Early detection program
- Levels of prevention
- Recent advances

■ DEFINITION BY WHO

❖ A disability is any condition of the body or mind (impairment) that makes it more difficult for the person with the condition to do certain activities (activity limitation) and interact with the world around them (participation restrictions).
   According to the World Health Organization (WHO), disability has three dimensions:
❖ **Impairment** in a person's body structure or function, or mental functioning; examples of impairments include loss of a limb, loss of vision or memory loss.
❖ **Activity limitation**, such as difficulty seeing, hearing, walking, or problem-solving.
❖ **Participation restrictions** in normal daily activities, such as working, engaging in social and recreational activities, and obtaining health care and preventive services.

Types of Disability

There are seven major types of disabilities:
1. Mental Retardation
2. Leprosy-cured
3. Blindness
4. Low Vision
5. Hearing Impairment
6. Locomotor Disability
7. Mental Illness.

CHAPTER 15: Early Identification and Intervention for Detection of Disability

■ LOCOMOTOR DISABILITY

Definition

"Locomotor disability" means a person's inability to execute distinctive activities associated with movement of self and objects resulting from affliction of musculoskeletal or nervous system or both.

■ EVALUATION OF DISABILITY

Guidelines for Evaluation of Permanent Physical Impairment (PPI) of Upper Extremities

Arm (Upper Extremity) Component

Total value of the arm component is 90%.

Principles of Evaluation of Range of Motion (ROM) of Joints

The value of maximum ROM in the arm component is 90%.

　　　　Shoulder—20%　　Elbow—20%　　Wrist—10%　　Hand—40%

Principles of Evaluation of Strength of Muscles

Numerical score of muscle power	Qualitative score	Loss of strength in %
0	Zero	100
1	Trace activity	80
2	Poor	60
3	Fair	40
4	Good	20
5	Normal	0

Principles of Evaluation of Coordinated Activities

- ❖ The total value for coordinated activities is 90%
- ❖ Ten different coordinated activities should be tested as given in the Form A. (Appendix II—assessment proforma for upper extremity)
- ❖ Each activity has a value of 9%.

Combining Values for the Arm Component

$a + b(90-a)/90$
where a = higher value and b = lower value
Reference—the Gazette of India: Extraordinary, 2018

Locomotor Disability

Hand Component

- ❖ Total value of hand component is 90%
- ❖ The functional impairment of hand is expressed as loss of prehension, loss of sensation and loss of strength.

Principles of Evaluation of Prehension

Total value of prehension is 30%.

It includes:
- **Opposition:** 8%
- **Lateral pinch:** 5%
- **Cylindrical grasp:** 6%
- **Spherical grasp:** 6%
- **Hook grasp:** 5%

Principles of Evaluation of Sensation

Total value of sensation in hand is 30%.

Principles of Evaluation of Strength

Total value of strength is 30%.

For shortening of upper extremity, addition weightage is as follows:

First 1"—No additional weightage
For each 1" beyond first 1"—2% additional weightage.

Additional weightage—a total of up to 10% additional weightage can be given to following accompanying factors if they are continuous and persistent despite treatment.

Combining Values of Hand Component

The final value of loss of function of hand component is obtained by summing up values of loss of prehension, sensation and strength.

Combining Values for the Extremity

Values of impairment of arm component and impairment of hand component should be added by using combining formula:

$$a + b(90-a)/90$$

where a = higher value and b = lower value.
Reference: The Gazette of India: Extraordinary, 2018

■ LOCOMOTOR DISABILITY

Guidelines for Evaluation of Permanent Physical Impairment in Lower Extremity

The measurement of loss of function in lower extremity is divided into two components, namely, **mobility** and **stability** components.

Mobility Component

Total value of mobility component is 90% which includes range of movement (ROM) and muscle strength.

Principles of Evaluation of Range of Movement

The value of maximum range of movement in mobility component is 90%.

| Hip—35% | Knee—35% | Ankle—20% |

Principle of Evaluation of Muscle Strength

The value for maximum muscle strength in the extremity is 90%.

Numerical score of muscle power	Qualitative score	Loss of strength in %
0	Zero	100
1	Trace activity	80
2	Poor	60
3	Fair	40
4	Good	20
5	Normal	0

Combining Values for Mobility Component

The values of loss of ROM and loss of muscle strength should be combined with the help of combining formula:

$$a + b(90-a)/90$$

where a = higher value, b = lower value.

Stability Component

- Total value of the stability component is 90%
- It shall be tested by clinical method as given in Form B (Assessment Proforma for lower extremity) in Appendix II (The Gazette of India: Extraordinary, 2018).

Extra Points

Extra points (% of impairment) are given for deformities, pain, contractures, loss of sensations and shortening, etc. Two types of shortening, i.e., true shortening and apparent shortening.

DISABILITY EVALUATION OF SPINE

Cervical Spine Injuries

Sl. No.	Cervical spine injuries	Percentage of PPI in relation to the spine
1.	25% or more compression of one or two adjacent vertebral bodies with No involvement of posterior elements, No nerve root involvement, moderate Neck rigidity and persistent soreness.	20%
2.	Posterior element damage with radiological evidence of moderate dislocation/subluxation including whiplash injury	
	• With fusion healed, no permanent motor or sensory changes	10%
	• Persistent pain with radiologically demonstrable instability.	25%
3.	Severe Dislocation:	
	• Fair to good reduction with or without fusion with no residual motor or sensory involvement	10%
	• Inadequate reduction with fusion and persistent radicular pain	15%

Cervical Intervertebral Disc Lesions

Sl. No.	Cervical Intervertebral disc lesions	Percentage of PPI in relation to spine
1.	Treated case of disc lesion with persistent pain but no neurological deficit	10%
2.	Treated case of disc lesion with pain and instability	15%

Thoracic and Thoracolumbar Spine Injuries

Sl. No.	Thoracic and thoracolumbar spine injuries	Percentage of PPI in relation to spine
1.	Compression of less than 50% involving one vertebral body with no neurological manifestation	10%
2.	Compression of more than 50% involving single vertebra or more with involvement of posterior elements, healed, no neurological manifestations persistent pain, fusion indicated	20%
3.	Same as (2) with fusion, pain only on heavy use of back	15%
4.	Radiologically demonstrable instability with fracture or fracture dislocation with persistent pain	30%

Lumbar and Lumbosacral Spine: Fracture

Sl. No.	Lumbar and/or lumbosacral spine fracture	Percentage of PPI in relation to spine
1.	Compression of 25% or less of one or two adjacent vertebral bodies, no definite pattern, no neurological deficit	10%
2.	Compression of more than 25% with disruption of posterior elements, persistent pain and stiffness, healed with or without fusion, inability to lift more than 10 kg.	20%
3.	Radiologically demonstrable instability in low lumbar or lumbosacral spine with pain	30%

Intervertebral Disc Lesion

Sl. No.	Intervertebral disc lesion	Percentage of PPI in relation to spine
1.	Treated case with persistent pain	10%
2.	Treated case with persistent pain and instability	20%
3.	Treated case with persistent pain and activities of lifting moderately modified	25%
4.	Treated case with persistent pain and stiffness, aggravated by heavy lifting necessitating modification of all activities requiring heavy weight lifting	30%

UPPER LIMB LEVELS PERCENTAGE OF AMPUTATIONS

Sl. No.	Level of upper limb amputation	% of permanent impairment in relation to that specific limb
1.	Forequarter amputation	100
2.	Shoulder disarticulation	90
3.	Transhumeral (above elbow) up to upper 1/3 of arm	85
4.	Transhumeral (above elbow) up to lower 1/3 of arm	80
5.	Elbow disarticulation	75
6.	Transradial (below elbow) up to upper 1/3 of forearm	70
7.	Transradial (below elbow) up to lower 1/3 of forearm	65
8.	Wrist disarticulation	60
9.	Hand through carpal bones	55
10.	Thumb through CM or through 1st MC joint	30
11.	Thumb disarticulation through metacarpophalangeal joint or through proximal phalanx	25
12.	Thumb disarticulation through interphalangeal joint or through distal phalanx	15
13.	Amputation through proximal phalanx or disarticulation through MP joint of: • Index finger • Middle finger • Ring finger • Little finger	 15 5 3 2
14.	Amputation through middle phalanx or disarticulation through PIP joint of: • Index finger • Middle finger • Ring finger • Little finger	 10 4 2 1
15.	Amputation through distal phalanx or disarticulation through DIP joint of: • Index finger • Middle finger • Ring finger • Little finger	 5 2 1 1

LOWER LIMB LEVELS PERCENTAGE OF AMPUTATIONS

Sl. No.	Level of lower limb amputation	% of permanent impairment in relation to that specific limb
1.	Hind quarter	100
2.	Hip disarticulation	90
3.	Transfemoral (above knee) up to upper 1/3 of thigh	85
4.	Transfemoral (above knee) up to lower 1/3 of thigh	80
5.	Through knee	75
6.	Transtibial (below knee) up to upper 1/3 of leg	70
7.	Transtibial (below knee) up to lower 1/3 of leg	60
8.	Through ankle	55
9.	Syme's	50
10.	Up to mid-foot (proximal to tarso-metatarsal joints level)	40
11.	Up to fore-foot (distal to tarso-metatarsal joints level)	30
12.	All toes	20
13.	Loss of first toe	10
14.	Loss of second toe	4
15.	Loss of third toe	3
16.	Loss of fourth toe	2
17.	Loss of fifth toe	1

Early Detection Program

❖ Early detection of disability is the basic approach to early intervention which is itself a continuous process.

Timing stages of development	Factor cause	Explanation
Prenatal (before birth)	• Genetic: single or multi-factorial	
	• Chromosomal defects	• Down syndrome in child

	• Infective agent:
	  – Viral
	  – Bacterial
	  – Protozoal
		• For examples
		  – Rubella in other/hepatitis haemophilia influenzas

	• Anoxia	• Hypnotic-ischemia encephalopathy • Intrauterine growth retardation
	• Nutritional	• Anemia
	• Maternal disease	• Hypertension, diabetes negative rhesus (Rh) factor in mother
	• Drugs, chemical, physical agent	• X-rays, radiation, exposure to pesticides

Contd...

CHAPTER 15: Early Identification and Intervention for Detection of Disability

Contd...

Timing stages of development	Factor cause	Explanation
Newborn	• Anoxia	• From long, difficult labor, cord wrapped around child's neck
	• Birth trauma	• Breech and other abnormal deliveries, forceps/suction cup delivery
Neonatal (immediately after birth)	• Prematurely, jaundice, hypoglycaemia, infection, anoxia	• Skin infection • Eye infection • Lack breastfeeding within first hours
Toddler/childhood	• Complication of infectious diseases	• Poliomyelitis, gastroenteritis with dehydration, measles, pertussis with encephalitis, inhalation of foreign body
	• Anoxia, meningitis, encephalitis, poisoning	• Lead in paints, battery acid, breathing in car exhaust • Chronic obstructive pulmonary disease (COPD)
	• Head injury, malnutrition	• Lack of vitamins (especially A), iodine
	• Environmental	• Lack of stimulation in the environment

❖ Early detection and early intervention will minimize and/or prevent the consequences of an impairment, ultimately preventing the impairment from becoming the disability.

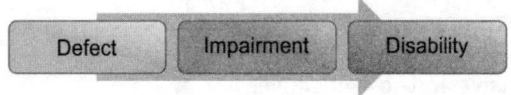

❖ Infant stimulation program (Child Development Centre) Model
  • Practical mother-oriented stimulation program
  • Objectives of early stimulation are:
    ❖ Stimulating the child through the normal developmental channel.
    ❖ Prevention of developmental delay
    ❖ Prevention of asymmetries and abnormalities
    ❖ Detection of transient abnormalities and minimization of persistent abnormalities.

Early Intervention Program

Early intervention is a term, which broadly refers to a wide range of experiences and supports provided to children, parents and families during the pregnancy, infancy and early childhood period of development [Dunst, 1996].

Primary Reason for Early Intervention

❖ To enhance the child's normal development,
❖ To provide support and assistance to the family,
❖ To maximize the child's and family's benefit to society.

Aim of Early Intervention

❖ Early identification of infants at risk

- Early identification of developmental delays
- Enhancement of normal development
- Cost-effective
- Psychological support to the family
- Early detection and prevention of secondary handicaps
- Minimizing the effects of the handicapping condition.

Nature of Population Requiring Early Intervention

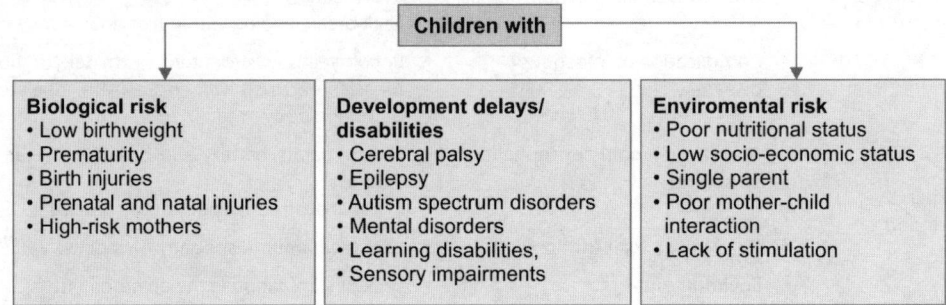

Biological risk
- Low birthweight
- Prematurity
- Birth injuries
- Prenatal and natal injuries
- High-risk mothers

Development delays/disabilities
- Cerebral palsy
- Epilepsy
- Autism spectrum disorders
- Mental disorders
- Learning disabilities,
- Sensory impairments

Enviromental risk
- Poor nutritional status
- Low socio-economic status
- Single parent
- Poor mother-child interaction
- Lack of stimulation

Developmental Screening

- The major goal of developmental screening is to reduce the time that elapses before any intervention begins.
- Accurate, comprehensive and cost-effective.
- Screening can occur through a variety of methods. They can include parent interviews, observations of the child, or the use of a specific instrument or checklist.

■ EARLY INTERVENTION STRATEGY

1. Parent involvement
2. Assessment

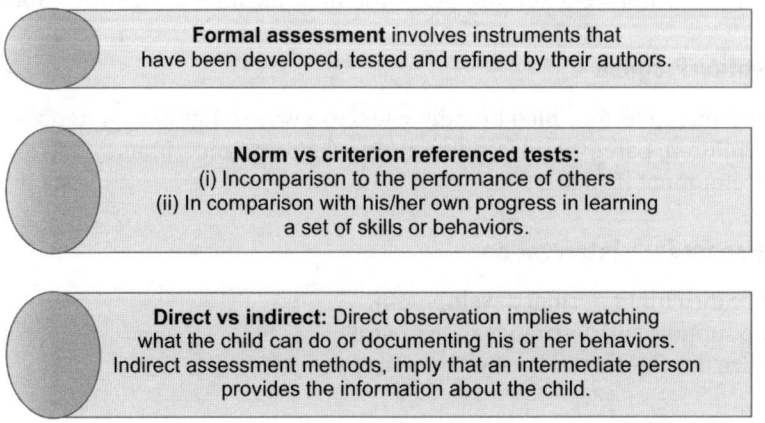

Formal assessment involves instruments that have been developed, tested and refined by their authors.

Norm vs criterion referenced tests:
(i) Incomparison to the performance of others
(ii) In comparison with his/her own progress in learning a set of skills or behaviors.

Direct vs indirect: Direct observation implies watching what the child can do or documenting his or her behaviors. Indirect assessment methods, imply that an intermediate person provides the information about the child.

CHAPTER 15: Early Identification and Intervention for Detection of Disability

Early Intervention Service Approach

The Multidisciplinary Approach

* The approach to early intervention now is multidisciplinary where each professional individually provides services to the child.
* In multidisciplinary teams, professionals from several disciplines work independently of each other (Fewell, 1983).

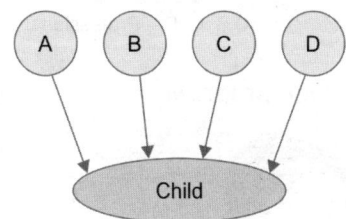

Multidisciplinary approach

The Interdisciplinary Approach

* Interdisciplinary approach defines a process where professionals from different but related disciplines work together to assess and manage problems by actively participating in mutual decision-making.
* Interdisciplinary teams are composed of parents and professionals from several disciplines.

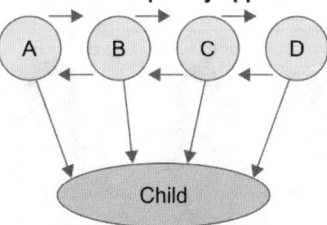

The interdisciplinary approach

A, B, C, D – Professionals

Transdisciplinary Approach

* In the transdisciplinary approach, each professional provides management plan to the case manager in consultation with the other team members.
* One of the members may be elected as a **case manager** who will deal with the child.
* The case manager may be a **rehabilitation worker**.
* This approach is holistic in nature and provides better case management and resource management (time and money).

Transdisciplinary approach

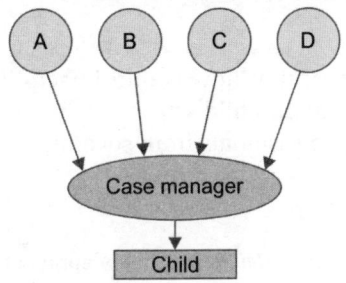

A, B, C, D – Professionals

Activities of early intervention program

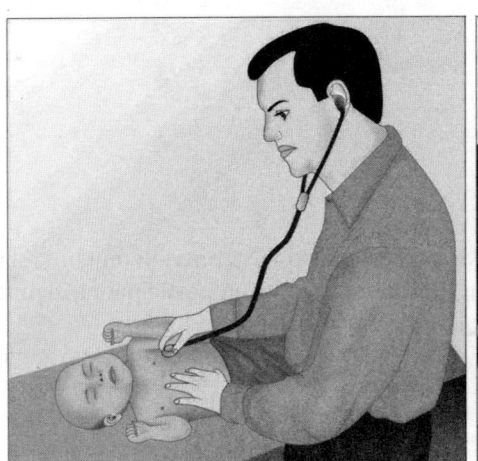

Medical examination

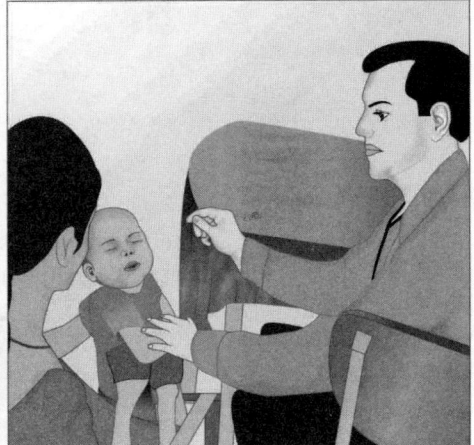

Parent councelling

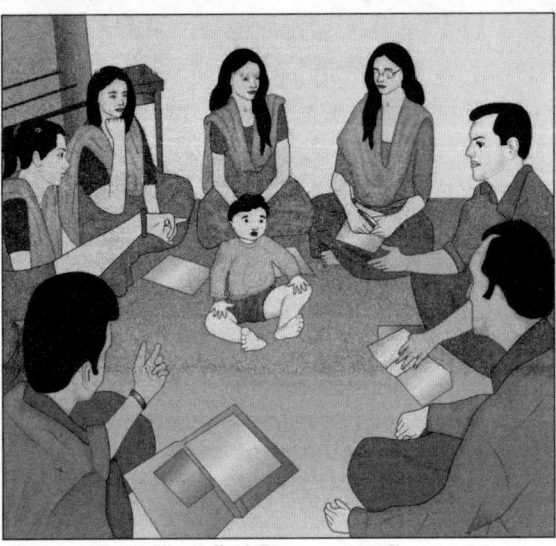

Transdisciplinary approach

Service Delivery Models in Early Intervention

Target Child-centered	The therapist works with the child directly to bring about the desired changes on a one-to-one basis.
Parent-centered	The interventionist works with the parents to produce effective and long-lasting changes in the child.
Family-centered	The focus is on the family.
Frequency of follow-up	The efforts and time spent on intervention may vary greatly giving rise to different type of services, daily, weekly or monthly. It depends on the need of the child, availability of professionals, the distance of the center and the cost of intervention.
Models of services Home-based programs	The programs are operated at home wherein one of the parents or any other family member or the caregiver participates in intervention.
Center-based programs	Programs are carried out in the centre—an institute, daycare centre or a community centre where services are provided by professionals/trained personnel.
Home-cum-center-based	Programs are carried out both at home and in the center. The professionals do carry out home visits to extend services.
Parent consultation model	Here parents take consultation from professionals but carry out the program at home.

Admission: Client Sources for Early Intervention

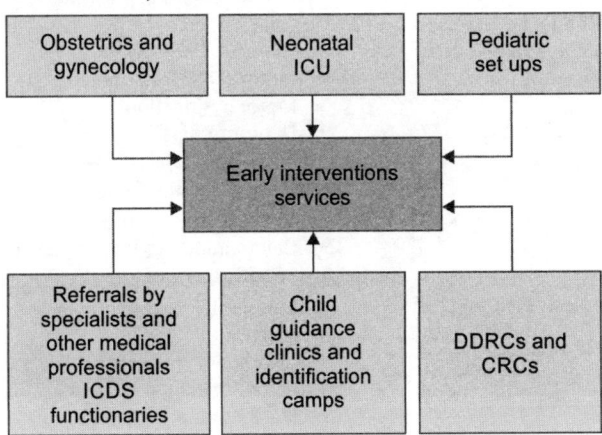

Details of Service Provision

The procedure to be followed from registration to the intervention is depicted below diagrammatically.

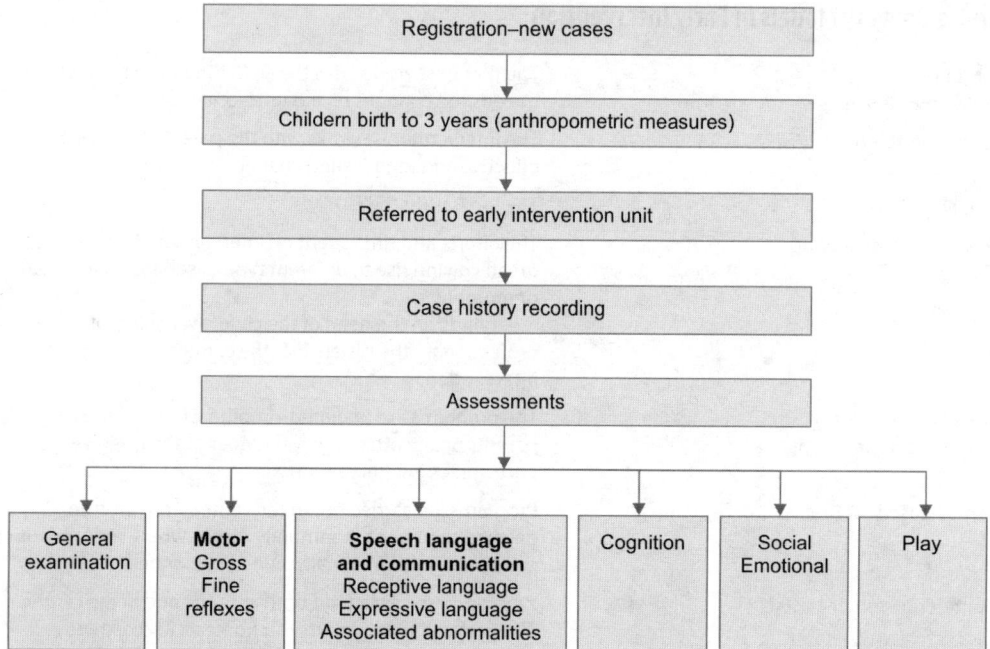

Role of Physiotherapist in Early Intervention

Physiotherapy interventions foster motor development in the child using Neurodevelopmental techniques. The emphasis of this technique is on facilitating movement under a normal postural tone.

■ PHYSIOTHERAPIST

1. Assessment	◆ Motor skills/development ◆ Motor dysfunction ◆ Neuromotor ◆ Musculoskeletal
2. Intervention	◆ Design adaptive equipment and mobility devices ◆ Motor intervention ◆ Gait training ◆ Specific therapies
3. Community and teamwork	◆ Interdisciplinary planning ◆ Referral ◆ Awareness programs ◆ Parent training programs ◆ Master training programs ◆ Case management

■ BIBLIOGRAPHY

1. Kumar M. National Policy for Persons with Disabilities. Ministry of Social Justice and Empowerment; 2006 Feb 10.
2. Rosenbaum P, Stewart D. The World Health Organization International Classification of Functioning, Disability, and Health: a model to guide clinical thinking, practice and research in the field of cerebral palsy. In Seminars in pediatric neurology. WB Saunders. 2004;11(1):5-10.

Section 4 Elderly Individuals and their Services

CHAPTER 16

Health Care and Fitness

Ashish Wasudeorao Bele

LEARNING OBJECTIVES

Through this chapter, the reader will be able to:
- Identify the different components of the health care delivery system
- Identify and understand the legal rights and benefits related to health
- Enumerate the different components of fitness training and importance of fitness at community level
- Discuss the strategies of health fitness for women and geriatric

■ NATIONAL HEALTHCARE DELIVERY SYSTEM

Introduction

Health is the general condition of person in all aspects. It is also a level of functional and metabolic efficiency of an organism, often implicitly human. Health has been declared a fundamental human right. This implies that the state has responsibility for health of its people. National governments all over the world are striving to expand and improve the health care services. Health care is the treatment and management of illness and preservation of health through services offered by the medical, dental, complementary and alternative medicine, pharmaceutical, clinical sciences, nursing and allied health professions. The widely accepted definition of health is that given by the World Health Organization (1948) in the preamble to its constitution, which is as follows: "Health is a state of complete physical, mental and social wellbeing and not merely an absence of disease or infirmity".[1]

Disease is defined as "An abnormal condition of an organism that impairs bodily functions associated with specific symptoms and signs".

Public Health

Public health is "The science and art of preventing disease, prolonging life and promoting health through the organized effort and informed choices of society, organizations, public and private, communities and individual. It is characterized by the deals with preventive rather than curative aspect of health and population level, rather than individual level of health issues".

Health Care

Health is influenced by number of factors such as adequate food, housing, basic sanitation, healthy lifestyle, protection against environmental hazards and communicable diseases, the frontiers of health extend beyond the narrow limits of medical care. Health care is defined as a, "multitude of services rendered to individuals, families or communities by the agents of the health services or professions, for the purpose of promoting, maintaining, monitoring or restoring health".[1] It is important to provide such services by the health professionals who help to diagnosed, cure the diseases along with educate the patient and also rehabilitate them. Medical care is the main component of health care which provide hospital care to domiciliary (Home) care with the help of medical professional including Physician, Physiotherapist etc.[1]

Characteristics of Health Care

- ❖ **Appropriateness:** It is nothing but the relevance which look after the services related to the human needs, prioritize and policies.
- ❖ **Comprehensiveness:** It involves the preventive, curative and promotional services.
- ❖ **Adequacy:** It is nothing but when the services are as per requirement.
- ❖ **Availability:** It is when the administrative unit population and the health facilities are proportionate.
- ❖ **Accessibility:** It is related to the geographic, economic or cultural accessibility.
- ❖ **Affordability:** The health care should be affordable when the cost is within the individual and state means.
- ❖ **Feasibility:** Health care should be well efficient of certain procedures, manpower, logistic support and material resources.[1]

Health System

Health services are designed to meet the health needs of the community through the use of available knowledge and resources. The health services are delivered by the '**health system**' which constitute the management sector and involves organizational matters like planning, determining priorities, mobilizing and allocating resources, translating policies into services, evaluation and health education.[1]

Components of the Health System

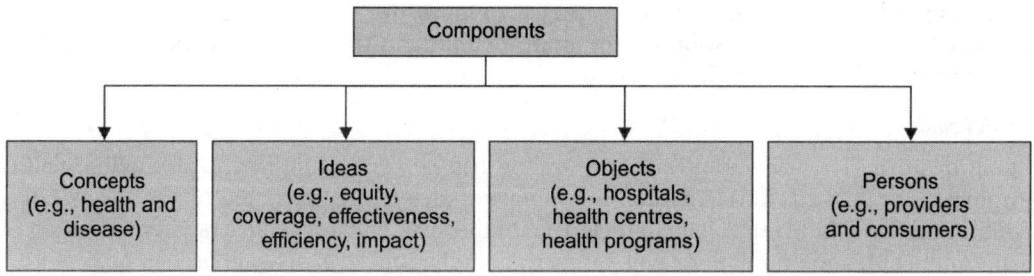

Levels of Health Care

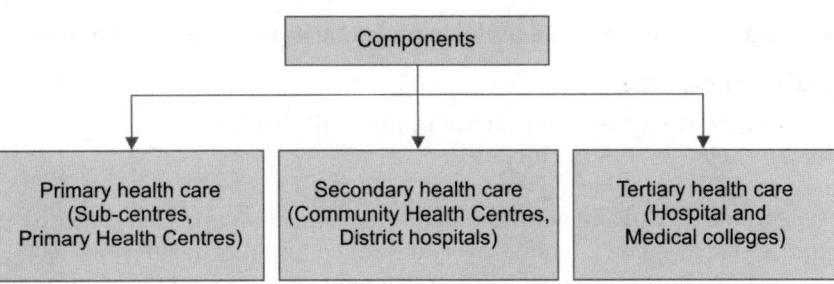

Primary Health Care

The primary health care concept highlighted in 1978 at international conference in Alma-Ata, USSR. It has been defined as: "Essential health care based on practical, scientifically sound and socially acceptable methods and technology made universally accessible to individuals and families in the community through their full participation and at a cost that the community and the country can afford to maintain at every stage of their development in the spirit of self-determination". This is the first level of health care where the individual and health system comes into contact.[1]

Principles of Primary Health Care

It includes:
- Equitable distribution.
- Community participation
- Intersectoral coordination
- Appropriate technology provided by Subcenters.
- **Primary health centres:** Auxiliary Nurse Midwife (ANM), Accredited Social Health Activist (ASHA), Anganwadi Worker (AWW), *Village Health Guide* (VHG), Traditional birth attendants (TBA), Local Dais.[2]

Elements of Primary Health Care

It includes:
- MCH services including family planning
- Immunization
- Provision of essential drugs
- Prevention and control of local endemic diseases
- Treatment of common illnesses and injuries
- Safe water supply and basic sanitation
- Provision of food supply and nutrition
- Health Education about prevailing health problems and its prevention and control.[2]

Primary Level Health Care Schemes

There are certain schemes which are useful in providing health care to community.

Village Health Guide Scheme (VHG)

- ❖ VHG were mostly women and chosen from community itself.
- ❖ Guidelines for selection of VHG included:
  - Permanent member of local community
  - Should be able to read and write and minimum education up to 6th standard
  - Should be able to spend 2-3 hours every day for community health work
  - After selection short training at PHC for 200 hours and stipend of ₹ 200/month during training
  - After completion of training, they receive a working manual and kit of simple medicine.

Duties Assigned to Health Guides

Treatment of simple aliments and refer in time if required:
- ❖ First aid
- ❖ MCH
- ❖ Health education and sanitation

Local Dais

Rural health scheme undertaken this program which focuses to train all categories of traditional birth attendants (dais) in obstetrics skills and also improves their knowledge in elementary concept of MCH and sterilization. Training session last for 30 days and stipend of ₹ 200 paid to each dai during training. They have being train at PHC, SC, MCH centre. Once they have completed the training, they have received a delivery kit and certificate. Training of one local dai in each village is the national target.

Anganwadi Worker (AWW)

- ❖ Under ICDS scheme, one AWW has been selected for 400–800 population from the community. They have been trained for 4 months in various aspect of health, nutrition, child development and honorarium of ₹ 1500/month.
- ❖ Services included:
  - Health check-up
  - Growth chart monitoring
  - Immunization
  - Supplementary nutrition
  - Health education
  - Non formal pre-school education
  - Referral beneficiaries
  - Nursing mothers
  - Pregnant women
  - Women in reproductive age
  - Adolescent girls
  - Children below 6 years of age.

Accredited Social Health Activist (ASHA)

- Under the National Rural Health Mission (NRHM) cadre was created which included women.
- Selection criterias for ASHA workers:
  - Resident of village: Married/Widow/Divorced/Separated
  - Age group: 25–45 years
  - Literate woman with formal education up to 10th Class.
  - Good communication skills
  - Leadership qualities
  - Representation from disadvantaged population/marginalized groups.
  - Family and social support.
- They have trained for knowledge and then provided with drug kit to deliver first contact health cares. They received performance-based incentives for promoting immunization and referral services for RCH and other health programs.

Roles and Responsibilities of ASHA Workers

- Create awareness
- Counsel
- Mobilize the community
- Escort/Accompany
- Community level curative care
- Information of Birth/death/unusual health problems/outbreaks
- Coordinate with other health and sanitation workers.[7]

Primary Level Health Care Centres

Subcentres (SC)

Subcenters are first contact between primary health care and community which lies in peripheral. It must include in general areas, 1 per 5,000 populations and in difficult/tribal and hilly areas, it should be 1 per 3,000 populations.[2] Required staffed in each SC includes, at least one auxiliary nurse midwife (ANM)/female health worker and one male health worker (further details are given in recommended staffing structure under the Indian Public Health Standards (IPHS)). There is a provision for one additional ANM on a contract basis under National Rural Health Mission (NRHM).[3]

Role of Sub-centre

- Provision of maternal and child health care.
- Prevention of malnutrition and common childhood diseases.
- Implementation of family planning and contraception.
- Monitoring water quality and disinfection of water resources.
- Provision of adolescent health care and school health services.
- Promotion of sanitation curative services for minor ailments.
- Implementation of community needs assessment.
- Periodic surveillance to be done and reported to PHC every week.

Role of Physiotherapy at Subcentres

- Under the programme (NPHCE), Physiotherapy is one of the important components.
- Physiotherapy provides Health Education related to healthy ageing.
- Physiotherapy also provides care to home bound/bedridden elderly.
- Physiotherapy assessment and management includes application of suitable callipers and supportive devices.[4]

Primary Health Centres (PHCs)

Primary health centre is the first contact point between the village community and the medical officer. Establishment of primary health centre (PHC) is with a population of 30,000 people and in hilly/difficult to reach/tribal areas with a population of 20,000. Primary Health Cares were likely to provide integrated preventive and curative health care to the rural community population which emphasized on the preventive and promotive aspects of health care. State Governments are established and maintained the PHCs under the Minimum Needs Program (MNP)/Basic Minimum Services (BMS) Program. As per minimum requirement, staff of the PHC included a medical officer with 14 paramedical and other staff. Under NRHM, there is a provision for two additional staff nurses on a contract basis. It acts as a referral unit for 5-6 SCs and consist 4-6 beds for indoor patients. Healthcare promotion and curative services are the primary activities of PHCs.[3]

Role of PHC

As per the outline in the Alma-Ata declaration, it covers 8 essential elements in Primary Health Care which includes:
- Provision of medical care.
- Implementation of MCH including family planning.
- Provision of safe water supply and basic sanitation.
- Prevention and control of locally endemic diseases.
- Collection and reporting of vital statistics.
- Health education.
- Relevant National Health Programs.
- Implementation of referral services.
- Training of health guides, health workers, local dais, and health assistants.
- Facilitation of basic laboratory services.

Types of PHCs

There are two types of PHCs as follows:
1. **Type A PHC:** PHC with delivery load of less than 20 deliveries/month.
2. **Type B PHC:** PHC with delivery load of 20 or more deliveries/month.[2]

Manpower at PHCs

Sl. No.	Staff	Number
1.	Medical officer	01
2.	Pharmacist	01
3.	Nurse–midwife	01
4.	Health educator	01
5.	Health worker ANM	01
6.	Health assistant (Male and Female)	02
7.	Clerks	02
8.	Laboratory technicians	01
9.	Driver	01
10.	Class IV	04
	TOTAL	**15**

Physiotherapy Services in Primary Care

Physiotherapists are well skilled and have competencies which are beneficial to community individuals and populations across the progression of care, including health promotion and illness prevention, self-management, treatment and rehabilitation. Physiotherapists can involve in assessment and treatment of persons life-long those have illness, injury or disability affecting the musculoskeletal, neurological, cardiovascular and pulmonary systems; they also plays important role to promote wellness and increased quality of life through education, specialized programming and a holistic approach to health care.

Role of Physiotherapists in Primary Health Care

- Physiotherapist plays an important role in assessment, diagnosis, and treatment of patients having musculoskeletal complaints.
- Also focused on education, exercise programs and self-management.
- They involve in education, assessment, diagnosis, and management of incontinence and pelvic pain conditions.
- Involves in assessment and management of neurological conditions like stroke, Parkinson's disease, etc.
- System navigation assistance for those who need to access physiotherapy and other services in the community.
- Assessment of mobility aids and also provide assistance in allowing funding options for devices.
- Involved in outreach programs in community including awareness camp, falls prevention programs, etc.

- Provision of specialist care for musculoskeletal, neurological, cardiovascular and respiratory conditions in collaboration with other health care specialist like Orthopaedician, Neurophysician, etc.
- Assessment and management of back pain including education, providing self-management program, community-based treatment programs referral and identification of need for additional diagnostics, specialist referral.
- Assessment, treatment, education, counselling, self-management programs for increasing the activities of patients for those have obesity, pre-diabetes, diabetes, arthritis and other chronic diseases.
- For chronic conditions patients Physiotherapist facilitate linkages with community programs, assessment of appropriateness of programs including pain management, providing counselling on safe participation.
- Physiotherapist those are included as palliative care, involved in assessment management of pain and mobility issues related to cancer.
- Providing support and education to caregivers those are involved in assistance of patients in chronic diseases. Plays an important role in prevention of injury programs for caregivers.
- Return to work programs.
- Counselling, patient-centric self-management and lung health programs which teaches the skill to patient for managing their acute periods like in chronic cardiorespiratory conditions such as asthma, COPD and deconditioning after illness.
- Involves in osteoporosis education and management programs.
  - Physiotherapists may also refer the patient for certain diagnostics (e.g., X-rays, CAT scans, ultrasound, MRI, specific laboratory tests), through delegation or medical directives, provided that they are within the scope of practice of physiotherapy.[5]

Auxiliary Nurse Midwife (ANM) (HWF)

ANM usually posted at Sub-centre and PHC. They provided primary health care to community and forms important link between health services and community. Their first priority is to provide Reproductive and Child Health services. They are usually 1 per 5000 Population and 1 per 3000 in hilly/tribal areas.

Functions of ANM

- ANM provides maternal and child health services.
- They facilitate family planning.
- They used to provide immunization services.
- They are facilitating ASHA.
- They also provide the maintenance of registers.

Secondary Health Care

More complex problems dealt at this level. This care involves the district hospitals and community health centres which comprises essentially preventive and curative services. This is the first referral level in the health system (FRUs).[1,2]

Community Health Centre (CHC)

CHC is required to be formed by four medical specialists i.e. surgeon, physician, gynecologist/obstetrician and pediatrician, they are supported by 21 paramedical and other staff.

State Government established and maintained Community health centres (CHCs) under the MNP/BMS program in the area with a population of 1,20,000 people and with a population of 80 000 in the hilly/difficult to reach/tribal areas. CHC has been provided with 30 beds for indoor patients with an operation theatre, X-ray machine, labour room, standby generator and laboratory facilities (Pathology). It serves as a referral centre for PHCs and also provides facilities for obstetric care and specialist consultations. As on 31st March, 2017, there were 5,624 CHCs functioning in the country and as on 31st March 2019, there are **5335 CHCs** functional in rural areas of the country.[2,3,6]

Role of CHC

- It has 30 indoor beds with an operation theatre, X-ray machine, labour room, pathological laboratory facilities and standby generator.
- Provision of 24 hour delivery service care of routine and emergency cases in surgery and medicine.
- Provided with essential and emergency obstetric care.
- Provided with family planning services.
- Facilitates safe abortion services.
- Facilitation of newborn care
- Provision of routine and emergency care of sick children.

District Level

It is a principal unit of administration in India under a District Collector. There are 6 types of administrative area within each district, included: Sub-divisions, Municipalities and corporation, Tahsils (Talukas), Villages, Community development block, Panchayats. It provides a 3 tier system of rural local self-government in India, linking village to the district. Panchayat is at village level, Panchayat samiti is at the block level and Zilla parishad is at district level.[2]

First Referral Units (FRU)

- An existing facility (district hospital, sub-divisional hospital, CHC) can be declared a fully operational first referral unit (FRU) only if it is equipped to provide round-the-clock services for emergency obstetric and newborn care, in addition to all emergencies that any hospital is required to provide.
- It should be noted that there are three critical determinants of a facility being declared as a FRU:
  - Emergency obstetric care including surgical interventions such as caesarean sections;
  - Care for small and sick newborns; and
  - Blood storage facility on a 24-h basis.

Tertiary Health Care

It is second referral level of health care in India. This level included super specialist care. This care is provided by the regional/central level institutions. These institutions provide highly specialized care with planning and managerial skills and teaching for specialized staff. In addition, the tertiary level supports and complements the actions carried out at the primary level. It includes hospitals.[1]

Hospitals

The hospitals might be Rural Hospitals, Subdivisional Hospitals which includes Subdivisional Health Centre, District Hospitals includes District Health Centre, Specialist Hospital and Teaching Hospitals.

Health Insurance

ESI (Employee State Insurance): It provides medical care for Sickness, Maternity and Pension for dependent on death due to employment injury.

CGHS (Central Government Health Scheme): Facilities provided under this scheme include OPD care through network of dispensaries, Supply of necessary drugs, Laboratory and X-ray investigation, hospitalization services at government and recognized private hospitals, antenatal, natal, postnatal services, family welfare services, emergency treatment.

Other Agencies

- **Defence medical services:** This agency provide medical care for defense personnel and their families, provide Armed Force Medical services and services are integrated and comprehensive.
- **Health care of railway employees:** Health care provided through railway hospitals, health units, clinics, provision of Environmental sanitation supervised by health inspector, facilitates Health checkup at entry and yearly interval and provide specialist services at divisional hospital.

Agencies Other Than Public Health Sector

Private agencies : Provide large share of health services, it is mainly curative in nature, mainly congregate in urban areas and available to those who can pay.

Indigenous system of medicine: It include Ayurveda, Siddha, Homeopathy, Unani, etc. It provide the bulk of medical care to rural people.

Voluntary health agencies: It includes Indian Council for Child Welfare and Indian Red Cross Society.

■ LEGAL RIGHTS AND BENEFITS RELATED TO HEALTH

- According to the World Health Organization's Constitution of 1946 "the best attainable standard of health as a fundamental right of every human being".
- Understanding health as a human right imposes a legal obligation on states to provide timely, acceptable, and affordable high-quality health care, as well as the underlying determinants of health such as safe and potable water, sanitation, food, housing, health-related information and education, and gender equality.
- According to a rights-based approach to health, health policies and programmes must prioritise the needs of the poorest people first in order to achieve more justice, a principle mirrored in the newly adopted 2030 agenda for Sustainable Development and Universal Health Coverage.[1]
- The right to health must be exercised without regard to race, age, ethnicity, or any other status factor. States must take action to correct any discriminatory law, practice, or policy under the principles of non-discrimination and equality.

- Significant engagement is a feature of rights-based methods. National stakeholders, including non-state actors such as non-governmental organisations, must be included meaningfully in all aspects of programming, including assessment, analysis, planning, implementation, monitoring, and evaluation.
- "The right to the highest attainable standard of health" implies a clear set of legal obligations on states to ensure appropriate conditions for the enjoyment of health for all people without discrimination.
- The right to health is one of a number of internationally recognized human rights standards, and it is inextricably linked to the other rights. This means that the realization of other human rights, such as food, shelter, job, education, information, and participation, is both important to and dependent on the realization of the right to health.
- Principles for setting and evaluating health policy and service delivery, targeting discriminatory practices and unjust power relations that are at the heart of inequitable health outcomes.
- In pursuing a rights-based approach, health policy, strategies and programmes should be designed explicitly to improve the enjoyment of all people to the right to health, with a focus on the furthest behind first. The core principles and standards of a rights-based approach are detailed below.
- The right to health, as with other rights, includes both freedoms and entitlements:
  - Freedoms include the right to control one's health and body (for example, sexual and reproductive rights) and to be free from interference (for example, free from torture and non-consensual medical treatment and experimentation).
  - Entitlements include the right to a system of health protection that gives everyone an equal opportunity to enjoy the highest attainable level of health.

Core Components of the Right to Health

The right to health (Article 12) was specified in General Comment 14 of the Committee on Economic, Social, and Cultural Rights, which is in charge of ensuring that the Covenant is followed.[7] The right includes the following core components:
- **Availability:** Refers to the need for a sufficient quantity of functioning public health and health care facilities, goods and services, as well as programmes for all. Availability can be measured through the analysis of disaggregated data to different and multiple stratifiers including by age, sex, location and socio-economic status and qualitative surveys to understand coverage gaps and health workforce coverage.
- **Accessibility:** Requires that health facilities, goods, and services must be accessible to everyone. Accessibility has four overlapping dimensions:
  - Non-discrimination
  - Physical accessibility
  - Economical accessibility (affordability)
  - Information accessibility.
  - Assessing accessibility may require analysis of barriers—physical financial or otherwise—that exist, and how they may affect the most vulnerable, and call for the establishment or application of clear norms and standards in both law and policy to address these barriers, as well as robust monitoring systems of health-related information and whether this information is reaching all populations.
- **Acceptability:** Relates to respect for medical ethics, culturally appropriate, and sensitivity to gender. Acceptability requires that health facilities, goods, services and programmes

are people-centred and cater for the specific needs of diverse population groups and in accordance with international standards of medical ethics for confidentiality and informed consent.
- **Quality:** Facilities, goods, and services must be scientifically and medically approved. Quality is a key component of Universal Health Coverage, and includes the experience as well as the perception of health care. Quality health services should be:
Safe—avoiding injuries to people for whom the care is intended;
Effective—providing evidence-based healthcare services to those who need them;
People-centred—providing care that responds to individual preferences, needs and values;
Timely—reducing waiting times and sometimes harmful delays.
Equitable—providing care that does not vary in quality on account of gender, ethnicity, geographic location, and socio-economic status.
Integrated—providing care that makes available the full range of health services throughout the life course
Efficient—maximizing the benefit of available resources and avoiding waste.[8]

Law for Universal Health Coverage (UHC)

For all aspects of health, there are binding rules that govern the rights and responsibilities of governments, health workers, companies, civil society and a country's population. Together these rules make up the legal framework, or legal architecture for health. They take many forms including: statutory laws, regulatory and administrative laws, contracts, case law, and customary laws. Who is involved in making these rules, and the form they take, differs from country to country.

Health laws are used to formalize commitment to goals, such as the goal of universal health coverage, creating a drive for action. To enable cooperation and achieve health goals, people use law to create different organizations (such as hospitals) and relationships (such as contracts for providing health services). In turn, organizations (whether health ministries, the private sector or civil society) have mandates, policies and strategies based on legal rules that guide their work.

There are also many rules that structure what health organizations and individuals should do, and what they may not do. This interaction between different health laws results in health system functions being carried out and health products and services being delivered.[9]

Right To Health: Indian Legislations

- Health being one of the most important fundamental right needs extra protection by specific legislations. Our Constitution also requires the State to ensure health and nutritional well-being of all people. Since independence the main emphasis has been the health care sector. This has been made possible by enacting various legislations.
- There are different legislations in India protect health as a human right of the citizens. The main source of law in our country is the Constitution, which itself provides for health care of the people. The Preamble to our Constitution, serves the following two purposes:
  - It indicates the source from which the Constitution derives its authority;
  - It also states the objects, which the Constitution seeks to establish and promote.[10]

Criminal Law and Health

The Indian Penal Code and the Code of Criminal Procedure by its various provisions protects the health of the people. The Indian Penal Code being a substantive law punishes various acts which influence the health of the people. The Code of Criminal Procedure also throws some light on the health aspect.[10]

- **Indian Penal Code, 1860:**
  - Indian Penal Code applies to any offence committed by any person anywhere in India and on any Indian registered ship or aircraft.
  - *Section 84* of the code exempts a man who is mentally unhealthy at the time of commission of crime.
  - *Section 88* of the Code exempts medical practitioners who while treating a patient cause death. It reads as "Nothing which is not intended to cause death, is an offence by reason of any harm which it may cause, or be intended by the doer to cause, to be known by the order to be likely to cause, to any person for whose benefit it is done in good faith, and who has given a consent, whether express or implied, to suffer that harm, or take the risk of that harm."
  - *Section 89* of the Code exempts a person who causes any harm when the act is done in good faith for the benefit of child less than 12 years of age, or of unsound mind, by or by consent of the guardian or other person having lawful charge of that person.
  - *Section 92* of the Code exempts a person from any harm caused to a person for the act done in good faith for benefit of a person without consent.
  - *Chapter XIV* of the Code specifically deals with offences affecting the public health, safety, convenience, decency and morals. Section 269 punishes any person who unlawfully or negligently does any act which is, and which he knows or has a reason to believe to be, likely imprisonment with or without fine.
  - **Consumer Law applicable to health services:**
    - The Consumer Protection Act, 1986: The Preamble of the Act states "an act to provide for better protection of interests of consumers and for that purpose to make provision for the establishment of consumer councils and other authorities for the settlement of consumers' disputes and matters connected therewith." Any patient who is provided with deficient medical services can take action before the District Forum.[10]
- **Environment and Health:**
  - Environment and health intricately linked. Environmental factors contribute significantly to health burden. In India, 60 per cent of malaria, almost all gastrointestinal and respiratory diseases, and significant proportion of organ specific, skin diseases, are caused because of poor environmental conditions. Environmental regulation is largely enacted and enforced with human well-being and public health as its focus.
  - Environmental laws were first enacted in the 1970s. For instance, when parliament enacted the Water Act of 1974, it adhered to the pattern of numerous other Indian statutes and created yet another agency-administered licensing system—this time to control effluent discharges into water. A breach of the act invited judge to imposed penalties.
  - The Environmental laws may be classified into three topics included Environment Protection Laws; Resource Management and Administration of Environment laws.[10]
- **Medical Laws:**
  - In the sphere of medicine and health, India has a plethora of regulations. The Poisons Act and the Dangerous Drugs Act, respectively, were passed in 1919 and 1930. The Opium Act was passed in 1878, and it was a long time ago.
  - *The 1940 Drugs and Cosmetics Act:* The Act regulates the importation, manufacturing, distribution, and sale of pharmaceuticals and cosmetics. The Act stipulates that The Drugs and Magic Remedies (Objectionable Advertisements) A person is prohibited from

participating in the publication of any advertisement relating to any medication under the Drugs and Magic Remedies Act 73.
- *The Narcotic Drugs and Psychotropic Substances Act of 1985* is a federal law that prohibits the use of narcotic drugs and psychotropic substances.
- *The Epidemic Diseases Act, 1897:* The Act was passed to provide for the better prevention of the spread of Dangerous Epidemic Diseases.
- *The Transplantation of Human Organs Act, 1994:* The Act aims to provide for the regulation of removal, storage and transplantation of human organs for therapeutic purposes and for the prevention of commercial dealings in human organs. The Act defines "therapeutic purpose" as a systematic treatment of any disease or the measures to improve health according to any particular method or modality; and "Transplantation" means the grafting of any human organ from any living person or deceased person to some other living person for therapeutic purposes.
- *Legislations for the conduct of Medical Profession*: Apart from these all legislations there are following legislations governing the conduct of medical profession:
  - Indian Medical Council Act, 1956
  - Indian Medicine Central Council Act, 1970
  - Indian Nursing Council Act, 1947
  - Dentist Act, 1948
  - The Pharmacy Act, 1948
  - The Homeopathy Central Council Act, 1973
- These all legislations broadly deal with the setting of Medical Councils at national and state levels and empower them with the powers, inter alia, to lay down minimum standards for medical education, enrolment of doctors and also regulate their profession by formulating the Code of Medical Ethics.[10]

❖ **Occupational Health Laws:**
  - Labour and Industrial Law legislations in India dates back to nearly 150 years. *Employees' State Insurance Act, 1948:* The Employees' State Insurance Act is a legislation which aims at bringing about social and economic justice to the poor labour class of the land. It aims at the labour welfare. The Employees' State Insurance Act, 1948, is designed to provide security to the industrial worker. The object of the Act is to introduce social insurance by providing certain benefits to employees in case of sickness, maternity, disablement or death due to employment injury.
  - *The Factories Act, 1948:* The Factories Act, 1948 is a social legislation which has been enacted for occupational safety, health and welfare of workers at work places and to provide congenial atmosphere, healthy and clean surroundings to the workers during the working hours and for the improvement of industrial efficiency.
  - *Maternity Benefit Act, 1961:* With the increase in the number of women employees there was a need of doing social justice to women workers employed in mines, factories and plantation. The Act was basically meant for maternity leave and benefits to women employees.
  - *The Mines Act, 1952:* This Act is aimed for the regulation of labour and safety in mines. It seeks to regulate the working conditions in mines by providing for measures required to be taken for the safety and security of workers employed therein and certain amenities for them. It prohibits employment of persons below eighteen years of age and employment of women below ground and above ground except between the hours of 6 am and 7 pm.

- *The Plantation Labour Act, 1951:* The object of the Act is to provide for the welfare of labour and to regulate the conditions of work in plantation. Plantation means any land which is used or intended to be used for growing tea, coffee, rubber and other plants and includes offices hospitals, dispensaries, schools and any other premises used for any purpose connected with such plantation.
- *Workmen's Compensation Act, 1923:* The Workmen's Compensation Act is one of the earliest measures taken up for the benefit of labourers and it is social insurance legislation.[10]

❖ **Women and Health Laws:**
- Women have always obtained an inferior status in our society. They are often ignored and are considered to be as child producing machines. The legislators have done a great task by enforcing laws protecting health of women.
- *Re-conception and Pre-Natal Diagnostic Techniques (Regulation and Prevention of misuse) Act, 1994:* The Act is aimed for the regulation of the use of prenatal diagnostic techniques for the purpose of detecting genetic or metabolic disorders or chromosomal abnormalities or certain congenital malformations or sex-linked disorders and the prevention of the misuse of such techniques for the purpose of prenatal sex determination leading to female foeticide.
- *The Medical Termination of Pregnancy Act, 1971:* By the passing of the Act of 1971 it has made abortions to be legal under certain circumstances. It is a health care measure which helps to reduce maternal morbidity and mortality resulting from illegal abortions. Permits Medical termination of pregnancy (MTP) only under certain conditions which are as follows:
  - MTP can be carried out in case of contraceptive failure, rape, threat to mother's life, and grave injury to her physical and mental health, risk of the child being born with congenital abnormalities.
  - MTP can only be conducted at approved hospitals i.e. Government hospitals and other hospitals and centers specifically approved by the authorities after ensuring availability of essential surgical facilities.
  - MTP can only be performed by doctors trained for the purpose and by postgraduates in Gynecology and Obstetrics.
  - Certification approval is needed by one doctor when pregnancy is below 12 weeks and by two doctors when it is between 12 to 20 weeks. Beyond 20 weeks, no termination is permissible.
  - Written approval of the lady or the guardian in case of a minor is to be obtained before carrying out the MTP.[10]

❖ **Children and Health:**
- *The Child Labour (Prohibition and Regulation) Act, 1986:* The Act was enacted to prohibit the employment of children in specific occupations and to control the working conditions of children in other occupations. An individual who has not reached the age of fourteen is considered a child under the Act. Employing someone under the age of 18 or breaking the Act's restrictions are both prohibited.
- *The Infant Milk Substitutes, Feeding Bottles, and Infant Foods (Regulation of Production, Supply, and Distribution) Act of 1992* regulates the production, supply, and distribution of infant milk substitutes, feeding bottles, and infant foods. Breastfeeding has been a part of our culture since the dawn of humanity. However, due to aggressive advertising of infant formulas and packaged cereal diets in modern times, our babies have been robbed of this God-given gift, resulting in increasing infant illness, malnutrition, and mortality.

The Indian government recognized this as a huge public health issue and created the aforementioned regulation to prevent such behaviours. With the passage of the Infantial Breast Milk Substitutes Act, India became one of the few Asian countries to fully apply the International Code of Marketing of Breast Milk Substitutes.[10]

- *The Juvenile Justice (Care and Protection) Act, 2000:* The purpose of the Act is to consolidate and amend the law relating to juveniles in conflict with the law and children in need of care and protection by providing proper care, protection, and treatment by catering to their developmental needs, and by adopting a child-friendly approach in adjudication and disposition of matters in the best interest of children and for their ultimate rehabilitation through various institutions established under the Act.[10]

❖ **Food Laws and Health Measures:** Food plays a very important role in protecting the health of a human being. The following legislations have been discussed relating health and food laws:
  - *The Food Safety and Standards Act, 2006:* The Act passed on 23rd August 2006 is aimed to consolidate the laws relating to food and to establish the Food Safety and Standards Authority of India for laying down science-based standards for articles of food and to regulate their manufacture, storage, distribution, sale and import, to ensure availability of safe and wholesome food for human consumption and for matters connected therewith and incidental.
  - *The Prevention of Food Adulteration Act, 1954:* The first step towards the menace of adulteration of food, drink and drug was taken under the Indian Penal Code, 1860. Section 272 to 276 included the provisions of offences relating to public health and safety.[10]

❖ **Disability and Law:** *The Mental Health Act of 1987* was enacted to protect people with mental illnesses. The public's perception of those suffering from mental illness has shifted dramatically, and it is now recognized that such sickness should not be stigmatized because it is curable, especially when detected early. As a result, mentally ill people should be treated like any other sick people, and their surroundings should be as normal as possible.[10]

❖ **The Persons with Disabilities (Equal Opportunities, Protection of Rights and Full Participation) Act, 1995 Revised in 2016:** The purpose of this Act is to assign responsibilities to the federal and state governments to provide services, create facilities, and provide support to people with disabilities to the extent that their resources allow, in order ensuring that they have equal opportunities to participate as productive and contributing citizens of this country to the full extent of their abilities.[10]

❖ **The National Trust (For Welfare of Persons with Autism, Cerebral Palsy, Mental Retardation and Multiple Disabilities) Act, 1999:**
  - The Trust's mission is to offer comprehensive care to people with mental retardation and cerebral palsy, as well as to manage the Trust's assets. The Trust also supports programmes that foster independence and address the issues of exceptional individuals who are not supported by their families. Grants, gifts, benefactions, requests, and transfers will be accepted by the Trust.
  - *India's Rehabilitation Council Act (RCI, 1992):* The Act was enacted to establish the Rehabilitation Council of India, which is responsible for regulating rehabilitation professional training and maintaining a central rehabilitation registry, among other things.[10]

❖ **The International Covenant on Civil and Political Rights (ICCPR), 1966** also sets certain human rights to health. "Every human being has an intrinsic right to life," says Article 6 of the Covenant. The right to life encompasses all that makes life worthwhile and meaningful, including health services supplied by the states parties. "No one should be subjected to torture or to cruel, brutal, or degrading treatment or punishment," reads Article 7. This Article focuses on the fact that no one should be exposed to medical or scientific research without his or her free permission.[10]

- **International Covenant on Economic, Social and Cultural Rights, 1966** lays down a number of human rights which directly protects the health of the people. The covenant under Article 7 lays recognizes the right of everyone to enjoy just and favourable conditions of work which ensure safe and healthy working conditions. It is vital because a standard of living includes health facilities availed by an individual. "The enjoyment of the maximum attainable degree of physical and mental health," according to the law.[10]
- **Convention on the Elimination of All Forms of Racial Discrimination 1965** under Article 5 ordains the "States Parties undertake to eliminate racial discrimination and to guarantee the right of everyone, without distinction as to race, color, or national or ethnic origin, to equality before the law, the right to public health, medical care, social security and social services".[10]
- **The Convention on the Rights of the Child, 1989** under Article 24 reads as "States Parties recognize the right of the child to the enjoyment of the highest attainable standard of health and to facilities for the treatment of illness and rehabilitation of health...."[10]
- **Convention against Torture and Other Cruel, Inhuman or Degrading Treatment or Punishment, 1987 (Torture Convention or CAT)** defines the term "torture" in order to preserve people's health. It specifies that the term 'torture' refers to any act of intentionally inflicting severe pain or suffering on a person, whether physical or mental, for the purpose of obtaining information or a confession from him or a third person, punishing him or a third person for an act he or a third person has committed or is suspected of having committed, intimidating or coercing him or a third person, or for any reason based on discrimination of any kind, when such pain or inflicted by or at the instigation of or with the consent or acquiescence of a public official or other person acting in an official capacity.[10]
- **The Convention for the Suppression of the Traffic in Persons and of the Exploitation of the Prostitution of Others** is also signed and ratified by a number of countries. The convention was entered in to force on 25th July 1951.[10]
- **The Standard Minimum Rules for the Treatment of Prisoners** which was adopted by the First United Nations Congress on the Prevention of Crime and the Treatment of Offenders, held at Geneva in 1955 lays down certain principles relating to the treatment of prisoners which directly affect the health of the prisoners.[10]
- **United Nations Rules for the Protection of Juveniles Deprived of their Liberty** was adopted by General Assembly resolution 45/113 of 14 December 1990. The rules define a juvenile as every person under the age of 18, the relevant rules for the protection of health are provide under the heads physical environment and accommodation, medical care and notification of illness, injury or death the guardian.[10]
- **Principles of Medical Ethics relevant to the Role of Health Personnel, particularly Physicians, in the Protection of Prisoners and Detainees against Torture and Other Cruel, Inhuman or Degrading Treatment or Punishment:** Principle 1 lays down that Health personnel, particularly physicians, charged with the medical care of prisoners and detainees have a duty to provide them with protection of their physical and mental health and treatment of disease of the same quality and standard as is afforded to those who are not imprisoned or detained.[10]
- **Declaration on the Rights of Mentally Retarded Persons** was proclaimed by General Assembly resolution 2856 (XXVI) of 20 December 1971: The Declaration on the Rights of

Mentally Retarded Persons calls for national and international action to ensure that it will be used as a common basis and frame of reference for the protection.[10]

- **Principles for the protection of persons with mental illness and the improvement of mental health care** was adopted by General Assembly resolution 46/119 of 17 December 1991: The principles have to be applied without discrimination of any kind. Certain rights have been laid down for persons with mental illness.[10]

- **Universal Declaration on the Eradication of Hunger and Malnutrition** was adopted on 16 November 1974 by the World Food Conference convened under General Assembly resolution 3180 (XXVIII) of 17 December 1973; and endorsed by General Assembly resolution 3348 (XXIX) of 17 December 1974. It was declare that the elimination of hunger and malnutrition is included as one of the objectives in the United Nations Declaration on Social Progress and Development, and the elimination of the causes that determine this situation are the common objectives of all nations.[10]

- **Declaration on the Rights of Disabled Persons** was proclaimed by General Assembly resolution 3447 (XXX) of 9 December 1975: The term "disabled person" is defined as any person unable to ensure by himself or herself, wholly or partly, the necessities of a normal individual and/or social life, as a result of deficiency, either congenital or not, in his or her physical or mental capabilities.[10]

- **Constitution of the World Health Organization:** In accordance with the United Nations Charter, the States Parties to this Constitution declare that the following principles are fundamental to the happiness, harmonious relations, and security of all people:
  - The enjoyment of the best attainable standard of health is one of every human being's fundamental rights, regardless of race, religion, and political belief, economic or social situation.
  - The health of all peoples is fundamental to the attainment of peace and security and is dependent upon the fullest cooperation of individuals and States.
  - The achievement of any State in the promotion and protection of health is of value to all.
  - Unequal development in different countries in the promotion of health and control of disease, especially communicable disease, is a common danger. Healthy development of the child is of basic importance; the ability to live harmoniously in a changing total environment is essential to such development. Governments have a responsibility for the health of their peoples, which can be fulfilled only by the provision of adequate health and social measures.[10]

- **Alma Ata Declaration:**
  - The World Health Organisation and United Nations Children Fund organised an International conference on "Health for All and Primary Health Care" at Alma Ata, Kazakhstan (CIS) from 6th to 12th September 1978.
  - It proclaimed the need for urgent action by all—the governments, health and development workers, and the world community to protect and promote the health of people of the world.
  - The conference reaffirmed that health, which is a state of complete physical, mental and social well-being and not merely the absence of disease or infirmity, is a fundamental human right. The attainment of the highest possible level of health is an important, worldwide, social goal, whose realisation requires the action of many other social and economic sectors in addition to the health sector.[10]

PRINCIPLES OF FITNESS TRAINING

Fitness

- Fitness is a general term which is used to describe the ability to perform physical work for prolonged period. Performing physical work generally requires musculoskeletal flexibility cardiorespiratory functioning, muscular strength and endurance.
- Optimum body composition is also to be considered when describing fitness. A key to become physically fit included that individuals must engage in some form of physical activity regularly which uses large muscle groups and also challenges the cardiorespiratory system.
- Activities that can be improve general fitness status included walking, running, swimming, cycling, stair climbing, cross-country skiing, and/or training with weights.
- Fitness levels can be described on a progression from poor to maximum which is based on amount of energy expenditure during the attempt of physical work. These ratings are often based on direct or indirect calculation of the body's maximum oxygen consumption (VO_2 max). Oxygen consumption can be affected by age, gender, heredity, inactivity, and disease.[11]

Strength

Muscle strength is a broad term that refers to the ability of tissue (contractile) to produce tension and a resultant force based on the demands placed on the muscle. It can be measured as cross-sectional area.[11]

Endurance

- Endurance refers to the ability of a person to perform low-intensity, repetitive, or sustained activities for a prolonged period of time. Cardiopulmonary endurance (total body endurance) utilizes the large muscles of the body and associated with repetitive and activities such as walking, cycling, swimming etc.
- To promote health it is important to implement contemporary approaches to wellness which usually focused on many aspects of life. For Examples, regular exercises to develop a fitness level that facilitates the involvement in recreational activities participation along with the balanced diet for optimal function.[12]

Components of Fitness

- **Aerobic fitness:** The word "aerobic" means "with oxygen." During aerobic or cardiorespiratory endurance exercises, the heart, lungs, and blood vessels works together to supply oxygen to muscles. Aerobic exercises included walking, jogging, running, cycling, swimming, dancing, hiking, and sports such as tennis and basketball.
- **Flexibility:** Flexibility refers to the full range of motion of a joints. It is very important to maintain flexibility to prevent Lack of flexibility which occurs due to disuse, injury or aging which ultimately affects the activities of daily living, can limit your ability to carry out daily activities. Lack of flexibility can be overcome by comprehensive stretching program.
- **Neuromotor exercise:** Neuromotor exercise training or functional fitness training, includes the activities that helps to improve balance, coordination, gait, agility, and proprioception (perception of physical location within space). The activities included combinations of neuromotor, resistance, and flexibility including yoga, tai ji (tai chi), exercises.[13]

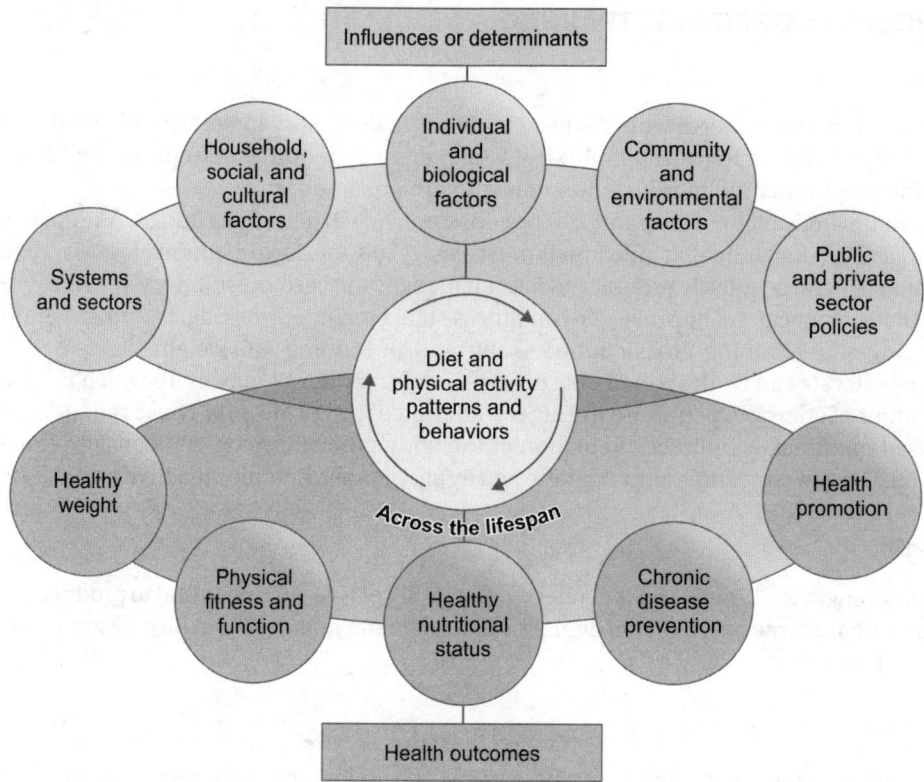

Figure16.1: Diet and physical activity, health promotion, and disease prevention across the lifespan.
(*Source:* US Department of Health and Human Services and US Department of Agriculture, 2015)

- **Body composition:** Body composition is defined the makeup of body. The body is made up of two tissues includes lean tissue (including muscle) and fatty tissue. Typically, body composition focuses on the relative amounts of fat compared to muscles. For example, measurement of overall body weight.
- **Diet and nutrition:** The word "diet" refers to what you eat, not a particular weight loss plan. A healthy eating pattern includes vegetables, fruits, grains (with at least half being whole grains), fat-free or low-fat dairy, and a variety of protein foods (e.g., seafood, lean meats and poultry, eggs, legumes, nuts, seeds, soy products) while limiting saturated and trans fats, added sugars, and sodium.
- **Sleep and stress management:** In addition to the mentioned areas of physical wellness, sleep and stress also influence the health and have the significant impact.

Influence of Sleep

Lack of adequate sleep adversely affects the relationships, productivity, and physical health. So sleep is very important for the improvement of many dimensions of wellness and quality of life as it provides the energy and alertness necessary to handle daily challenges. Adults typically need sleep between 7 and 8 hours per night.

Influence of Stress

- Most of the people suffered from acute and chronic stress from any source including, losing your car keys or handling a customer complaint at work etc. These stresses ultimately leads

to symptoms include irritability, anxiety, tension headache, muscular tensions, digestive system problems, and other physiological responses such as higher blood pressure, faster heart rate, sweating, and even shortness of breath or chest pain, feelings of being overloaded etc. The exercise role in stress reduction is not that much clear, but it has been observed that the active people handles and overcome the stress more effectively than sedentary people.
* Proper scheduling of activities to reduce the effect of stressful situations, avoid procrastination by completing activities before the deadline, relaxed deep breathing to counteract the fast and shallow breathing that is common experience during stress, limiting alcohol consumption and regular talk with family and friends regarding the stressful events will helps you "get it off your chest" and because you might receive helpful suggestions.

Exercise Prescription and Program[13]

Warm-up Period

* The purpose of the warm-up period is important to enhance the numerous adjustments that must take place before physical activity. The basic purpose of the warm-up to increase muscle and core temperature without causing fatigue or reducing energy stores, so should be gradual.
* A 5 to 10-minute period of total body movement exercises, such as calisthenics, and walking slowly, Gentle stretching etc. to be recommended specially in order to planning for flexibility and resistance training.[11,12]

Mode

* The prescribed exercise program should be focused on one or more modes, or types, including walking, jogging, running, hiking, cycling, rowing, and swimming.[11,12,13] Activities such as walking, jogging, running, cycling, swimming, rowing, aerobic dancing, box stepping, and hiking are good endurance activities.
* As far as the resistance training is concerned, the ACSM has included resistance training in its recommendations for a general health and fitness program. The maximum amount of weight one can lift successfully only one time is the 1-repetition maximum, or 1RM.
* Certain recreational activities are important to any comprehensive exercise program which includes hiking, tennis, handball, squash etc. to improve health and fitness by promoting enjoyment and relaxation.[13]
* **Exercise frequency:** The frequency of exercise participation is an important factor. Three to five days per week of exercise for the optimal gain is prescribed mostly. Initially the exercises should be limited to three or four days per week and increased up to five or more days per week only if the activity is enjoyed and as per the physical tolerance.[13]
* **Exercise duration:** As per the several studies the exercise periods varies from 5–10 min per day to 20–30 min per day (optimal amount: greatest return for time invested, and the specified time refers to the time during which one is at one's appropriate exercise intensity).[13]
* **Exercise intensity:** Exercise intensity is one of the most important factors. For most people, intensity should be at least 50% to 60% VO_2max. However, health benefits might also be occurred at intensities lower than those needed for aerobic conditioning in some people and can also occur at very high intensities.[13]
* **Rest periods:** The length of the rest period between sets and exercises is also important in order to avoid fatigue, energy recovery like in muscular strength, heavier weights and longer rest periods of 2 to 3 minutes are needed, whereas in order to achieve muscular endurance, lighter weights, higher repetitions, and shorter rest periods of 30 to 60 seconds are required.[12]

❖ **Cool-down:** The cool-down brings the body systems back to resting levels as it helps to transition the body from the higher demands of the conditioning phase to the lower levels of physiological demand seen at rest also helps to avoid sudden pooling of blood.[12] 5-10 minutes of calisthenics and static stretching exercises are appropriate.[11]

■ STRATEGIES OF HEALTH FITNESS FOR WOMEN AND GERIATRIC

Strategies of Health fitness for women:

- ❖ Recent researches have shown repeatedly that women have specific and distinct physiological processes that usually extend beyond the obvious considerations of anatomy and hormones, including differences in symptoms of heart attack and metabolism of medications. Although pregnancy is a time when there is of tremendous musculoskeletal, physiological, and emotional change.[11]
- ❖ Women's health and fitness are two important aspects of life for ladies everywhere. It should not be feasible to underestimate the benefits of eating right, exercising right and the peace and harmony it brings to your mind and body. It is very important to have nutritious food, hydrating yourself, getting enough sleep, and in general – taking care of yourself for a women to get in shape physically and mentally.[14]
  - **Keep calm and hydrate:** Staying hydrated leads to healthy physical and mental functioning. Drinking lots of water during the day is important to prevent dehydration and also to keep the women to keep fit from the inside out. Hydrating is also crucial to weight loss or maintenance because it will helps to reduce the feeling of hunger and eat less during meal times.
  - **Maintain a healthy weight:** Most of the women have a great concern about the weight gain and weight loss in order to healthy weight is important for overall well-being. Increase in weight significantly increases the risk of several chronic diseases and can affect the quality of your life. So, in order to achieve healthy weight women should have a good combination of healthy food, get enough sleep, and exercise regularly.
  - **Exercise:** There are various causes of heath in women including heart disease which can be under control with exercise. In order to keep the heart functioning properly it is recommended for women to exercise for 30 minutes per day. Aerobic exercises like walking, jogging, bicycling and dancing are good for women's health.
  - **Nutrition:**
    - ◆ As women are mostly concern about their families and putting family's needs first and also too busy to adhere to a set diet leads to negligence of own dietary needs. It is must to eat as close to a natural food diet as possible include fresh vegetables, fruits, whole grains, meat, fish, poultry, low-fat dairy products, and lots of **nuts**.
    - ◆ Also with the increasing age, women need lots of calcium to build healthy bones and teeth to keep them strong, good sources of calcium include dairy products, grains, leafy green vegetables, tofu, and cabbage are highly recommended.
    - ◆ Apart from calcium, Zinc and Magnesium are two other minerals that are most needed by women's bodies. Consume Zinc, to boost up immune system which prevents the thinning of hair and acne. Magnesium helps in sleep, bone health, and may also help in relieving premenstrual symptoms, anxiety, and migraines.
  - **Strengthening of support circle:** Several research studies show that in order to surviving health problems, increasing level of happiness and to live longer, it is important for women to have social circles of friends and family. The best way to build a support circle is to be a part of someone else's support circle.

- **Getting relaxed from stress:** It has been known that due to some responsibilities during the every phase of life, women have lots of stress and it is very difficult for them to cope up with. It is important to get relaxed from the stress and it can possible by engaging in an hour-long yoga session or even unwind by reading favorite magazine.
- **Regular check-ups:** Health screenings are an important way to help recognize problems in the body. So it is highly recommended for women to have a yearly check-up with a primary care doctor to stay on the safer side of things.
- **Sleep solves everything:** Sleep is one of the best things women can get with all the busy schedules, cooking, and running around they do. Sufficient **sleep** increases the productivity, improves the mental and physical state of body and overall wellbeing. It has been recommended to have a minimum of 6-7 hours which is vital.
- **Giving time to yourself:** One of the best health and fitness tips for women is to make time for "just you". A daily dose of just 10 minutes for yourself is every day that will keep you feeling you are very best which helps women to get stressed-out.

Recommendations for Fitness Exercise for Pregnant and Postnatal Women[11]

NOTE: These recommendations are for pregnant women with no maternal or fetal risk factors.

- 15 to 30 minutes/session, daily for a week is strongly recommended for all women with mild to moderate exercise, for both strength and cardiopulmonary benefits
- Because of decreased oxygen supply, pregnant women should modify exercise intensity according to their tolerance. Use of the Borg scale of perceived exertion is more appropriate in this population, with exertion between 12 and 14 suggested during pregnancy. It has been advisable to stop exercising once get fatigue.
- Contact sports, anything with a high-risk of abdominal trauma or falling, high-altitude activities (greater than 6000 ft), and scuba diving activities should be avoided as the fetus is at increased risk of decompression sickness during scuba diving.
- Non-weight-bearing aerobic exercises such as stationary cycling, swimming, or water aerobics are recommended as these activities minimizes the risk of injury throughout pregnancy and the postpartum period.
- Look for the risk of falling for the woman if she safely unable to maintain balance because of the shifting and increasing weight, that could result in falling and injury to herself or the fetus. So, she has been given modified exercises.
- Adequate caloric intake for nutrition, adequate fluid intake, and appropriate clothing for heat dissipation has to be implemented.
- There should be gradual resumption of pre-pregnancy exercise routines during the postpartum period. In order to reduce symptoms and duration of incontinence, initiation of pelvic floor exercises immediately postpartum is highly recommended.
- Breastfeeding women can be reassured that moderate exercise does not impair quantity of breast milk or infant growth. There may be a short-term increase in lactic acid secreted in breast milk after exercise; if the baby appears to eat less after an exercise session, this can easily be remedied by nursing before exercise.[11]
- Safe activities during pregnancy included Walking, Jogging, Cycling, Stairmaster, Swimming, Aqua-fitness, Rowing, Yoga, Pilates, Spinning, Muscular/strength training, Elliptical/cross trainer machine, Boxing conditioning training—non-contact.[15]
- **Activities to avoid:** Rollerblading, Cross-country skiing, Water skiing, Scuba diving, Skating, Soccer, Basketball, Obstacle courses, Contact activities such as hockey, football, rugby

or broomball, Parachuting, repelling or rock climbing, Rucksack marches and casualty evacuation.[11]
- **Recommended postnatal exercises:** Walking, Swimming (once bleeding stopped), Gym programs—maintain posture, light weights, no breath holding, postnatal abdominal and pelvic floor exercises, low impact aerobics or a postnatal class and low intensity water aerobics classes (once bleeding stopped).[16]

Strategies of Health Fitness for Geriatric

- It is important to prescribe exercises to older adults as it has a simultaneously impact and mediate chronic disease, many impairments, functional deficits, quality of life, and cognition and prevent the negative sequelae associated with sedentary lifestyles.[13]
- **CDC Physical Activity Guidelines for older adults:** To achieve the recommended amount of physical activity all geriatrics should engage in at least one of the following options on a regular basis:

Option 1
- 2 hours 30 minutes (150 minutes) of moderate-intensity aerobic activity (i.e., brisk walking) every week.
- Muscle strengthening exercises (moderate) which involves all major muscle groups (legs, hips, back, abdomen, chest, shoulders, and arms) for 2 or more days a week.

Option 2
- Vigorous-intensity aerobic activity (i.e., jogging or running) for 1 hour 15 minutes (75 minutes) of every week.
- Muscle strengthening exercises which involves all major muscle groups (legs, hips, back, abdomen, chest, shoulders, and arms) for 2 or more days a week that works.

Option 3
- It involves an equivalent mix of moderate- and vigorous-intensity aerobic activity.
- Muscle strengthening exercises which involves all major muscle groups (legs, hips, back, abdomen, chest, shoulders, and arms) for 2 or more days a week that works. (http://www.cdc.gov/physicalactivity/everyone/guidelines/olderadults.html)

Types of Fitness Exercises for Geriatrics[13,17]

Aerobic Exercise
- Aerobic exercise is indicated for those patients having lack the ability to sustain activity for a desired period of time due to decreased cardiovascular efficiency. The body's capacity to absorb, deliver, and utilize oxygen can be increased by aerobic exercises.
- **Contraindications and safety:** Resting heart rate greater than 100 bpm, systolic blood pressure higher than 200 mmHg, and/or diastolic blood pressure higher than 120 mmHg are absolute contraindications for aerobic exercise. Patients need to be reported as they have light headedness, dizziness, profuse sweating, or nausea before, in between and after exercise.

Aquatic Exercise
- The older adults those cannot tolerate the stresses of land-based exercises recommended for Aquatic exercise which allows the application of the physical stress theory. The buoyancy of

the water allows the exercise for older adults having a deconditioning or with significant joint pathology by decreasing the forces needed to move and decreasing the compressive forces within the joint while offering hydrostatic support to the upright position.
- **Contraindications and safety:** It should be carefully monitored the patient walking over wet slippery surfaces, going up and down ladders or steps when entering or leaving the pool and while in the water. Occasionally, the older adults may develop an allergic skin reaction to the chemicals in the water that should be carefully looked for. Resting heart rate greater than 100 bpm, systolic blood pressure higher than 200 mmHg, and/or diastolic blood pressure higher than 120 mmHg are absolute contraindications for aquatic exercise.

Strengthening Exercise

- It is a normal physiological process in geriatrics to deteriorate strength. Loss of strength can be associated with loss of function. The minimum training stimulus for strengthening exercise is 60% of a 1 RM. Slowness of movement, a hallmark of frailty, should be addressed with a combination of strength and power training.
- **Contraindications/Safety:** It is important for older adult not to hold his or her breath during exercise.

Stretching Exercises

- In order to promote adaptation of to a more lengthening of the shortened muscles which need to achieve better posture and movement patterns, stretching is recommended. Stretching intervention is strongly indicated in limitation of joint range of motion which can be lead to pain syndromes, painful postures, abnormal movement patterns, and loss of function.
- Even stretching indicated when losses of motion have not yet led to pain or disability like the pectoralis minor muscle, a muscle that commonly shortens because of typical, sedentary posture, has the potential to lead to shoulder impingement and pain by decreasing the subacromial space which needs to be lengthen.
- **Contraindications:** The stretching is absolutely contraindicated in the presence of joint instability in order to avoid further progression of instability.

Plyometrics

- Plyometric exercise uses the stretch reflex of the muscle spindle and the elastic energy that is stored in a stretched muscle to enhance an immediate reciprocal contraction in that muscle.
- It involves eccentric (lengthening) contraction followed by a concentric (shortening) contraction of the same muscles. For example, rapid squatting followed by a ballistic contraction to achieve a jumping motion. In this, energy is stored in the gastrocnemius as the ankle dorsiflexes and in the quadriceps as the knee flexes.
- Plyometrics may also help in bone formation, according to Wolff's law, by increasing the compressive forces that the bone is required to absorb. It has been shown that, jumping reduces fall risk in long-term-care residents when combined with strengthening, stretching, and aerobic conditioning.
- **Tai Chi:** Tai Chi is a form of marshal arts having multiple forms and styles (ranges from the classic 109 postures to as few as 42). Tai Chi focuses on the complete movements and the sequence of postures credited with both the mental calm and the cognitive benefits. Tai Chi useful in the chronic conditions such as arthritis, cancer, cardiovascular disease, and diabetes and decreases stress, lessens depression, improves mental health and cognitive function by improving balance and fitness, thus decreasing falls and lessening fall risks.

SUMMARY

Health is the general condition of person in all aspects. It is also a level of functional and metabolic efficiency of an organism, often implicitly *human*. Health has been declared a fundamental human right. This implies that the state has responsibility for health of its people. National governments all over the world are striving to expand and improve the health care services. Health care is the treatment and management of illness and preservation of health through services offered by the medical, dental, complementary and alternative medicine, pharmaceutical, clinical sciences, nursing and allied health professions.

Health care is defined as a, "multitude of services rendered to individuals, families or communities by the agents of the health services or professions, for the purpose of promoting, maintaining, monitoring or restoring health".[1] It is important to provide such services by the health professionals who help to diagnosed, cure the diseases along with educate the patient and also rehabilitate them. There are three levels of health care included Primary, secondary and tertiary health care. Primary Health Centres—Auxiliary Nurse Midwife (ANM), Accredited Social Health Activist (ASHA), Anganwadi Worker (AWW), *Village Health Guide (*VHG), Traditional birth attendants (TBA), Local Dais. Community health centres and sub-centres also plays an important role in health system. It is also important to provide legal rights and health benefits to people related to health. There are certain laws like medical laws, women and child health law, laws for labourer, occupational health law, persons with disability law etc. implemented by the government which provide human right to health.

Fitness is one of the major components in order to keep the healthy life. There are certain principles of which facilitates the fitness to community people. As the women and geriatrics are important and concerned part of the community, it is important to give special emphasis to this group. Women's health and fitness are two important aspects of life for ladies everywhere. It should not be feasible to underestimate the benefits of eating right, exercising right and the peace and harmony it brings to your mind and body. It is very important to have nutritious food, hydrating yourself, getting enough sleep, and in general—taking care of yourself for a women to get in shape physically and mentally. Fall prevention and intervention is the main part of rehabilitation, so there are numerous strategies that provides fitness health. It is important to prescribe exercises to older adults as it has a simultaneously impact and mediate chronic disease, many impairments, functional deficits, quality of life, and cognition and prevent the negative sequelae associated with sedentary lifestyles.

REFERENCES

1. Park K. Park's Textbook of Preventive and Social Medicine, 23rd edition; 2015.
2. Chaturvedi S. A document on "Healthcare Delivery System In India". Available on: https://ucms.ac.in/Lectures-C 2020/Health%20care%20delivery%20sysytem%20in%20india-2020.pdf.
3. Chokshi M, Patil B, Khanna R, Neogi SB, Sharma J, Paul VK, et al. Health systems in India. Journal of Perinatology. 2016;36:S9-S12; doi:10.1038/jp.2016.184.
4. Kumar P. Role of physiotherapy in primary health care: Opportunities and challenge. Conference Paper at 2nd International Conference and workshop on Physical Therapy AIIMS 2013. Available on: https://www.researchgate.net/publication/262179007_Role_of_Physiotherapy_in_Primary_Health_Care_Opportunities_and_Challenge.
5. Ontario Physiotherapy Association. Physiotherapists in primary health care. Available on: https://opa.on.ca/wp-content/uploads/Physiotherapists-Primary-Health-Care.pdf.
6. PEO Evaluation Studies. Functioning of Community Health Centres (CHCs). Available on: https://niti.gov.in/planningcommission.gov.in/docs/reports/peoreport/peo/peo_chc.pdf

7. Office of the United Nations. High Commissioner for Human Rights. The *Right to Health*. Fact Sheet No. 31. World Health Organization. Available on: https://www.ohchr.org/documents/publications/factsheet31.pdf.
8. Human rights and health. World Health Organization. 29 December 2017. Available on: https://www.who.int/news-room/fact-sheets/detail/human-rights-and-health.
9. Health Law. World Health Organization. Available on: https://www.who.int/health-topics/health-laws-and-universal-health-coverage#tab=tab_1.
10. Chapter V Right to Health: Indian legislations and International documents. Available on: http://qi.nhsrcindia.org/sites/default/files/Chapter%205-Right%20to%20Health%20Indian%20Legislations%20%26%20International%20Documents.pdf/
11. Kisner C. Therapeutic Exercise Foundations and Techniques. Fifth Edition. ISBN-13: 978-0-8036-1584-7 ISBN-10: 0-8036-1584-1.
12. Bushman B. ACSM's Complete Guide to Fitness and Health, 2nd edition; 2017. Available at: https://www.pdfdrive.com/acsms-complete-guide-to-fitness-health-2nd-edition-e191748236.html.
13. Larry Kenney W, Wilmore J, Costill D. Physiology of Sport and Exercise. Fifth Edition. ISBN-10: 0-7360-9409-1 (print) ISBN-13: 978-0-7360-9409-2 (print)
14. Navya. 12 Health and Fitness Tips Every Woman Should Follow. Healthifyme. March 7, 2020. Available on: https://www.healthifyme.com/blog/12-health-and-fitness-tips-every-woman-should-follow/
15. Guide to Fitness during and after pregnancy in the CF. Canadian Forces Personnel Support Agency.
16. Pre-and-Post-Natal-Exercise-Guidelines. Fitness Australia. Available on: https://bp-fitnessaustralia-production.s3.amazonaws.com/uploads/uploaded_file/file/219/Pre-and-Post-Natal-Exercise-Guidelines.pdf.
17. Guccione AA. Geriatric Physical Therapy, 3rd edition. Mosby, Inc., an affiliate of Elsevier Inc. Publication. ISBN: 978-0-323-02948-3.

CHAPTER 17

Geriatric Rehabilitation

Shyam D Ganvir, Pratima Sarwadikar

LEARNING OBJECTIVES

Through this chapter, the reader will be able to:
- Understand the concepts of elderly
- Understand the concepts of geriatrics
- Gain an introduction to geriatric rehabilitation
- Discuss the examination and how to measure the functional impairment in elders
- Various screening methods used in geriatric assessment
- Ask about the presence or absence of falls
- Screen patients for gait impairment and
- Screen patients for cognitive impairment
- Screen patients for major depressive illness

■ INTRODUCTION

Geriatric rehabilitation aims to improve or restore the motor function, sensorial and cognitive status of elderly having a loss or disability due to a disease, which may be an acute or chronic condition. However, elderly people living independently in the community or in the institutions may gain the benefits of geriatric rehabilitation in the concept of preventive measures and social rehabilitation. Thus, we may briefly define the geriatric rehabilitation as an approach of multidisciplinary interventions to upgrade the functional level and the overall quality of life as well as the life satisfaction of elderly.[1]

The geriatric assessment is a multidimensional, multidisciplinary assessment designed to evaluate an older person's functional ability, physical health, cognition and mental health, and socioenvironmental circumstances.[1]

It is usually initiated when the physician identifies a potential problem. Specific elements of physical health that are evaluated include nutrition, vision, hearing, fecal and urinary continence, and balance. The geriatric assessment aids in the diagnosis of medical conditions; development of treatment and follow-up plans; coordination of management of care; and evaluation of long-term care needs and optimal placement. The geriatric assessment differs from a standard medical evaluation by including nonmedical domains; by emphasizing functional capacity and quality of life; and, often, by incorporating a multidisciplinary team. It usually yields a more complete and relevant list of medical problems, functional problems, and psychosocial issues.[1]

The Comprehensive Geriatric Assessment

As the elderly patient has multiple health problems that may exist together, it is necessary to thoroughly evaluate these problems that would have a bearing on comprehensive management. Accordingly, in addition to the psychiatric evaluation, many geriatricians recommend a Comprehensive Geriatric Evaluation. This is a process of multidisciplinary evaluation in which the multiple problems of older persons are evaluated, and the resources and strengths of the person are catalogued, the need for services assessed, and a coordinated care plan is developed to focus interventions on the person's problems.[5]

The **goals** of comprehensive geropsychiatric assessment are:
- To improve diagnostic accuracy
- To guide the selection of interventions to restore or preserve health
- To recommend an optimal environment for care
- To predict outcomes
- To monitor clinical change over time.

The setting: Structured comprehensive geriatric assessment may be done in many institutional settings, including acute care, psychiatric, or rehabilitation hospitals and nursing homes, and in ambulatory settings, including outpatient or freestanding clinics, the offices of psychiatrists and primary care physicians, or in the patient's home. It has often been applied to elderly persons at critical transition points in their lives, including actual or threatened decline in health and functional status, impending change in living environment, bereavement, or other unusual stress.[5]

Process: Comprehensive geropsychiatric assessment is initiated by a referral from one of many sources. In addition to the patient the process often includes family members and other important persons in the individual's environment. It is conducted by a core team that consists at a minimum, of a psychiatrist, nurse, and social worker, each with special expertise in caring for older people. The specific activities and contributions of each team member may vary considerably, and flexibility in roles may facilitate the assessment process.[5]

The assessment begins with a case-finding approach that utilizes screening instruments and techniques. Based on these initial findings, a more detailed assessment is frequently undertaken. This in-depth assessment often requires the participation of many other professions. These may include audiology, clinical psychology, dentistry, nutrition, occupational therapy, optometry, pharmacy, physical therapy, speech pathology, and the clergy. Support from other medical disciplines, such as neurology, ophthalmology, orthopaedics, physiotherapy, surgery, and urology, is commonly needed. Self-rating scales completed by the patient or caregivers may provide some aspects of geropsychiatric assessment. Such information may lead to different insights than those obtained through external assessment performed by one member of the health care team.[5]

Comprehensive Geriatric Assessment [Reuben, 2003] comprises of the following components:
- Physical health
- Mental health
- Functional status
- Social and economic status
- Environmental characteristics

1. **Physical health**: A careful **history** is obtained from the patient and others with significant knowledge of the patient. Special attention is directed to the use of prescription and non-prescription medications and clues to the presence of malnutrition, falling, incontinence, and immobility. Data is gathered on smoking, exercise, alcohol use, immunization status and sexual function. Also important is information regarding the patient's personal strengths, values, perceived quality of life, acceptability of interventions, and expected outcomes from his or her health care.

   The **geriatric physical examination** is performed with emphasis on identification of specific diseases or conditions for which curative, restorative, palliative, or preventive treatment may be available. Special attention is directed toward visual or hearing impairment, nutritional status, and conditions that may contribute to falling or difficulty in ambulation. Laboratory tests and other diagnostic studies are obtained as indicated.

   The geriatric exam starts as soon as the patient is first seen (observations are made about the patient's appearance, speech, ability to move around, etc.) and continues after the formal exam is completed, (i.e., does the patient have problems with dressing himself/herself, finding the way back to the car). Elderly patients may require additional time to undress and transfer to the examining table for the physical examination; they should not be rushed. The examining table is adjusted to a height that the patient can easily access; a footstool facilitates mounting. The patient must not be left alone on the table. Portions of the examination may be more comfortable if the patient sits in a chair. The patient may want a relative or aide in the room during the examination. Preliminary assessment of the patient's functioning can be made by observing personal hygiene. The patient's general appearance is described, (e.g., comfortable, restless, malnourished, inattentive, pale, dyspnoeic, cyanotic). If the patient is examined at bedside, use of a water mattress, a sheepskin, bedside rails (partial or full), restraints, a urinary catheter, or an adult diaper is noted. During measurement of height and weight, patients with balance problems may need to grasp grab bars placed near or on the scale. When the temperature is recorded, hypothermia can be missed if the thermometer does not measure low temperatures. The absence of fever does not exclude infection. The pulse and blood pressure (BP) are checked in both arms. The pulse is taken for 60 seconds and any irregularity noted. Because many factors can alter BP, several measurements are taken under resting conditions. As per the complaints of the patient examinations of other systems like respiratory, GIT, Skin, Eyes, Ears, Nose, Oropharyngeal, Neck/Thyroid, Lymphatic, Breasts, Heart, Peripheral Vascular, Abdomen, Musculoskeletal and Pelvic/Rectal may be carried out.

   The **neurological examination** for an elderly patient, similar to that for any adult, assesses cranial nerves, motor function and sensory function. However, non-neurological disorders that are common among the elderly may complicate the neurological examination. For example, diminished sight and hearing may impede the assessment of cranial nerves, and peri-arthritis of the shoulder due to hemiplegia may interfere with the assessment of motor function.

   Signs detected during the examination must be considered in light of the patient's age, history, and other findings. Symmetric findings unaccompanied by functional loss, other neurological signs, and complaints may be a result of aging. The physician must decide whether these findings justify a detailed evaluation for a neurological lesion. Patients should be re-evaluated periodically for functional changes, asymmetry, or new complaints. Normal age-related changes seen on neuro exam are decreased lower extremity vibratory sensation, diminished knee jerk, diminished or absent ankle jerk.

Look for cortical release signs such as grasp, palmomental, glabellar, and snout reflexes. Focused on looking for neurological deficits that may be a sign of neurological disease (CVA, Parkinson's, etc.). Difficulty may be encountered in sensory exam if patient has altered mental status or aphasia.

2. **Mental health**: Cognitive, behavioural, and emotional status is evaluated. Detection of dementia, delirium, and depression is particularly important. A range of assessment instruments is available for this purpose. For some patients a detailed psychiatric interview, a neurobehavioral consultation or comprehensive neuropsychological testing is indicated.
3. **Social and economic status**: Evaluating the social support network includes identifying present and potential caregivers and assessing their competence, willingness to provide care and acceptability to the older person. This information may be obtained by questionnaires, structured interviews, or other methods. The degree of caregiver stress and the caregiver's support network also are considered. Areas of special importance to the individual, such as cultural, ethnic, and spiritual values, are noted. The individual's own assessment of the quality of life is recorded. The clinician evaluates the economic resources of the elderly person, which often determine access to medical and personal care and influence options for living arrangements.
4. **Functional status**: There are several components to a comprehensive assessment of an older person's ability to function. Physical functioning is usually measured by the ability to accomplish basic activities of daily living (ADL) including eating, bathing, toileting and dressing. Other components of functional well-being are behavioural and social activities that require a higher level of cognition and judgment than physical activities. These instrumental activities of daily living (IADL) include preparation of meals, shopping, light housework, financial management, medication management, use of transportation and use of the telephone. Functional status (ADL and IADL) is probably most accurately evaluated by direct observation of the patient by family or health professionals in the home or a simulated homelike environment. However, surprisingly accurate information is also obtained by standardized questionnaire or self-report.
5. **Environmental characteristics**: Evaluating the patient's physical environment is essential. Home visits and questionnaires are used to determine the safety, physical barriers, and layout of the home as well as access to services, such as shopping, pharmacy, transportation, and recreation facilities.[5]

Physical Health

The geriatric assessment incorporates all facets of a conventional medical history, including main problem, current illness, past and current medical problems, family and social history, demographic data, and a review of systems. The approach to the history and physical examination, however, should be specific to older persons. In particular, topics such as nutrition, vision, hearing, fecal and urinary continence, balance and fall prevention, osteoporosis, and polypharmacy should be included in the evaluation. **Table 17.1** is an example of a focused geriatric physical examination.

Table 17.1: Components of geriatric physical examination.

Signs	Physical sign or symptom	Differential diagnoses
Vital signs		
Blood pressure	Hypertension	Adverse effects from medication, autonomic dysfunction
	Orthostatic hypotension	Adverse effects from medication, atherosclerosis, coronary artery disease
Respiratory rate	Increased respiratory rate greater than 24 breaths per minute	Chronic obstructive pulmonary disease, congestive heart failure, pneumonia
Temperature	Hyperthermia, hypothermia	Hyper- and hypothyroidism, infection
Heart rate	Bradycardia	Adverse effects from medication, heart block
	Irregularly irregular heart rate	Atrial fibrillation
General	Unintentional weight loss	Cancer, depression
	Weight gain	Adverse effects from congestive heart failure medication
Head	Asymmetric facial or extraocular muscle weakness or paralysis	Bell palsy, stroke, transient ischemic attack
	Frontal bossing	Paget disease
	Temporal artery tenderness	Temporal arteritis
Eyes	Hearing loss	Acoustic neuroma, adverse effects from medication, cerumen impaction, faulty or ill-fitting hearing aids, Paget disease
Mouth, throat	Gum or mouth sores	Dental or periodontal disease, ill-fitting dentures
	Leukoplakia	Cancerous and precancerous lesions
Neck	Carotid bruits	Aortic stenosis, cerebrovascular disease
	Thyroid enlargement and nodularity	Hyper- and hypothyroidism
Cardiac	Fourth heart sound (S4)	Left ventricular thickening
	Systolic ejection, regurgitant murmurs	Valvular arteriosclerosis
Pulmonary	Barrel chest	Emphysema
	Shortness of breath	Asthma, cardiomyopathy, chronic obstructive pulmonary disease, congestive heart failure
Breasts	Masses	Cancer, fibroadenoma
Abdomen	Pulsatile mass	Aortic aneurysm
Gastrointestinal, genital/rectal	Atrophy of the vaginal mucosa	Estrogen deficiency
	Constipation	Adverse effects from medication, colorectal cancer, dehydration, hypothyroidism, inactivity, inadequate fiber intake
	Fecal incontinence	Fecal impaction, rectal cancer, rectal prolapse
	Prostate enlargement	Benign prostatic hypertrophy
	Prostate nodules	Prostate cancer
	Rectal mass, occult blood	Colorectal cancer
	Urinary incontinence	Bladder or uterine prolapse, detrusor instability, estrogen deficiency

Contd...

Contd...

Signs	Physical sign or symptom	Differential diagnoses
Extremities	Abnormalities of the feet	Bunions, onychomycosis
	Diminished or absent lower extremity pulses	Peripheral vascular disease, venous insufficiency
	Heberden nodes	Osteoarthritis
	Pedal edema	Adverse effects from medication, congestive heart failure
Musculoskeletal	Diminished range of motion, pain	Arthritis, fracture
	Dorsal kyphosis, vertebral tenderness, back pain	Cancer, compression fracture, osteoporosis
	Gait disturbances	Adverse effects from medication, arthritis, deconditioning, foot abnormalities, Parkinson disease, stroke
	Leg pain	Intermittent claudication, neuropathy, osteoarthritis, radiculopathy, venous insufficiency
	Muscle wasting	Atrophy, malnutrition
	Proximal muscle pain and weakness	Polymyalgia rheumatica
Skin	Erythema, ulceration over pressure points, unexplained bruises	Anticoagulant use, elder abuse, idiopathic thrombocytopenic purpura
	Premalignant or malignant lesions	Actinic keratoses, basal cell carcinoma, malignant melanoma, pressure ulcer, squamous cell carcinoma
Neurologic	Tremor with rigidity	

Geriatric Rehabilitation for Specific Conditions

Geriatric rehabilitation covers the complex approaches of the congenital or acquired diseases or impairments of the elderly. These may be a postoperative physical therapy and rehabilitation intervention after a femoral neck fracture, cerebrovascular attack or a vascular problem; or may be an approach such as to relieve the pain, to improve the strength of the elderly who have chronic musculoskeletal or neurologic problems. Rehabilitation is an essential component of geriatric care and therapy and it can make a critical difference in the life quality of elderly people. The goal of rehabilitation in older people is the development of physical independence and the ability to do as many as possible daily living activities.

The general indications of geriatric rehabilitation are:
* Acute reversible or partially reversible insults e.g., amputation
* Chronic progressive disabling diseases e.g., ostheoarthritis, Parkinson disease
* Acute disabling event due to a chronic disease e.g., stroke due to cerebrovascular disease or hip fracture due to osteoporosis.

Patients unlikely to benefit from rehabilitation are:
* The terminal care patients
* Medically unstable patients, requiring frequent medical review, investigations or changing treatments
* Irrecoverable mental changes, rehabilitation being a cooperation and learning process
* Acute febrile illnesses or exacerbation of chronic diseases
* Neoplasias

- ❖ Cachectic states,
- ❖ Pacemaker wearers
- ❖ Hemorrhagic states
- ❖ Chronic diseases at the limit of organ failure.

Principles of Geriatric Rehabilitation

- ❖ The first principle of geriatric recovery is of the elderly patients have to be known for a better implementation of the recovery therapy, the most important being:
    - Progressively diminishing of the capacity to adapt due to the physiological involution that characterizes senescence: Physiological aging is a degenerative progressive process with functional decline of all systems that must be taken into account when a recovery program is established for a condition that left infirmity, physical, mental or intellectual sequelae. For example, Lung deficiency with decreased pulmonary, Cardiac deficiency decreasing the capacity of adaptation to effort, Nervous deficiency with decreased nerve conduction, prolonged reaction time and, consequently, significantly reduced speed of movements, Muscular hypertonia and loss of muscle strength, Osteoporosis with an increased risk of fractures and trophic damage of periarticular structures and with an increased risk of stretching, rupture, and limited mobility, Sensory deficit etc.
    - *Increasing individual variations:* There are important differences between elderly individuals, so age is a relative criterion. Biological age should be taken into account more than the chronological age. Also there are differences at the same person between the rate of aging of various organs and systems.
    - *Presence of the comorbidities:* Comorbidities (arthritis, diabetes, hypertension, congestive heart failure) can interfere with the rehabilitation process by delaying or interrupting services and therefore require a systematic approach to screening, prevention and management of those conditions. The presence of a disabling condition in the context of physiological decline and comorbidities can make elderly patients to become incapable of even basic autonomy (such as washing, performing daily activities, getting dressed, eating, going to the toilet).
- ❖ The many dimensions of geriatric rehabilitation require a multidisciplinary care team formed by physician, physiotherapist, psychologist, rehabilitation nurse, social worker, nutritionist, optometrist, and, if necessary, orthotist or prosthetist. The health professionals who work with geriatric patients should have a basic geriatric training, knowledge of clinical and geriatric psychology and appropriate bioethics and special human qualities: tact, patience, calm and understanding.
- ❖ Efficient communication between the care team and the patient and also between the team members is an important principle of geriatric rehabilitation. The practitioner must ensure that the patient understands how physical therapy can help the prognosis of his disabling condition, how to perform each exercise and he must motivate the elderly to continue the exercises for the long-term.
- ❖ Another principle is the conscious and active participation of the patient in the recovery process. The patient and his family are in the centre of the rehabilitation team. Because of the chronic nature of many disabilities in elderly (arthritis, diabetes, hypertension, congestive heart failure), at some point, the patients and their families will have to take over their own rehabilitation program including self-monitoring and personal control over prevention and management practices.

- ❖ A basic principle of geriatric rehabilitation is the individualization of the treatment with adaptation of the physiotherapy programs for each patient regarding the following aspects:
  - Age-related functional deficiencies
  - Coexisting diseases and the associated treatment
  - Remaining capacity, reserves and ability to adapt to exercise
  - Previous physical training.
- ❖ Periodic team meetings in order to review the progress of the patient, to adjust the goals or to establish new goals are an important rule of rehabilitation in elderly patients.
- ❖ Geriatric rehabilitation should be started as soon as possible starting with postural education and early mobilization in order to prevent the immobilization syndrome with stiffness, contractures, ankyloses, deformations, osteoporosis, muscle atrophy.
- ❖ Grading effort is another principle of rehabilitation. If the patient was immobilized in bed, the recovery begins with postural education and respiratory gymnastics and afterwards, exercises with the unaffected extremity are performed. As the patient improves the sitting balance, he will get out of bed and transfer to an armchair, and as he improves general strength, coordination and balance, he will regain the standing position.
  Increased stability will allow walking recovery, initially with the aid of walking support (bars, crutches, frames). Simultaneously, autonomy in daily living activities will be initiated (eating without help, getting dressed, going to the toilet).
- ❖ Therapeutic exercises, broadly conceived, are designed to improve physical functioning of the geriatric patients and to optimize strength, balance and endurance.
  The exercise program respects the principle: The following exercises are prohibited in geriatric patients:
  - Exercises requiring maximal and submaximal muscular efforts
  - Isometric exercises
  - Extended efforts with the glottis closed
  - Anaerobic exercises
  - Exercises with heavy weights
  - Exercises with the head down below the trunk
  - Exercises with sudden changes of position.

Geriatric Orthopedic Rehabilitation

Orthopedic rehabilitation is based on a sequence of events proceeding from the acquisition of pathology (acute or chronic diseases, or injury) to the generation of impairments manifested at the level of organs and body systems (e.g., a decrease in muscle strength, flexibility, aerobic capacity and cognitive capacity), which leads to functional limitations at the level of the organism as a whole (e.g., restrictions in walking, stair climbing, general mobility skills and balance), and finally to disability (e.g., difficulty or inability to manage daily activities of personal care, household chores, and employment and leisure activities within the context of the environment and its challenges).

Osteoarthritis

Osteoarthritis (OA) as a highly prevalent, progressive, degenerative disease is causing functional impairment and/or disability. It is associated by pain, impaired muscular stabilization and reduced range of motion, and the progressive loss of functions. However, flexibility exercises are important to decrease stiffness, increase joint mobility, and prevent soft tissue contracture.

Strength training is an essential part of rehabilitation for people with osteoarthritis. Resistance training may reverse many age-related physiological changes and can enhance the function by improving the strength of muscles that supports affected joint. Isometric exercises are preferred improve muscle strength and static endurance and are better options if the joint is inflamed or unstable.

Osteoporosis

The physical inactivity/sedentary life style and impaired neuromuscular function are among the risk factors of osteoporosis besides the genetic features and smoking. A negative correlation has been reported between the strength of back extensor muscle and thoracic kyphosis in the women with osteoporosis. It was showed that the relative risk for compression fractures was 2.7 times lower in women (56 years and above) trained with the extensor exercises compared to control group. Specific balance training can also be helpful to manage the osteoporosis among elderly, because patients with osteoporosis and kyphosis maintain their balance with an increased use of hip joints movements.

■ REHABILITATION FOR SPECIFIC CONDITIONS

There are important age-related differences in rehabilitation for nearly every condition treated with rehabilitation, primarily because of the high prevalence of multiple comorbid conditions in the older population and age-related changes in physiology of a variety of organ systems that impact physical function. One study showed that medical comorbidity scores higher than 5 on the Cumulative Illness Rating Scale predicts greater length of stay and less gain in functional status, and 60% of geriatric patients receiving rehabilitation have scores of 6 or more. Greater lengths of stay and lower functional outcomes have been reported for older patients for most conditions in which this has been examined. For example, among patients with spinal cord injury, it was found that length of stay is 58 days and the gain in score on the Functional Independence Measure is 27.8 among patients aged 60 and over, but the length of stay is 43 days and the gain on the Functional Independence Measure is 38.2 among patients aged 18 to 39. Unfortunately, age-specific differences in outcomes have not been examined for all conditions treated with rehabilitation. For example, a National Institutes of Health consensus statement on rehabilitation of persons with traumatic brain injury states that little attention has been paid to the needs of high-risk age groups (e.g., elderly persons), and it recommends research to examine the consequences and effects of rehabilitation after traumatic brain injury in elderly persons. In addition, data are lacking on the disabling impact of specific medical conditions in the older population as a whole or for particular subsets (e.g., nursing-home patients). Given the lack of empirical data to guide the selection of conditions to cover, the conditions reviewed herein were selected on the basis of prevalence in the older population along with likely utility and importance of rehabilitation to condition-specific outcomes.[2]

■ ARTHRITIS AND RELATED MUSCULOSKELETAL PROBLEMS

Rehabilitation interventions are used widely to treat arthritic conditions. Research into their effectiveness is of great importance, and rehabilitation treatment of arthritic conditions is an active area of research. However, an important caveat in reviewing the literature and an important priority for research on rehabilitative treatment of arthritic conditions is to specify the underlying pathophysiology and the joint being studied. Otherwise, important findings may be overlooked. For example, two recent reviews of exercise for osteoarthritis showed conflicting results. Although differing methods may account for the discrepancies, another possibility is that the less conclusive analysis included studies of both the hip and the knee whereas the more conclusive study examined the knee alone. From an anatomic point of view, it is likely that exercise is not as effective for a deep ball-and-socket joint like the hip as it is for a more mobile joint like the knee, where the muscles and tendons provide considerable support to the joint, and exercises that strengthen the muscles therefore are likely to affect the biomechanical function of the joint. Thus, a review that combines studies of the two joints might come up with inconclusive results, not because of the ineffectiveness of the intervention but rather because of the effectiveness differential.

Similarly, it might make sense at first glance to review painful musculoskeletal conditions of a given joint as a general group. However, there likely are important differences in response to therapy, depending on the underlying cause of the musculoskeletal disorder. Consider, for example, osteoporosis and osteoarthritis of the spine, with spinal stenosis as the specific example of the latter. Spinal stenosis is a consequence of bony hypertrophy and narrowing of the central neural canal. There is little reason to believe that exercise would reduce bony hypertrophy; if anything, just the opposite would result. Moreover, it is difficult to envision how alterations in the strength or mechanics of the paraspinous muscles would affect the central canal. On the other hand, the underlying pathophysiology of osteoporosis likely would be affected beneficially by weight-bearing exercise; moreover, pain from the flexion deformities seen after compression fractures in spinal osteoporosis might well respond to flexibility and strengthening exercises for the paraspinous muscles. Indeed, one recent review of exercise for low back pain distinguished among major disease categories and found important differences in outcomes.

A number of studies of exercise, assistive technology, and orthotics show that these can be effective strategies to reduce disability due to diverse musculoskeletal disorders, although the specific type and amount of exercise and the most useful devices and orthotics depend on the specific joints affected and the underlying disorder(s). We lack comparisons of home-based versus clinic-based exercise for arthritic conditions.

What is the difference in short- and long-term efficacy of exercise therapy for osteoarthritis of the knee from a one-time PT evaluation with recommendations for home exercise versus PT in the clinic three times weekly for 3 to 4 weeks? Does the amount and kind of patient education when prescribing a mobility aid affect outcome? Which patients prescribed a cane would benefit from seeing a physical therapist for gait training, and which patients need no more assistance than that available from untrained staff at a local medical supply store?

■STROKE

Post-stroke rehabilitation can be provided in a rehabilitation hospital, a subacute rehabilitation unit, a skilled nursing facility, or via home health or on an outpatient basis. Guidelines published in 1995 by the Agency for Health Care Policy and Research (renamed: Agency for Healthcare Research and Quality) as well as guidelines published in 2003 by the Veterans Health Administration suggest that choice of rehabilitation setting be dictated by the severity of the patient's impairment, the availability of family and social support, and the patient's or family's preferences. The research evidence on settings for stroke rehabilitation and use of massed activity to treat stroke-related deficits are discussed above, in the section on interventions.

Studies have shown surprising plasticity in the adult brain. Currently, investigators are studying not only massed activity but also combinations of exercise and pharmacologic treatment (e.g., sympathomimetic) in an attempt to enhance the responsiveness of the brain to interventions designed to facilitate motor recovery via neuronal plasticity.

This research has not targeted the older population per se, but since strokes are common in the older population, the work is pertinent to geriatric rehabilitation. Investigation into interventions to mold and enhance neural plasticity is a very exciting area of research in stroke rehabilitation, and work in this area that focuses on older persons will be needed. A number of comorbid conditions can have important effects on stroke outcomes. Kelly-Hayes and Paige provide a review of psychosocial factors important to stroke recovery. For example, depression is common after stroke and is associated with poor functional outcomes, and treatment of stroke-related depression may improve cognitive function post-stroke. Stroke patients with dysphagia are at risk for malnutrition, which can adversely affect functional outcomes. One study showed that early nutritional support in these patients reduces mortality. Malnutrition may also adversely affect functional recovery by reducing endurance, interfering with rebuilding muscle strength, and increasing the risk of pressure ulcers and infectious complications.

■ CARDIAC DISEASE

The federal guidelines for cardiac rehabilitation note that elderly patients are referred for cardiac rehabilitation less frequently than younger persons, but that they likely would benefit from exercise-based cardiac rehabilitation. However, there is little hard evidence of this because most cardiology clinical research has not specifically examined the older population. In addition, the effect of comorbid cardiopulmonary disease on rehabilitation outcomes for other conditions needs further study in light of data suggesting that, for example, cardiac disease in combination with arthritis produces more disability that either condition alone. We have good evidence that there are important age-related changes in cardiac function, and cardiac disease is common in the older population.

■ HIP FRACTURE

The goals of hip fracture rehabilitation are to restore functional ambulation and independent self-care; however, many people have substantial decline in physical function after hip fracture despite surgery and rehabilitation. Several studies have shown that high-intensity postoperative PT may prevent postoperative complications and promote better functional outcomes. However, a review suggests that definitive proof of the merits of early, high-intensity PT after acute hip fracture is lacking. A prospective case series of nearly 600 patients aged 65 and over with hip fracture who were allowed full weight bearing showed that, after 1 year or more, 5.3% of those treated by internal fixation suffer loss of fixation or nonunion and 0.6% of those treated with hemiarthroplasty require revision. However, a Cochrane Review concludes that there is insufficient evidence to determine the effects of early weight-bearing after the internal fixation of an intracapsular proximal femoral fracture. The merits of postoperative ambulation restrictions like "partial weight-bearing" or "touch-down weight-bearing" need further study, as older adults may have difficulty comprehending these instructions if they have cognitive deficits or postoperative delirium, and such restrictions in turn may interfere with optimal postoperative PT.[1]

■ AMPUTATION

Amputation in older persons usually occurs in the setting of severe peripheral vascular disease, often in association with longstanding diabetes mellitus, sometimes complicated by hypertension or tobacco abuse. Comorbid disease, including cardiopulmonary disease, stroke, retinopathy, and prior amputation, are common and may affect the functional outcome (as does the level of amputation). Premorbid functional limitations and comorbid conditions must be considered both preoperatively in determining the level of amputation and the ability to tolerate repeated surgery, and postoperatively in determining the goals for rehabilitation. There are recent advances in design of artificial limbs that increase biomechanical efficiency, but at considerable financial cost. Andrews, as well as Cutson and Bongiorni, provide recent reviews of rehabilitation for the older amputee. The cost-benefit trade-offs for older patients differ markedly from those seen with younger persons, for whom amputation usually is traumatic but the cardiovascular and musculoskeletal systems are otherwise intact.

■ DECONDITIONING, SARCOPENIA, AND FRAILTY

Deconditioning occurs with a decrease in activity level for whatever reason, and typically it includes loss of strength, loss of flexibility, and metabolic and hemodynamic abnormalities (e.g., calcium wasting, orthostatic hypotension). Deconditioning may occur with disuse because of pain, incoordination, or any other cause of decreased physical activity. A common cause of deconditioning is enforced immobility as a consequence of acute illness or hospitalization. Early mobilization during hospitalization and regular participation in exercise during hospitalization and after discharge are thought to be the most helpful interventions to prevent and treat deconditioning. However, evidence for the efficacy of exercise among acutely ill older patients is just beginning to appear. Deconditioning is thought to be one of the factors underlying the sarcopenia and frailty sometimes found with aging. Treatment of sarcopenia and related frailty is an active area of research in geriatrics. Research on deconditioning, sarcopenia, and frailty is highly pertinent to geriatric rehabilitation in that exercise, alone or in combination with other treatments (e.g., growth hormone, nutritional support), is being used as a treatment for sarcopenia; moreover, deconditioning, sarcopenia, and frailty can adversely affect rehabilitation outcomes. The evidence on exercise interventions is reviewed in the intervention section of this chapter. However, some evidence supports the concept that sarcopenia is a complex condition due to the interaction of multiple factors, both hormonal and environmental. The efficacy of rehabilitation treatment for sarcopenia likely will be enhanced as the complex physiologic abnormalities underlying this condition are better understood.

■ FALLS

"Falls" is a diagnosis not often mentioned in connection with rehabilitation, but rehabilitation interventions are among those often used to prevent falls. The most commonly used rehabilitation interventions in falls prevention programs are various types of exercise and home assessment with environmental modification. A review of randomized trials of falls prevention interventions identified 23 studies that included exercise, 9 studies of home assessment and surveillance, 1 study of hip protectors, and no studies of footwear. The authors concluded that the majority of exercise studies suggest a decrease in falling, with balance training appearing to be the most effective exercise intervention, and they concluded that the majority of home assessment studies showed benefit as well. A Cochrane review of 18 falls prevention trials and one planned meta-analysis concludes that the evidence does not support the effect of exercise alone in establishing protection against falls, but that the evidence does support the use of exercise as one of multiple interventions specifically targeting identified risk factors in individual patients. An editorial by Tinetti, identifies two research needs on falls: Research that focuses intently on single interventions (as opposed to the multifocal interventions previously tested) to better establish the potency of each intervention and to establish its utility for subgroups of patients and research that would enable implementation in clinical practice of the results of this research. The American Geriatrics Society, the British Geriatrics Society, and the American Academy of Orthopaedic Surgeons recently issued a research agenda for falls and identified the following priorities: cost-effectiveness studies of falls-prevention strategies; examination of risk stratification to identify persons most at risk and persons who would benefit the most; treatment interventions for specific subgroups of patients, including hospitalized patients and those with cognitive impairment; identification of the most effective elements of exercise programs (e.g., types of exercise, duration, frequency); identification of patient groups most likely to benefit from home safety assessment; and examination of the merits of mobility aids for falls prevention.

PAIN

Acute, chronic, and acute-on-chronic pain problems are common in older patients. This is not surprising, given the prevalence of musculoskeletal problems and malignancies in this age group. Unfortunately, pain may be under-recognized in older patients, especially those with cognitive disorders. Currently, the management of pain in older patients includes the use of medications, injections, exercise, physical modalities like heat or cold, behavioural approaches, assistive devices, and orthotics. However, we know little about which interventions are most effective.

Geriatric Neurologic Rehabilitation

Congenital or acquired childhood diseases as cerebral palsy (CP), spina bifida, poliomyelitis; adult life diseases as multiple sclerosis, Parkinson 's disease, amyotrophic lateral sclerosis or diseases that can be seen in any age as stroke or spinal cord injuries result with increased physical, mental, psychosocial consequences of aging. Dementia, especially Alzheimer disease conduce physical disabilities that result with dependency to bed. Thus, the geriatric neurologic physiotherapy and rehabilitation approaches are important to provide an improvement in function or to delay the eventual deterioration of elderly due to the ongoing pathology.

Table 17.2: Assessment in neurologic rehabilitation.

- History and sociodemographic features and environmental factors (age, marital status, lifestyle before the disease, living environment, the aspects of the patient and the family to stroke and rehabilitation, their expectations, support of family and relatives, where to live after discharge)
- Motor function assessment (Motor Assessment Scale, Motor Function Measure),
- Balance (Berg Balance Assessment)
- Mobility (Rivermead Mobility Index)
- Activities of Daily Living Assessment (Barthel Index, functional independence measure - FIM)
- Neurophysiologic approaches (Rood, proprioceptive neuromusculer facilitation-PNF, Brunnstrom, Bobath, Margaret-Johnstone Techniques)
- Muscle strength and impairments (gross motor test, manual muscle test- MMT, myometric tests, grip power, pinch power test)
- Range of motion (goniometric tests)
- Muscle shortenings and deformities (hand deformities, knee flexors contracture, equinovaruos)
- Respiration (frequency, depth, type-diaphragmatic or chest respiration)
- Pain (McGill pain test, visual perception scale)
- Skin (pressure sores) and sensation (touch, hot-cold, point-dull)

Table 17.3: Geriatric rehabilitation program for elderly with neurologic problems.

Aim	Intervention
Improving motor control	Neurofacilitation technique: Bobath, Brunnstrom, Rood, PNF techniques, FES, biofeedback
Chest physiotherapy	• Respiratory control, respiratory exercises • Coughing and force expiratory exercises • Bronchial hygiene and its training • Mobility exercises
Balance and weight-bearing exercises	• Neurofacilitation techniques • Mat exercises, exercises in-and-out of the parallel bar • Proprioceptive exercises • Balance and weight-bearing exercises in ADL
Prevention of trunk control	• Shoulder girdle and pelvic control • Trunk and abdominal strengthening and proprioceptive exercises • Improving the body awareness
Gait training	• Characteristics of gait (style, rhythm, speed, step number, step length etc.) • Exercises for the asymmetry of trunk • Kinesthetic exercises for step and breath control • Functional mobility exercises
Fall prevention	• Strengthening of pelvic muscles (hip flexors, gluteus maximus and medius), ankle joint muscles (tibialis anterior and peroneals, tensor fasia lata) • Appropriate shoe for in-and-outdoors • Home modifications • Shock absorbent pillows, carpet softening layers • Gait training
Orthotic approaches	• Positioning splints (antispasty splints for hand, foot) • AFO (night/day) • UCBL foot orthosis • Shoe modifications
Edema control	Elevation, lymphatic drainage

(AFO: Ankle Foot Orthosis; UCBL: University of California-Berkeley Lab)

An elderly person with *cerebral palsy (CP)* faces with physical changes in their functionality, especially regarding to their mobility besides the physiological changes occurring due to aging. The contractures and deformities may tend to increase the severity of their functional limitations as they become elderly. The knee and foot deformities as well as the hip dislocation, scoliosis and the pelvic obliquity are the most common conditions tend to increase, that all require special care of physiotherapy and rehabilitation, mainly for hygiene, positioning and transfers. The pain (mainly on hips, knees, feet, lumbar and cervical spine) is also another feature that should be considered in geriatric neurorehabilitation of persons with CP. Thus the family and the caregivers should be observant about the possibility of pain, even if, they do not complain, especially for the ones with communication and cognitive problems. Increased weakness of the muscles due to aging may cause bowel and bladder incontinence that limits their activity of daily livings and of course, their quality of life.[3]

If elderly with poliomyelitis have a post-polio syndrome (PPS) should be suggested to change their life style not to alleviate the symptoms as weakness, fatigue, and pain that may arise with physical activity, especially as the day progresses. Thus, the physical therapy and rehabilitation program should be planned according to the physical condition of the patient. However, the manifestations of general fatigue may result with increased sleep requirements and decreased concentration that the physiotherapist or the occupational therapist should take these in consideration while planning the treatment, as well as the activity program.

Thus, while planning the rehabilitation interventions and the exercise treatment programs, exercise items should be:

- Given in low intensity and low repetitions,
- Distributed in the day time when the elderly not feeling tired, mainly in the morning hours.

Stroke as a disease causes long-term disability in any age of life may result with more serious disabilities in elderly age. However, elderly having stroke weather in young or adult ages or in later ages, unfortunately, usually have less attention by the medical team regarding to their rehabilitation process. They are either discharged home after a short period of rehabilitation program or if they cannot live at home, are discharged for a nursing home. Although elderly care in nursing homes are very well organized, the inefficiency in rehabilitation programs are often common in institutional settings due to the administrative structures (such as, lack of time or staff, changes in treatment time table) or due to the features of the elderly person (such as decreased motivation, changes in physical features or environment). In this context, it is generally a common thought that the institutionalized elderly with stroke may have tendency to lose their gained activity level in the acute and subacute rehabilitation programs administered in the hospital.[3]

The main goal of geriatric rehabilitation of the patients with stroke is to achieve the most possible independent condition, physically, mentally and sensorial. Thus, the necessary compensation mechanisms are to be furnished in the area of supportive devices such as, orthoses, canes, walkers, wheelchairs etc., and assistive devices such as touch screens, ergo keyboards or pointing devices. However, aging negatively affects the outcome measures of the rehabilitation program, especially for the ones over 85 and more.

Geriatric Rehabilitation in Spinal Cord Injuries

Spinal cord injuries either occurred in early or in advanced ages result with decreased quality of life and limited social inclusion of the elderly. This may be due to the decline in physical, cognitive and sensorial conditions and also the consequences of the cardiovascular or respiratory diseases that are commonly seen in advanced ages, reported that the incidence of wheelchair usage and dependency in activities of daily living as well as the bowel and bladder incontinence are higher among the elderly than the younger ones having more or less the same level of spinal cord injuries. They may also be affected much more seriously from the bed sores and the disturbances of the venues return that these features should be taken in consideration as a part of the rehabilitation program. Accordingly, besides the individualized rehabilitation programs aiming to maintain the physical condition of the elderly, group therapy programs emphasizing on the activities of daily living, recreation and leisure improve their independence level and social interactions.

Geriatric Rehabilitation in Diseases of Older Ages

The aims of the rehabilitation program of the person with *Parkinson's disease, Multiple sclerosis or Amyotrophic lateral sclerosis (ALS)* that are mostly seen in older ages, include generally to prevent and upgrade their functional level and the quality of life as much as possible. However, according to the special characteristics of the diseases, there are certain treatment approaches that need to be emphasized on during the regular physiotherapy and rehabilitation program. For instance, the balance and coordination exercises are important in the rehabilitation of the elderly with Parkinson's disease to achieve better equilibrium in the movements of the body, not only for the lower extremities for better gait cycle and for prevention of falls, but also for the upper extremities for daily living (as basic, instrumental and advanced activities of daily living-ADL), recreative and leisure activities. Resting periods between the exercises are important during the rehabilitation program of the patients with multiple sclerosis; especially the afternoon fatigue should be taken in consideration by the physiotherapist.

Geriatric Rehabilitation in Dementia

If elderly is diagnosed with dementia, special care must be given during the rehabilitation program regardless of the degree of dementia. The physiotherapy and occupational therapy are among the effective approaches to decrease the severity or to delay the physical and social consequences of dementia. Thus, while planning the exercise programs to improve the functional levels of elderly with dementia, the specific approaches should be focused on to support them cognitively and to foster their memory on the given tasks and/or on the previously learnt activities. In this context, the motor learning procedures can be considered as effective tools of the cognitive approaches in geriatric rehabilitation are among the effective approaches to decrease the severity or to delay the physical and social consequences of dementia. Thus, while planning the exercise programs to improve the functional levels of elderly with dementia, the specific approaches should be focused on to support them cognitively and to foster their memory on the given tasks and/or on the previously learnt activities. In this context, the motor learning procedures can be considered as effective tools of the cognitive approaches in geriatric rehabilitation.

During the exercise program, the skills of the activity of daily living, especially the instrumental type such as the ability to use telephone, shopping, housekeeping, laundry, food preparation etc., and the mobility at indoors and outdoors are aimed to be improved. However, these are embedded with exercises to support or stimulate the cognitive functions and abilities of the elderly for example on their memory, attention, the visiospatial functioning, reasoning and learning-recalling the new information skills. During these exercises their cognition can be stimulated through their possibly diminished executive functioning skills as planning, judgment and insight. For this purpose, the exercises are assessed according to their aims and consequences, by means of providing the media for elderly to find a relation between the reason and the result of the tasks. For example, during the dressing exercises, the elderly can be encouraged to find out the reason of the task that is to *put on a sweater*, and then, the result of it that is *for not to have a cold*. On the other hand, more sophisticated exercise patterns can be preferred by the therapist according to the need of the elderly, such as they may be guided in selecting one of the tasks; deciding on the next task can be done; deciding on a task for her/his partner during the activity; selecting an exercise for her/his partner or for the group in a group treatment; selecting an exercise according to the day or the time, such as deciding to have a walk by the sea in a nice weather or to have an indoor exercise program in a cold weather. The elderly may be involved much more actively into the exercise programs by having the responsibility of counting the repetition by grouping the tasks according to the number of repetitions, the affected area on body or the features of the exercises as strengthening, stretching, and coordination and so on. Then, one more step further in exercise regime is to demand from the person to remember, define and execute the task for example according to the planned schedule written on the board or on the refrigerator.

Overall, the variety of different mental activities can be selected by the therapist to guide the person to fulfill the planned functions. However, the family and the caregivers should be included into the practices and they must be aware of that many repetitions and trials are needed for the success. Thus, the patience and motivation of the medical team, the elderly person, her/his family and the caregivers are noteworthy.

Balance Problem and Fall Prevention in the Elderly

The risk of falling and suffering injury increases dramatically especially in elderly. In frail institutionalized populations, almost threefold higher incidence of falls has been noted. Even falls which result in no physical injury often have serious social and psychological consequences.

It was implied that 40% of 90% ambulatory nursing home patients fell two or more times in the previous 6 months. One in 10 falls results in serious injury and is the cause of mortality in 40% of injury-related deaths in adults over age 65. Serious injuries commonly resulting from falls include fractures of the femoral neck, limbs, and vertebrae, and subdural hematoma. With advancing age, changes related to normal aging, and those associated with diseases and their treatments, can affect the integrity and function of the musculoskeletal, vestibular, central, and peripheral nervous systems. These effects are further compounded by a reduced capacity for plasticity and repair in the elderly. Postural insufficiency, gait disorders and fear of falling have been observed after falling in frail older patients. Remaining on the ground for more than one hour after a fall is a marker of muscle weakness, illness, and social isolation in the elderly that increases the outcome effects of the fall. They may experience decreased confidence in their physical capabilities and reduced physical activities. Thus, in geriatric rehabilitation the main goal is actually the prevention of fall that is depending on many factors, including both extrinsic and environmental factors and intrinsic factors or personal factors. Although some falls may have a single cause, most falls are believed to result from a combination of factors. Not all risks can be eliminated, but the modification of even one risk factor can be a worthwhile therapeutic goal in geriatric rehabilitation. For example, strengthening exercises for the antigravity muscles, stretching exercises for the shortened tight hamstring muscles may increase the confidence of elderly while walking or stair climbing.

For a comprehensive approach to elderly in rehabilitation a thorough physical assessment including examination of strength, power, balance, posture, and gait is essential. These assessments also include evaluation of the coordination of general body, as well as the vision, hand and leg movements, sensation and proprioception. The gait assessment tests evaluating the dynamic balance and the quality of walking, including normal gait, tandem walking as well as dual task activities, such as walking while carrying an object or head movements during walking are to have a detailed information about the elderly. Several performance-based assessments of daily living activities and computerized dynamic posturography tests are also to understand their physical capacity and balance quantitatively.[3]

General Exercise Prescription for the Elderly

The skeletal muscle strength begins to decline at approximately age 45 and is associated with a 30–40% decrease in strength by the age 80 years. This loss of muscle mass not only causes a reduction in strength but may be responsible for as much as 30% of the decline in maximal rate of O_2 consumption (VO_2 max). The loss of skeletal muscle mass below a critical threshold (sarcopenia) leads to a functional impairment and frailty. As the population surveys suggest muscle loss is common and highly correlated with the decreased function in older adults.

Approximately 8% of men and 10% of women had values of muscle mass below two standard deviations of young adult values (class II sarcopenia). It has been established that sarcopenia, characterized by diminished muscle mass, strength, and power, is a key common denominator in the development of frailty.

Regular participation in physical activity and/or exercise is not only integral to the maintenance of good health and functional independence in older adulthood, but also serves as a primary role in the prevention of numerous chronic diseases (e.g., type 2 diabetes, cardiovascular disease, osteoporosis, certain types of cancer) and cognitive decline. Conversely, inactivity doubles the risks of developing a disability that will adversely affect mobility as well as the ability to perform even the most basic activities of daily life. This downward spiral in physical function ultimately heightens the risk of both the loss of functional independence and falls.[4]

It has been identified that the general body exercises have a potential to influence on functional balance and mobility in geriatric inpatients. It is possible that these frail elderly would have benefit from the resistance exercises for the leg muscles. However, ankle exercises directed at increasing ankle ROM may have an influence on reducing falls in this population. Additionally, it has been concluded that the ankle ROM exercises have potential increase on the effectiveness of clinical and community interventions designed for improving balance and reducing falls in elderly women.

Although the general principles of exercises and their relative adaptations are similar in different age groups, there are particular differences especially for the exercise programs aiming to improve cardiorespiratory fitness, flexibility as well as resistance training.

In this context, it is important to know whether the elderly is having a systemic disease or not for the physiotherapist during planning the physiotherapy program. Thus, to design a safe and an effective exercise prescription for elderly, the physiological changes in aging as well as the possibility of the active or latent processes of the systemic diseases should be considered. On the other hand, the necessary consultations should be realized before the initiation of the treatment program.

Resistance Training for Elderly

Resistance training has potential to increase muscular strength, power, and endurance of elderly, improve mobility and prevent falls and fractures. Thus, resistance training is effective, especially, on frail elderly to improve their physical fitness that the followings are the guidelines of resistance training recommended for elderly. The resistance training sessions should be closely supervised and monitored, especially the first a few sessions until the elderly is acquainted. It should begin with minimal resistance to allow for the adaptation of the connective tissue elements. The followings are the important features of a resistance-training program planned by the physiotherapists for elderly.

- The exercises should be performed as a set of 8 to 10 exercises mainly for all the major muscle groups.
- A set of exercise should involve 10-15 repetitions that elicit a perceived exertion rating at the level of 12 to 13, which corresponds to somewhat hard.
- The multi-joint (as opposed to single-joint) exercises should be performed.
- The exercises should be performed in range of motion that is within a pain-free arc, which means the maximum range of motion that does not elicit pain or discomfort.
- First the number of repetitions should be increased then the amount of resistance for achieving a safe overload.

- When returning from a layoff of more than 3 weeks, it should be started with the resistance of 50% or less than the previous training intensity, and then the resistance should be increased gradually.
- The participants should be instructed to maintain their normal breathing pattern while exercising.
- Routine activities (e.g., domestic work, gardening, walking) may help to maintain muscular strength.[4]

Flexibility Exercises for Elderly

A well-planned program of stretching can counteract the usual decline in the flexibility of elderly people, may improve balance and agility. Thus, the flexibility exercises have potential to enhance their functional capacity and reduce the injury potential (e.g., risk of muscle strain, falls). Exercises should be planned for the major joints in the body and for the back, upper trunk and neck region with mild stretching. Yoga and Tai-Chi may be helpful in improving or maintaining the flexibility of the body that could be included into the rehabilitation program. In this regard, a general exercise prescription for achieving and maintaining flexibility of elderly may include the fallowing approaches:

- The flexibility exercises should be performed a minimum of 2 to 3 days/week
- Stretching should be performed till the end of the range of motion at a point of limitation.
- Tightness, however, without inducing any discomfort
- Performing static stretching exercises routinely for the major joints and the muscle
- Tendon units to increase the range of motion.
- Holding each stretch for 15–30 seconds to achieve the muscular adaptation.

Mode of Exercises

Although there are variety of exercise models as isometric, isotonic (eccentric, concentric) exercises for elderly, they should be selected specifically for not impose excessive orthopedic stress to the body. Isotonic exercises are preferred according to the needs of the elderly as passive, active, active assistive or resistive modes. However, the outdoor walking is an excellent mode of exercise for many elderly people that could be suggested safely. As an effective weight-bearing exercise it is also important for the psychosocial status of the elderly since they are naturally encouraged for the social interactions while walking outdoors with their peers or friends. Swimming, aquatic exercise and stationary cycle exercises may be especially advantageous for those with reduced ability to tolerate weight-bearing exercises.

The exercises should be accessible according to the physical and mental conditions of the elderly; however, they should be enjoyable as well, to improve their exercise habits. However, a group setting such as callisthenic exercises may provide important social reinforcement to improve their exercise adherence. Hence, if possible, the group exercises could be embedded into the exercise rehabilitation programs to challenge their participation.

Intensity of Exercises

It is important to remember that, the exercise intensity for the active elderly people should start at low level and gradually may progress according to their tolerance and preference individually for not to alleviate any medical problem and also for the promotion of long-term fitness. For instance, the measured peak hearth rate is preferable to an age predicted peak hearth rate when prescribing aerobic exercises because of the variability in peak hearth rate for the individuals above 65 years of age and also higher risk of underlying coronary disease.

Thus, initiating a program at less than 40% VO_2 max is not unusual. The exercises need not to be vigorous and continuous to be beneficial; a daily accumulation 30 minutes of moderate intensity of physical activity may efficiently provide health benefits.

Duration of Exercises

Exercise duration need not to be continuous to produce benefits, thus, those who have difficulty sustaining exercise for 30 minutes or who prefer shorter bouts of exercise can be advised to exercise for 10-minute periods at different times throughout the day. It is preferable for the elderly to increase exercise duration rather than intensity to avoid injury and ensure safety.

Frequency of Exercises

Physical activity performed at moderate intensity should be performed most days of the week. If exercise is undertaken at a vigorous level, it should be performed at least 2-4 days/week or at low-to moderate intensity on alternating days.

Exercises for Fall and Balance

It was documented that frail elderly people with a history of falls must benefit from vestibular rehabilitation programs in order to avoid the loss of functional capacities and disability. These specific rehabilitation programs are based on the basic motor patterns of training, including the practice of vestibular and balance exercises as well as gait training. This program can be intensified through a multidisciplinary approach, which requires the education of all the members of the team taking care of the elderly.

Vestibular rehabilitation is designed to restore homeostasis of the balance system. The goals of vestibular rehabilitation include decreasing dizziness, improving balance, and minimization the fall risk by improving vestibulo-ocular reflex accuracy, postural control, and occulomotor skills. Various techniques used in vestibular and balance rehabilitation therapy include adaptation exercises, habituation exercises, substitution exercises, balance exercises, gait and general conditioning exercises. The planned exercise program should be consistent with the patient needs, so that it is specific for each particular case.

It was demonstrated that the use of other forms of exercises such as Tai Chi is a good evidence as a medium for lowering fall risk among more sedentary community-residing elderly. Low, Ang et al. (2009) have reported in their systematic review that Tai Chi has the potential to reduce falls or risk of falls among the elderly, if they are relatively young and non-frail. The longitudinal study on the effects of Tai Chi exercise among elderly with osteoarthritis (OA) suggested that Tai Chi should be encouraged to maintain physical function and improve quality of life elderly people with OA.

Balance Training

Loss of balance is common in certain medical conditions that are associated with aging. This can contribute to falls and difficulty walking. Therefore, it is important for older adults to learn and consistently perform simple exercises that will improve their balance skills and help them feel more confident in their activities of daily living.[4]

Balance exercises are specific activities that help build lower extremity (leg) muscle strength as well as improve balance. Balance exercises are particularly beneficial in the older adult as they have been shown to help prevent falls. Each year, U.S. hospitals have 300,000 admissions for broken hips, and falling is often the cause of those fractures. Balance exercises can help an older adult stay independent by helping avoid disabilities that may result from falling.

- Single leg stand
- Tandem standing
- Tandem walking (Heel-to-Toe)
- Chair sitting and standing
- Standing hip raise

Cardiorespiratory Fitness Exercises for Elderly

Elderly people should be encouraged to do for at least 30 minutes of moderate-intensity physical activity on most and preferably, all days of the week. This can be accomplished with activities such as brisk walking, gardening, yard work, housework, climbing stairs, and active recreational pursuits. For those achieving this level, additional benefits may be obtained with longer – duration moderate – intensity physical activity or by substituting moderate with higher intensity physical activity. It is important to remember that the activities performed at a given Metabolic Equivalent Threshold (MET) value may represent greater relative effort in elderly than young people because of the decrease in peak MET's with age. On the other hand, the optimal mode of exercise for elderly can be influenced by the physiologic and psychosocial variables, such as work capacity, orthopedic problems, poor balance, and travel limitations. Thus, while planning an exercise program for the elderly, the mode, intensity, duration and frequency of the exercises should be specific in relation to their physiological and psychological conditions.[4]

General Exercises for Older People

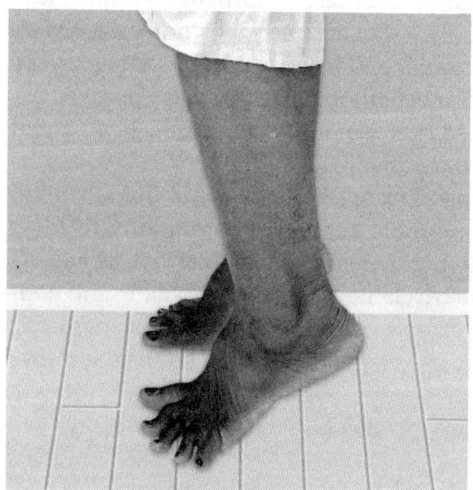

Figure 17.1: Heel raise.

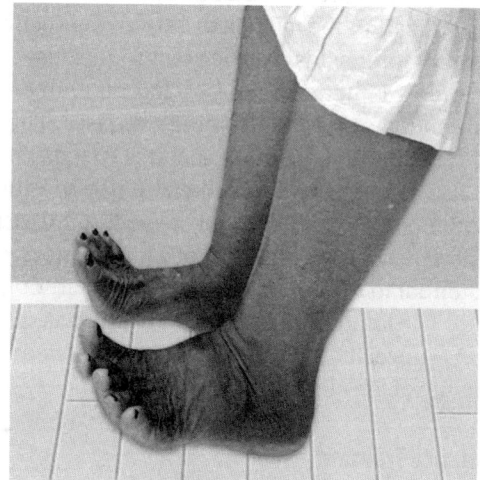

Figure 17.2: Toe raise.

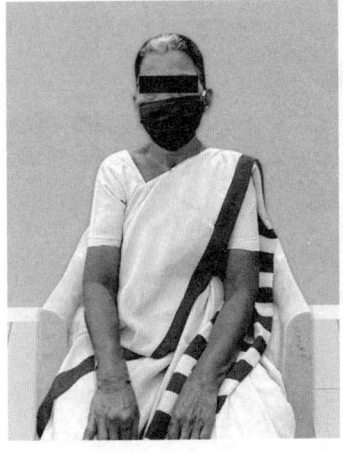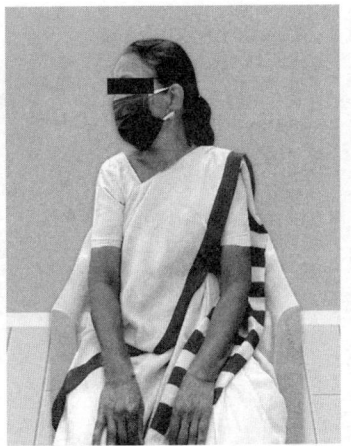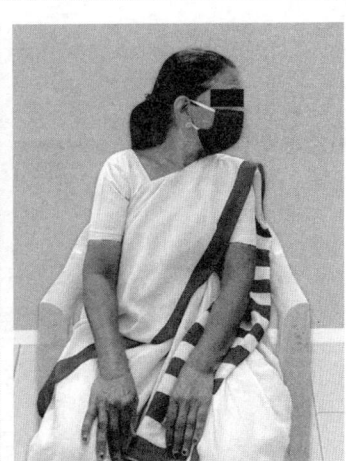

Figure 17.3: Neck rotation.

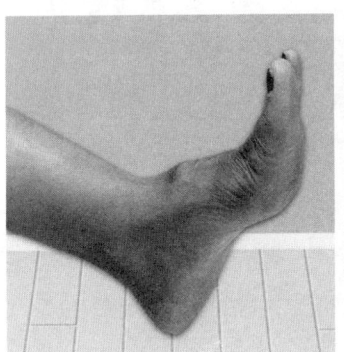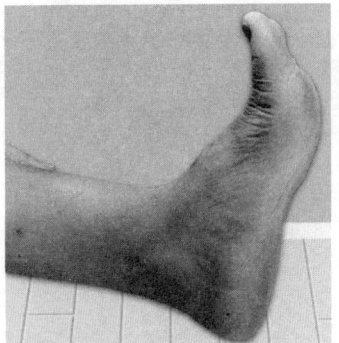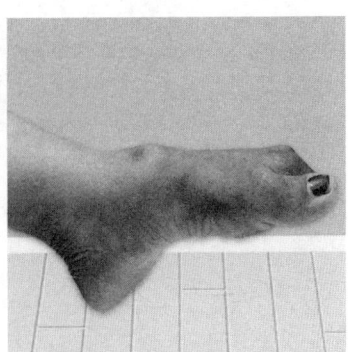

Figure 17.4: Ankle toe movements.

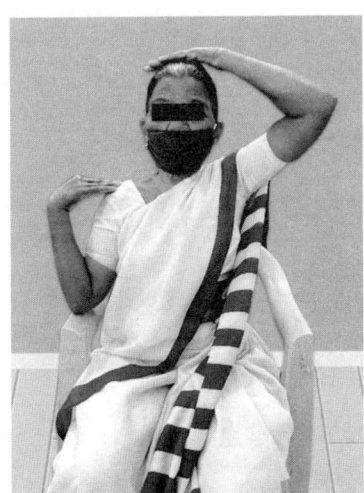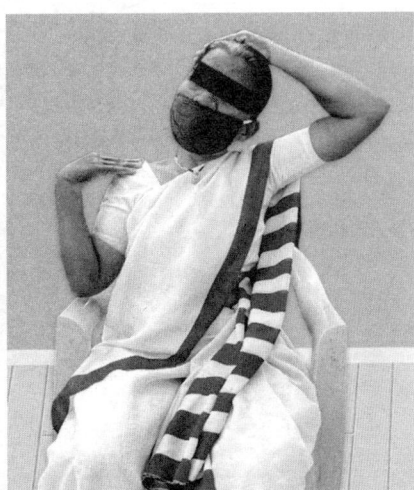

Figure 17.5: Self-neck stretching.

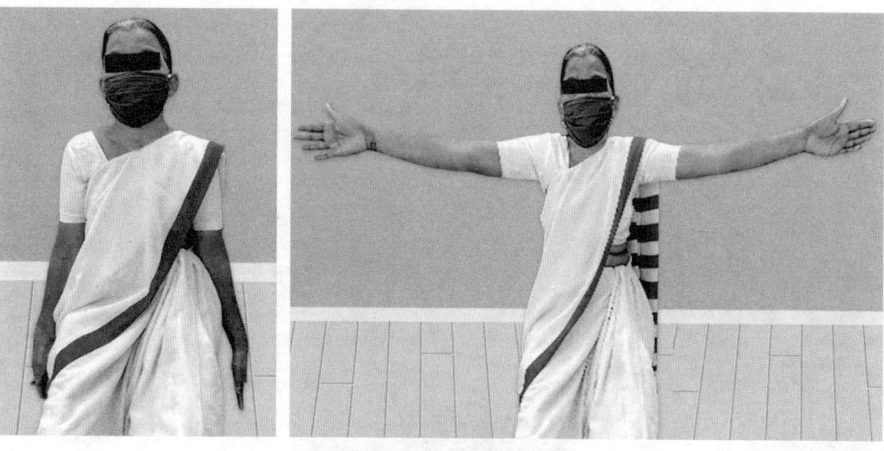

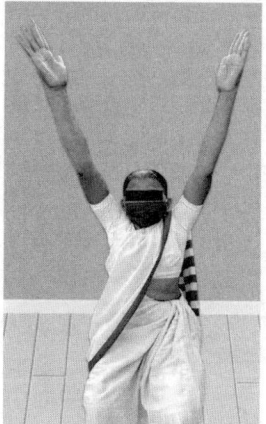

Figure 17.6: Arm raise.

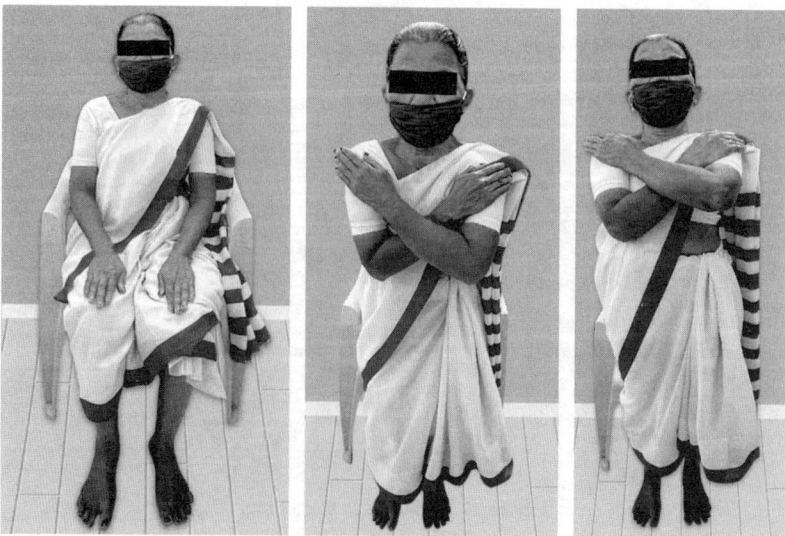

Figure 17.7: Sit to stand.

Geriatric Functional Assessment

Definition: Functional impairment is defined as difficulty performing, or requiring the assistance of another person to perform, one or more of the following Activities of Daily Living **(ADL):** ADLs are the essential elements of self-care. Inability to independently perform even one activity may indicate a need for supportive services.[5]

IADLs are associated with independent living in the community and provide a basis for considering the type of services necessary in maintaining independence.

Activities of Daily Living (ADLs): Bathing, Dressing, Toileting, Transfers, Grooming, Feeding.

Instrumental Activities of Daily Living (IADLs): Administering own medication, Grocery shopping, preparing meals, Using the telephone, Driving and transportation, Handling own finances, Housekeeping, Laundry.

Implications: ADL impairment is a stronger predictor of hospital outcomes (functional decline, length of stay, institutionalization, and death) than admitting diagnoses, Diagnosis-related Group, and other physiologic indices of illness burden. ADL impairment is also a risk factor for nursing home placement, emergency room visits, and death among community-dwelling adults.

Screening for Cognitive Impairment

Patients with suspected cognitive impairment should be screened for delirium and depression. Delirium is a disorder of attention, and should be considered in patients with waxing and waning attention or level of consciousness. Delirium is commonly a side effect of medications, and often unrecognized by clinicians.[5]

Clinical Implications

Many elderly patients seen by surgical and medical specialists and subspecialists have significant cognitive impairment, often undiagnosed. Unrecognized cognitive impairment is a risk factor for medication non-adherence, poor compliance with behavioural recommendations, difficulty navigating the health care system, and caregiver stress. The most common causes of cognitive impairment in elderly patients are dementia, depression, and delirium.

Screening Test

- Mini-Cog
- Min-Mental State Examination (MMSE) Score >=26
- 3-item recall at one minute
- Serial 7's
- Clock Drawing Test

Mini-Cog

Consisting of two parts: 3-item recall plus clock draw test (CDT).
- Instruct the patient to listen carefully as you name 3 unrelated objects and then to repeat the object names.
- Instruct the patient to draw the face of a clock, either on a blank sheet of paper, or on a sheet with the clock circle already drawn on the page. After the patient puts the numbers on the clock face, ask him or her to draw the hands of the clock to read a specific time, such as 11:20.

These instructions can be repeated, but no additional instructions should be given. Give that patient as much time as needed to complete the task. The CDT serves as the recall distractor.
- ❖ Ask the patient to repeat the 3 previously presented object names.
  Scoring give 1 point for each recalled word after the CDT distractor. Score 0–3. The CDT is considered normal if all numbers are present in the correct sequence and position, and the hands readably display the requested time.
  - A score of 0 indicates dementia (regardless of CDT results).
  - A score of 1 or 2 with an abnormal CDT indicates dementia
  - A score of 1 or 2 with a normal CDT indicates absence of dementia
  - A score of 3 indicates absence of dementia (regardless of CDT results).

Screening for Depression

More than 75% of older adults who commit suicide were suffering from a major depression; a physician had seen the vast majority within 1 month of suicide. Risk factors for late-life suicide include depression, comorbid physical illness, living alone, male gender, and alcoholism. Depression commonly accompanies major medical illness. Depression complicating medical illness can be particularly difficult to recognize, since somatic symptoms are more common presenting complaints of depressed elderly patients than among younger populations.[5]

Clinical Implications

One to two out of every five older inpatients suffer from depression. Depression lower patients' quality of life and contributes to poor adherence. Major and minor depression are treatable conditions in elderly patients, with response rates comparable to those in younger populations.

A number of tools exist to help screen for depression among older patients such as Geriatric Depression Scale, Beck Depression Inventory Scale.

Clinicians screen for depression older patients who:
- ❖ Are 80 years of age or older
- ❖ Complain of sleep disturbance, lack of energy, poor appetite, or "just feeling bad".
- ❖ Suffer a functional decline
- ❖ Have difficulty taking medications.

Evaluating Patients with Gait Instability or Falls

Walking disability increases with age, from about 6% of persons aged 65–69 years to about 40% among persons aged 85 or older. In older adults with diseases such as arthritis, 35% admit to difficulty in walking one-quarter mile.
- ❖ Between 30% and 40% of community-dwelling older persons fall each year.
- ❖ Among those who have fallen in the past year, the annual incidence of falls is close to 60%.
- ❖ About half of all persons in long-term care settings fall each year.

Clinical Implications

Complications resulting from falls are the leading cause of death from injury in older men and women. While most falls result in some soft tissue injury, 10 to 15% of falls result in a fracture or other serious injury. Falls are associated with subsequent decline in functional status, increased likelihood of nursing home placement, and increased use of medical services. Approximately

40–70% of fallers develop fear of falling. Of those elderly persons who fall, only half are able to get up without help.

Screening for Gait Instability/Risk of Falls: "Timed Get Up and Go" Test

Assessment

Screening for gait instability/risk of falls: "Timed Get Up and Go" test

Just before the test, open the exam room door and place a marker on the floor ten feet from the patient's chair.

To test the patient, give the following instructions:
- Rise from the chair
- Walk to the line on the floor (10 feet)
- Turn
- Return to the chair
- Sit down again

Use a standard armchair. Place the line ten feet from the chair. The score is the time taken in seconds to complete the task. The subject is encouraged to wear regular footwear and to use any customary walking aid. No physical assistance is given. Have the subject walk through the test once before being timed, to become familiar with the test. Explain to the patient that you will then time them and have them complete the test for a second time. Normal time required to complete test: less than 10 seconds. Further evaluation required if test not performed in 20 seconds. Patients who require more than 20 seconds for this test have limited physical mobility, may be at risk for falls and may require assistance from others for many mobility tasks including basic transfers.[5]

Clinical Applications

All older patients who are under the care of a health professional or caregiver should be asked at least once a year about falls or near-falls. Older persons who report a single fall should undergo the "Timed Up and Go" test. Those demonstrating no difficulty or unsteadiness AND who complete the test in 10 seconds or less need no further assessment. Those who require more than 20 seconds to complete the maneuver should undergo further evaluation. Those with scores between 10 and 20 seconds are at intermediate risk; further evaluation should be considered. Persons who have fallen more than once in the past year, have abnormalities of gait or balance, or both, should be referred to clinicians with skills and experience in gait and falls evaluation and management.[5]

■ REFERENCES

1. Morrison M. Physiotherapy in geriatric rehabilitation.
2. Exercise for Older Adults. Health Care Provider Edition.
3. Elsawy B, Higgins KE. The Geriatric Assessment.
4. Paraschiv C, Esanu I, Ghiuru R. General principles of geriatric rehabilitation. Romanian Journal of Oral Rehabilitation. 2015;7(1).
5. Geriatric functional assessment. Division of Geriatric Medicine Department of Internal Medicine; 2003.

CHAPTER 18

Elderly in India

Shyam D Ganvir, Abhijit D Diwate

LEARNING OBJECTIVES

Through this chapter, the reader will be able to:
- Define aging.
- Understand problems associated with aging.
- Learn about policy and programs for elderly in India
- Gain insight about legal backings and measures to be taken for elderly people.

■ AGING

- ❖ Aging is a continuous, irreversible, universal process, which starts from conception till the death of an individual.
- ❖ However, the age at which one's productive contribution declines and one tends to be economically dependent can probably be treated as the onset of the aged stage of life.
- ❖ National Elderly Policy defines person of 60+ age group as elderly.

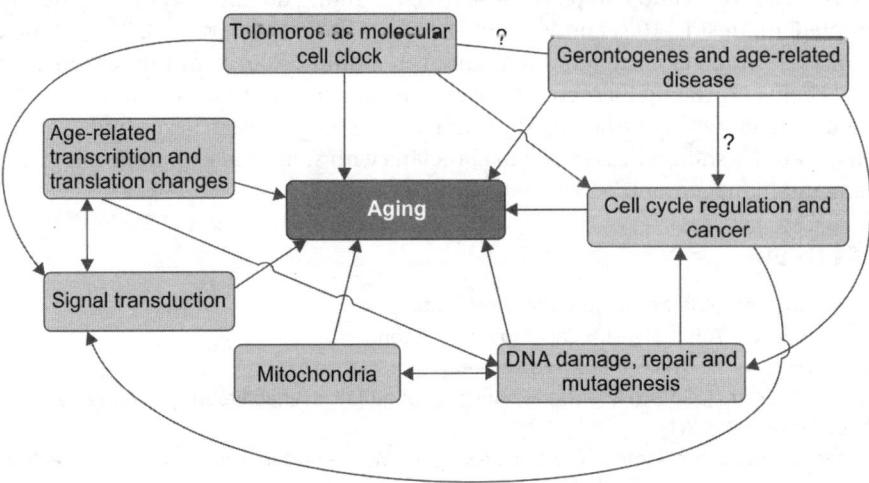

CHAPTER 18: Elderly in India

❖ In 1991, the book *Evolutionary Biology of Aging* offered the following definition of aging: *a persistent decline in the age-specific fitness components of an organism due to internal physiological deterioration* (Rose, 1991).

■ THEORIES OF AGING

Biological Theories

❖ Wear and tear theory
❖ Cellular theory
❖ Autoimmune theory
❖ Gene mutation theory
❖ Free radical theory

Psychosocial Theories

❖ Disengagement theory
❖ Activity theory
❖ Continuity theory

Population Figures on Aging

❖ Age division of Indian population (0-14) is 30.8%, (15-59) is 60.3%, (60+) is 8.6%. According to Population Census 2011, there are nearly 104 million elderly persons in India.
❖ It has increased from 5.5% in 1951 to 8.6% in 2011.
❖ Projected a rise up to 19% by 2050.
❖ As regards rural and urban areas, more than 73 million persons, i.e. 71% of elderly population resides in rural areas while 31 million or 29% of elderly population are in urban area.
❖ Between 2015 and 2050, the proportion of the world's population over 60 years will nearly double from 12% to 22%.
❖ By 2020, the number of people aged 60 years and older will outnumber children younger than 5 years.
❖ In 2050, 80% of older people will be living in low- and middle-income countries.
❖ The pace of population aging is much faster than in the past.
❖ All countries face major challenges to ensure that their health and social systems are ready to make the most of this demographic shift.

Feminiaation of Aging

❖ Among the challenges which India faces, UNPF report says the feminization of aging remained a key one.
❖ The sex ratio of the elderly has increased from 938 women to 1,000 men in 1971 to 1,033 in 2011 and is projected to increase to 1,060 by 2026.
❖ The report also noted that between 2000 and 2050, the population of 80-plus people would have grown 700% "with a predominance of widowed and highly dependent very old women" and so the special needs of such old women would need significant focus of policy and programs.

Problems Associated with Old Age

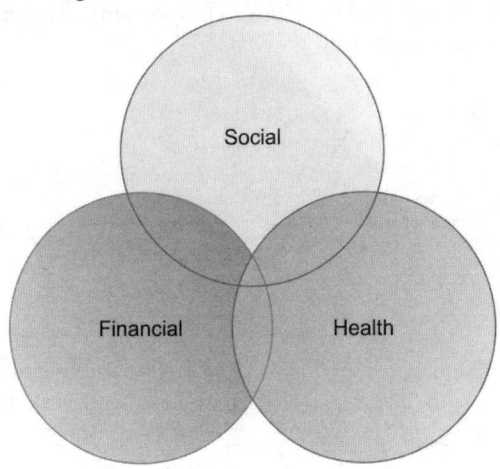

Social

- Indian society is undergoing rapid transformation under the impact of industrialization, urbanization, technical & technological change, education and globalization.
- Consequently, the traditional values and institutions are in the process of erosion and adaptation, resulting in the weakening of intergenerational ties that were the hallmark of the traditional family.
- Industrialization has replaced the simple family production units by the mass production and the factory.
- Negligence by kids towards their old parents.
- Disillusionment due to retirement.
- Feeling of powerlessness, loneliness, uselessness and isolation in elderly.
- Generational gap.

Financial

- Retirement and dependence of elderly on their child for basic necessity.
- Sudden increase in out of pocket expenses on treatment.
- Migration of young working-age persons from rural area have negative impacts on the elderly, living alone or with only the spouse usually poverty and distress.
- Insufficient housing facility.

Health

- Multiple disabilities among the elders in old age.
- Health issues like blindness, locomotor disabilities and deafness are most prevalent.
- Mental illness arising from senility and neurosis.
- Absence of geriatric care facilities at hospitals in rural area.

■ POLICY AND PROGRAMS FOR THE WELFARE OF ELDERLY IN INDIA

Administrative Setup

- The Ministry of Social Justice and Empowerment is the nodal Ministry for the welfare of senior citizens.

- The Ageing Division in the Social Defence Bureau of the Department of Social Justice and Empowerment develops and implements programs and policies for the senior citizens in close collaboration with State Governments, Non-Governmental Organizations and civil society. The programs for senior citizens aim at their welfare and maintenance, especially for indigent senior citizens, by supporting old age homes, day care centers, mobile medi-care units, etc. These programs are implemented through providing support for capacity building of Government/Non-Governmental Organizations (NGOs)/Panchayati Raj Institutions (PRISs/local bodies and the Community at large.

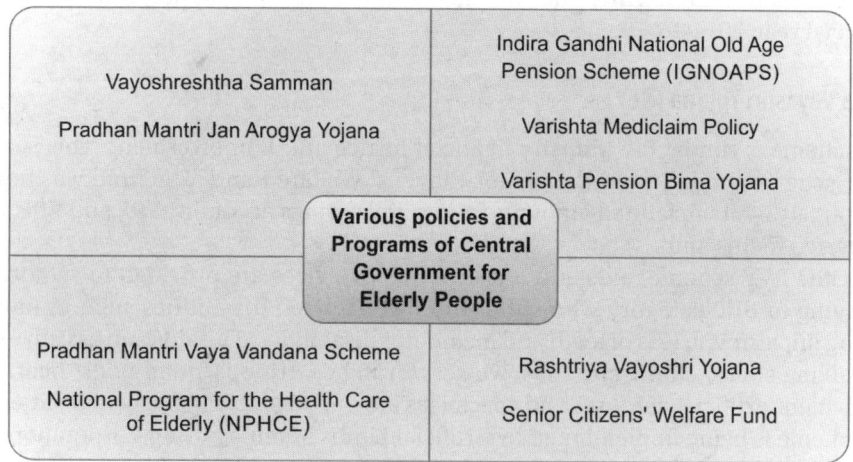

Integrated Program for Older Persons (IPOP)

Ministry of Social Justice and Empowerment is a nodal agency for the welfare of elderly people. The main objective of the scheme is to improve the quality of life of older persons by providing basic amenities like shelter, food, medical care and entertainment opportunities, etc.

The Ministry of Social Justice and Empowerment is implementing a Central Sector Scheme of Integrated Program for Older Persons (IPOP) since 1992 with the objective of improving the quality of life of senior citizens by providing basic amenities like shelter, food, medical care and entertainment opportunities etc. through providing support for capacity building of Government/ Non-Governmental Organizations/Panchayati Raj Institutions/Local bodies etc.

The Scheme was revised with effect from 01.04.2008 and 01.04.2015. Besides revising cost norms of financial assistance for existing projects, several innovative projects were added as being eligible for assistance under the Scheme during the 2008 revision. The following projects are being assisted under the IPOP Scheme:

- Maintenance of Old Age Homes;
- Maintenance of Respite Care Homes;
- Running of Multi Service Centres for Older Persons;
- Mobile Medicare Unit;
- Day Care Center for Care of Old Person with Dementia;
- Multifacility Care Center for Older Widows;
- Physiotherapy Clinics;
- Regional Resource and Training Center;

- Helplines and Counseling for Older Persons;
- Program for Sensitization Schools/College Student;
- Awareness Projects for Older Persons;
- Volunteers Bureau for Older Persons;
- Formation of Vridha Sanghas/Senior Citizen Associations/Self Help Groups;
- Any other activity, which is considered suitable to meet the objective of the Scheme.

In view of the rising cost of living index, the cost-norms of the IPOP Scheme has been revised w.e.f 01-04-2015. The average increase in cost norm ranges between 70–100%. Ministry of Social Justice and Empowerment has initiated online processing of proposals of NGOs from the financial year, 2014-15.

Rashtriya Vayoshri Yojana (RVY)

- This scheme is run by the Ministry of Social Justice and Empowerment. This is a central sector scheme funded from the Senior Citizens' Welfare Fund. The fund was notified in the year 2016. All unclaimed amounts from small savings accounts, PPF and EPF are to be transferred to this fund.
- Under the RVY scheme, aids and assistive living devices are provided to senior citizens belonging to BPL category who suffer from age-related disabilities such as low vision, hearing impairment, loss of teeth and locomotor disabilities. The aids and assistive devices, viz walking sticks, elbow crutches, walkers/crutches, tripods/quad pods, hearing aids, wheelchairs, artificial dentures and spectacles are provided to eligible beneficiaries.
- The scheme is being implemented by Artificial Limbs Manufacturing Corporation of India (ALIMCO), which is a public sector undertaking under the Ministry of Social Justice and Empowerment.

Indira Gandhi National Old Age Pension Scheme (IGNOAPS)

- The Ministry of Rural Development runs the National Social Assistance Programme (NSAP) that extends social assistance for poor households for the aged, widows, disabled, and in cases of death where the breadwinner has passed away.
- Under this scheme, financial assistance is provided to person of 60 years and above and belonging to family living below poverty line as per the criteria prescribed by Government of India. Central assistance of ₹ 200 per month is provided to person in the age group of 60-79 years and ₹ 500 per month to persons of 80 years and above.

Varishtha Pension Bima Yojana (VPBY)

This scheme is run by the Ministry of Finance. The Varishtha Pension Bima Yojana (VPBY) was first launched in 2003 and then relaunched in 2014. Both are social security schemes for senior citizens intended to give an assured minimum pension on a guaranteed minimum return on the subscription amount.

The Pradhan Mantri Vaya Vandana Yojana

- The Pradhan Mantri Vaya Vandana Yojana (PNVVY) was launched in May 2017 to provide social security during old age. This is a simplified version of the VPBY and will be implemented by the Life Insurance Corporation (LIC) of India.
- Under the scheme, on payment of an initial lump sum amount ranging from ₹ 1,50,000 for a minimum pension of ₹ 1000 per month to a maximum of ₹ 7,50,000/- for a maximum pension

of ₹ 5,000 per month, subscribers will get an assured pension based on a guaranteed rate of return of 8% per annum payable monthly/quarterly/half-yearly/annually.
- The Center will bear 75 percent of the total budget and the state government will contribute 25 percent of the budget, for activities up to district level.

■ INTERNATIONAL DAY FOR OLDER PERSONS (IDOP) AND NATIONAL AWARDS: VAYOSHRESHTHA SAMMAN

- The Ministry of Social Justice and Empowerment observes the International Day for Older Persons (IDOP) on 1st October every year in a befitting manner by organizing a series of events and programs dedicated to the senior citizens. The day is dedicated to acknowledge the contribution of senior citizens to the society and to sensitize the public at large about their problems and needs and to make our society more elderly friendly.
- In order to recognize the efforts made by eminent senior citizens and Institutions involved in rendering distinguished services for the cause of elderly persons, especially indigent senior citizens, the Ministry of Social Justice and Empowerment (Department of Social Justice and Empowerment) has prepared a new Scheme of National Awards for senior citizens to showcase the Government's concern for senior citizens and its commitment towards senior citizens with the aim of strengthening their legitimate place in the society. The Scheme of National Awards for senior citizens has been notified in the Gazette of India on 22.01.2013 and was given for the first time during 2013.
- Applications/nominations for National Award 2015 were invited through advertisements in National Dailies. The last date for inviting applications had been 15th May 2015 which was later extended till 31st May 2015. A function was organized at the Vigyan Bhawan, New Delhi wherein National Awards were conferred on eminent senior citizens and Institutions, from any part of the country, in recognition for their contribution towards the cause of the elderly on 1st October 2015. President of India, Shri. Pranab Mukherjee gave away the National Awards. The Award in each category shall carry a Citation, a Memento and also Cash Award in some of the categories as decided from time to time.
- In collaboration with a reputed NGO, this Ministry of Social Justice and Empowerment organized an Intergenerational Walkathon at the India Gate Lawns, Rajpath, New Delhi on the morning of 1st October 2015.

■ NATIONAL COUNCIL FOR OLDER PERSONS (NCOP)/ NATIONAL COUNCIL OF SENIOR CITIZENS (NCSRC)

- In pursuance of the National Policy for Older Persons (NPOP), a National Council for Older Persons (NCOP) was constituted in 1999 under the Chairpersonship of the Minister for Social Justice and Empowerment to oversee implementation of the Policy. The NCOP is the highest body to advise the Government in the formulation and implementation of policy and programmes for the aged.
- In order to have a definite structure as well as regional balancing, National Council for Older Persons (NCOP) has been reconstituted and renamed as National Council for Senior Citizens (NCSrC) vide a resolution dated 17-2-2012 which was published in the Gazette of India on 22-2-2012. The NCSrC will advise Central and State Governments on the entire gamut of issues related to welfare of senior citizens and enhancement of their quality of life. The NCSrC will meet at least twice a year.

■ THE NATIONAL POLICY ON OLDER PERSONS (NPOP)

- The National Policy on Older Persons (NPOP) was announced in January 1999 to reaffirm the commitment of the State to ensure the well-being of the older persons. The Policy envisages State support to ensure financial and food security, health care, shelter and other needs of older persons, equitable share in development, protection against abuse and exploitation, and availability of services to improve the quality of their lives.
- Keeping in view the changing demography of the senior citizens in the country over the last decade, the Ministry of Social Justice and Empowerment constituted a Committee to (i) assess the present status of various issues concerning senior citizens, in general, and implementation of NPOP, 1999, in particular, and (ii) draft a new NPOP keeping in view the emerging trends in demographic, socioeconomic, technological and other relevant fields. The new National Policy for Senior Citizens is under finalization.

■ BENEFITS EXTENDED BY OTHER CENTRAL MINISTRIES FOR THE WELFARE OF SENIOR CITIZENS

Ministry of Rural Development

The Ministry of Rural Development is implementing the Indira Gandhi National Old Age Pension Scheme (IGNOAPS) under which Central assistance is given towards pension @ Rs. 200/- per month to persons above 60 years and @ Rs. 500/- per month to persons above 80 years belonging to a household below poverty line, which is meant to be supplemented by at least an equal contribution by the States.

Ministry of Health and Family Welfare

The Ministry of Health and Family Welfare provides the following facilities for senior citizens of:
- Separate queues for older persons in government hospitals.
- Geriatric clinic in several government hospitals.
- The Ministry implemented the National Program for the Health Care for the Elderly (NPHCE) from the year 2010-11.

Objectives of the National Program for the Healthcare for the Elderly

- Provide preventive, curative and rehabilitative services to the elderly persons at various level of healthcare delivery system of the country
- Strengthen referral system
- Develop specialized man power and
- Promote research in the field of diseases related to old age

Major Components

- To establish geriatric department in all the existing 8 Regional Geriatrics Centres
- Strengthening healthcare facilities for elderly at various levels of 100 identified districts in 21 States of the country.
- Regional Institutions to provide technical support to geriatric units at district hospitals whereas district hospitals will supervise and coordinate the activities down below at CHC, PHC and subcenters.

Ministry of Finance

Health Insurance

Insurance Regulatory Development Authority (IRDA) vide letter dated 25.5.2009 issued instructions on health insurance for senior citizens to CEOs of all General Health Insurance Companies which, inter-alia, includes:
- Allowing entry into health insurance scheme till 65 years of age,
- Transparency in the premium charged
- Reasons to be recorded for denial of any proposals, etc. on all health insurance products catering to the needs of senior citizens. Likewise the insurance companies cannot deny renewability without specific reasons.

Tax Benefits

The Ministry provides the following facilities for senior citizens for the Assessment Year 2016-17:
- Income tax exemption for Senior Citizens of 60 years and above up to Rs. 3.0 lakh per annum.
- Income tax exemption for Senior Citizens of 80 years and above up to Rs. 5.0 lakh per annum.
- Deduction of Rs. 30,000 under Section 80D is allowed to an individual who pays medical insurance premium for his/her parent or parents, who is a senior citizen.
- An individual is eligible for a deduction of the amount spent or Rs. 60,000, whichever is less for medical treatment of a dependent senior citizen suffering from specified diseases. For senior citizens of 80 years and above the limit is Rs. 80,000.

Ministry of Home Affairs

Protection of Life and Property

Chapter V of the Maintenance and Welfare of Parents and Senior Citizens Act, 2007 provides for protection of life and property of senior citizens. State Governments are required to prescribe a comprehensive Action Plan for providing protection of life and property of senior citizens. The Ministry of Home Affairs, Government of India has also issued detailed advisories dated 27.3.2008 and 30.08.2013 to all the State Government/UTs, who are primarily responsible for prevention, detection, registration, investigation and prosecution of crime including crime against senior citizens as 13 "Police" and "Public order" are state subjects. The Ministry of Home Affairs in its advisories has advised the States/UTs to take immediate measures to ensure safety and security and for elimination of all forms of neglect, abuse and violence against old persons through initiatives such as identification of senior citizens; sensitization of police personnel regarding safety, security of older persons; regular visit of the beat staff; setting up of toll free senior citizens helplines; setting up of senior citizen security cell; verification of domestic helps, drivers, etc.

Ministry of Railways

Concession in Rail Fares the Ministry of Railways provides the following facilities to senior citizens:
- Separate ticket counters for senior citizens of age 60 years and above at various Passenger Reservation System (PRS) centres if the average demand per shift is more than 120 tickets;

- Provision of lower berth to male passengers of 60 years and above and female passengers of 45 years and above.
- 40% and 50% concession in basic rail fare for male (60 years) and female (58 years) senior citizen respectively.
- Wheel chairs at stations for old age passengers.

Ministry of Civil Aviation

The National Carrier, Air India under the Ministry of Civil Aviation provides air fare concession in up to 50% of basic fare of normal economy class for senior citizens who have completed 63 years of age on the date of commencement of journey and on production of proof of age (Photo-ID) and nationality.

Note: Information given in Section "H" of Part II has been taken from websites of Ministry of Social Justice and Empowerment and other Ministries as on 1 February 2016.

Legal Backings

- Article 41 and Article 46 are the constitutional provisions for elderly persons. Although directive principles are not enforceable under the law, but it creates a positive obligation towards the state while making any law.
- Section 20 of Hindu marriage and adoption Act, 1956 makes it obligatory provisions to maintain an aged parents.
- Under Section 125 of Criminal Procedure Code, the elder parents can claim maintenance from their children.
- The Maintenance and Welfare of Parents and Senior Citizens Act, 2007, seeks to make it legal for the children or heirs to maintain their parents or senior citizens of the family.
- Convention on the Rights of Older Persons is proposed in united nation.
- In 1982, the Report of the World Assembly on Aging (also known as "the International Plan on Aging") was published, which represented the first international debate on the rights of older persons and presented a plan for their implementation.
- The UNPF were tasked with implementing the Plan of the Second World Assembly which adopted "Madrid International Plan" on aging in 2002.

Relevant Constitutional Provisions

Article 41 of the Constitution

Article 41 of Directive Principles of State Policy has particular relevance to Old Age Social Security. According to Article 41 of the constitution of India, "the state shall, within the limits of its economic capacity and development, make effective provision for securing the right to work, to education and to public assistance in cases of unemployment, old age, sickness and disablement and in other cases of undeserved want."

Article 47 of the Constitution

Article 47 of the constitution of India provides that the state shall regard the raising of the level of nutrition and the standard of living of its people and improvement of public health as among its primary duties.

Some Other Constitutional Provisions

- Entry 24 in list III of schedule VII of constitution of India deals with the welfare of labour, including conditions of work, provident funds, liability for workmen's compensation, invalidity and old age pension and maternity benefits.
- Further, item 9 of the state list and item 20, 23 and 24 of concurrent list relates to old age pension, social security and social insurance, and economic and social planning. The right of parents, without any means, to be supported by their children having sufficient means has been recognized by section 125(1) (d) of the Code of Criminal Procedure 1973, and section 20 (1 & 3) of the Hindu Adoption and Maintenance Act, 1956.

■ LEGISLATIONS

Maintenance and Welfare of Parents and Senior Citizens Act, 2007

- The Maintenance and Welfare of Parents and Senior Citizens Act, 2007 was enacted in December 2007, inter alia, to ensure need based maintenance for parents and senior citizens and their welfare. The Act shall come into force in a State on such date as the State Government may, by notification in the Official Gazette, appoint. So far, all the States and UTs have notified the Act. The Act does not extend to the state of Jammu and Kashmir. Himachal Pradesh has its own Act for welfare of Parents and Senior Citizens.
- The Act provides for:
  - Maintenance of Parents/senior citizens by children/relatives made obligatory and justiciable through Tribunals
  - Revocation of transfer of property by senior citizens in case of negligence by relatives
  - Penal provision for abandonment of senior citizens
  - Establishment of Old Age Homes for Indigent Senior Citizens
  - Protection of life and property of senior citizens
  - Adequate medical facilities for Senior Citizens
- Consequent upon notifying the Act, State Governments/UT Administration are required to take the following necessary measures/steps for effective implementation of the Act:
  - Frame Rules under Section 32;
  - Appoint Maintenance Officers under Section 18 (1);
  - Constitute Maintenance Tribunals under Section 7 (1);
  - Constitute Appellate Tribunals under Section 15 (1).
- The status implementation of the Act is also discussed in Annual Regional Conferences held with the State/UT Social Welfare Departments/Ministers, as well as during the visit of senior Ministry Officers during their visit to the States/UTs.

Contributions to Society

- Elderly people carry immense experience of their personal and professional life, society at large need to channelize those experience for better tomorrow.
- They can provide a vital generational link for upcoming generations. It provides support and stability to families and society at large.

- Grandparents in joint families provide a crucial link for transferring values and morals to the younger generation in their initial years, thereby contributing towards upbringing of better human beings and responsible citizens.
- Acknowledging seniors' contributions would help to make ours a more age-inclusive that does not pit one generation against the other.
- Their deep cultural impressions and social experiences provide the necessary buffer against intolerance, violence and hate crimes which provides stability in society especially in the era of hate and crime. They can play a significant role in easing out societal tensions, both within and outside families through their insight and understanding.

What measures can be taken?

- Increasing the monthly pension of elderly to minimum of ₹ 2,000 per month.
- Under Pradhan Mantri Awas Yojana, Housing for the aged, particularly the aged poor, must be a priority.
- Assisted living facilities for indigent elderly, particularly those with age-related issues like dementia, needs policy focus.
- More tax benefits, or at least removing tax on deposit interest for seniors.
- Enhancing the geriatric care health infrastructure especially in rural area.
- Allocation of special budget for elderly population at both levels.
- Providing entertainment facilities like libraries and clubs at panchayat level.
- Appreciations for the contributions of elderlies at village level.

CONCLUSION

- Social security is the concurrent responsibility of the central and state governments as, mandated under Indian constitution, i.e., Well-being of senior citizens – Article 41 in particular and 46 in general of Indian constitution. In this regard, National Policy on Senior Citizen, 2011 was framed.
- For the welfare and care for the older persons, we must focus on the protection of already existing social support systems/traditional social institutions such as family and kinship, neighborhood bonding, community bonding and community participation must be revived and kins should show sensitivity towards elderly citizens.

REFERENCE

1. Government of India. Ministry of Statistics and Programme Implementation National Statistical Office; 2021.

CHAPTER 19

Wheelchair Management

Shyam D Ganvir

LEARNING OBJECTIVES

Through this chapter, the reader will be able to:
- Understand about wheelchair users and the problems faced by them.
- Gain insight about right of wheelchair users and benefits of wheelchair.
- Acquire knowledge about the wheelchair measurements and wheelchair user's needs.
- Understand in depth about pressure sore, its management, cushion and transfer board.
- Assess to different scales used to assess person with disabilities.

■ WHEELCHAIR USERS

Wheelchair users are people who already have a wheelchair or who can benefit from using a wheelchair because their ability to walk is limited. Wheelchair users include:
- Children, adults and the elderly; men, women, girls and boys;
- People with different mobility impairments, lifestyles, life roles and backgrounds;
- People living and working in different environments including rural, semi-urban and urban.

The needs of each wheelchair user will vary. However, they all need an appropriate wheelchair.

■ NEED FOR WHEELCHAIRS

About 10% of the global population, i.e., about 650 million people, have disabilities. Studies indicate that, of these, some 10% require a wheelchair. It is thus estimated that about 1% of a total population – or 10% of a disabled population—need wheelchairs, i.e., about 65 million people worldwide. In 2003, it was estimated that 20 million of those requiring a wheelchair for mobility did not have one. There are indications that only a minority of those in need of wheelchairs have access to them, and of these very few have access to an appropriate wheelchair.

■ RIGHTS TO WHEELCHAIRS

States Parties to the Convention on the Rights of Persons with Disabilities have the obligation "to take effective measures to ensure personal mobility with the greatest possible independence for persons with disabilities". This is a commitment to provide mobility aids, such as wheelchairs, that make personal mobility possible. In 1993, the Standard Rules on the Equalization of

Opportunities for Persons with Disabilities expressed the same commitment, demanding that countries ensure the development, production, distribution and servicing of assistive devices for people with disabilities in order to increase their independence and to realize their human rights. These two important international declarations create rights to wheelchairs because it is universally recognized that an appropriate wheelchair is a precondition to enjoying equal opportunities and rights, and for securing inclusion and participation. Personal mobility is an essential requirement to participating in many areas of social life, and wheelchairs are for many the best means of guaranteeing personal mobility.

Independent mobility makes it possible for people to study, work, participate in cultural life and access healthcare. Without wheelchairs, people may be confined to their homes and unable to live a full and inclusive life. We know that eliminating world poverty is not possible unless the needs of those with disabilities are taken into account. Without wheelchairs, these individuals are unable to participate in those mainstream developmental initiatives, programs and strategies that are targeted to the poor, such as are embodied in the Millennium Development Goals, the Poverty Reduction Strategies and other national developmental initiatives.

It is a vicious circle: lacking personal mobility aids, people with disabilities cannot leave the poverty trap. They are more likely to develop secondary complications and become more disabled, and poorer still. If they are children they will be unable to access the educational opportunities available to them, and without an education they will be unable to find employment when they grow up and will be driven even more deeply into poverty.

On the other hand, access to appropriate wheelchairs allows people with disabilities to work and participate in mainstream development initiatives that will reduce their poverty. Similarly, a wheelchair can enable a child to go to school, to gain an education and, when the time comes, to find a job.

The right to a wheelchair must be an essential component of all international endeavours to secure the human rights of people with disabilities.

■ BENEFIT OF WHEELCHAIRS

Wheelchair provision is not only about the wheelchair, which is just a product. Rather, it is about enabling people with disabilities to become mobile, remain healthy and participate fully in community life. A wheelchair is the catalyst to increased independence and social integration, but it is not an end in itself.

The benefits of using an appropriate wheelchair include those outlined below.

■ HEALTH AND QUALITY OF LIFE

In addition to providing mobility, an appropriate wheelchair is of benefit to the physical health and quality of life of the user. Combined with adequate user training, an appropriate wheelchair can serve to reduce common problems such as pressure sores, the progression of deformities or contractures, and other secondary conditions. A wheelchair with a proper cushion often prevents premature death in people with spinal cord injuries and similar conditions and, in one sense, is a life-saving device for these people. A wheelchair that is functional, comfortable and can be propelled efficiently can result in increased levels of activity. Independent mobility and increased physical function can reduce dependence on others. Other benefits, such as improved respiration and digestion, increased head, trunk and upper extremity control and overall stability, can be achieved with proper postural support. Maintenance of health is an important factor in measuring quality of life. These factors combined serve to increase access to opportunities for education, employment and participation within the family and the community.

■ECONOMY

A wheelchair often makes all the difference between being a passive receiver and an active contributor. Economic benefits are realized when users are able to access opportunities for education and employment. With a wheelchair, an individual can earn a living and contribute to the family's income and national revenue, whereas without a wheelchair that person may remain isolated and be a burden to the family and the nation at large. Similarly, a wheelchair that is not durable will be more expensive owing to the need for frequent repairs, absence from work and eventual replacement of the wheelchair. Providing wheelchairs is more cost-effective if they last longer. It is also more cost-effective if users are involved in selecting their devices and if their long-term needs are considered. For society, the financial benefits associated with the provision of wheelchairs include reduced healthcare expenses, such as those for treating pressure sores and correcting deformities. A study from a developing country reported that in 1997, 75% of those with spinal cord injuries admitted to hospital died within 18–24 months from secondary complications arising from their injuries. In the same place, the incidence of pressure sores decreased by 71% and repetitive urinary tract infections fell by 61% within two years as a result of improvements in healthcare training and appropriate equipment, including good wheelchairs with cushions.

Factors that Affect Selection of Wheelchair

- Level and completeness of injury
- Medical complications
- Functional skills
- Physical attributes
- Accessibility
- Previous life activities
- Transportation
- Funding

Wheelchair Measurements

Four measurements from the wheelchair user are needed to choose the best available size of wheelchair for that person. Each measurement relates to the wheelchair.

	Body Measurement		Measurement (mm)	Change body measurement to ideal wheelchair size	Wheelchair measurement (mm)
A	Hip width			Hip width = seat width	
B	Seat depth	L		B less 30-60 mm = seat depth (if length is different, use shorter one)	
		R			
C	Calf length	L		= top of seat cushion to footrests height or = top of seat cushion to floor for foot propelling	
		R			
D	Bottom of rib cage			= top of seat cushion to top of backrest (measure D or E - depending on the user's need)	
E	Bottom of shoulder blade				

SECTION 4: Elderly Individuals and their Services

How to Take Body Measurements

- Ask the wheelchair user to sit as upright as possible.
- The wheelchair user's feet should be supported on the floor or on foot-blocks if they cannot reach the floor comfortably.
- For all measurements, make sure the tape measure is held straight and the wheelchair user is sitting upright. Holding a clipboard/book on either side of the wheelchair user can help in obtaining an accurate measurement.
- Bend down to ensure you are viewing the tape measure at the correct angle.

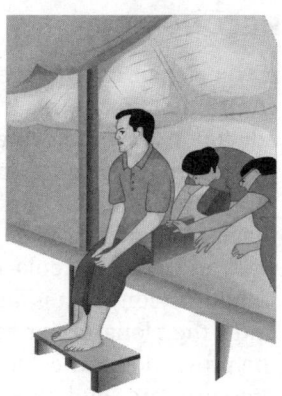

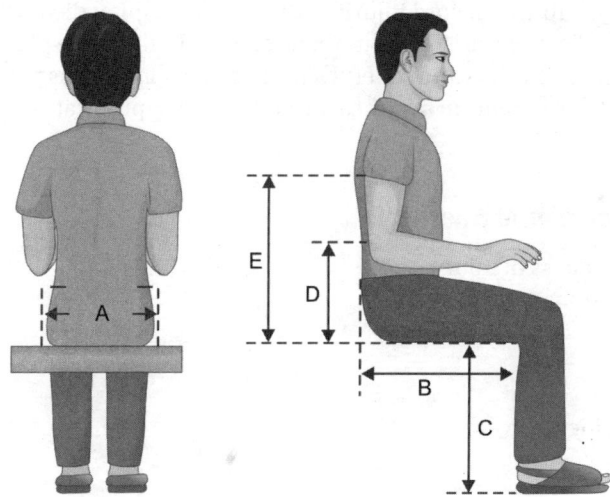

A	• Check there is nothing in wheelchair user's pockets before measuring. • Measure hips or widest part of thighs. • Holding two clipboards/books against each side of the wheelchair user can help in obtaining an accurate measurement.
B	• Place a clipboard/book at the back of the wheelchair user to help get an accurate measurement. • Measure from the back of the pelvis to the back of the knee in a straight line. • Always measure both legs. If there is a difference between the two legs, check that the wheelchair user is sitting up with the pelvis level. If there is still a difference, make the wheelchair prescription for the shorter side.
C	• Measure from the back of the knee to the base of the heel. • Make sure the wheelchair user's ankles are bent at 90 degrees (if possible). • Always measure both legs. • The wheelchair user should wear the shoes he/she wears most days (if any).
D	• Measure the seat to the bottom of the rib cage. • To help find the bottom of the rib cage, place hands on both sides of the pelvis. Gently squeeze hands inwards and slide hands upwards. The bottom of the rib cage is just above the waist.
E	• Measure from the seat to the bottom of the shoulder blade in a vertical line. • To help find the bottom of the shoulder blade, ask the user to shrug his/her shoulders.

CHAPTER 19: Wheelchair Management

■ PARTS OF WHEELCHAIR

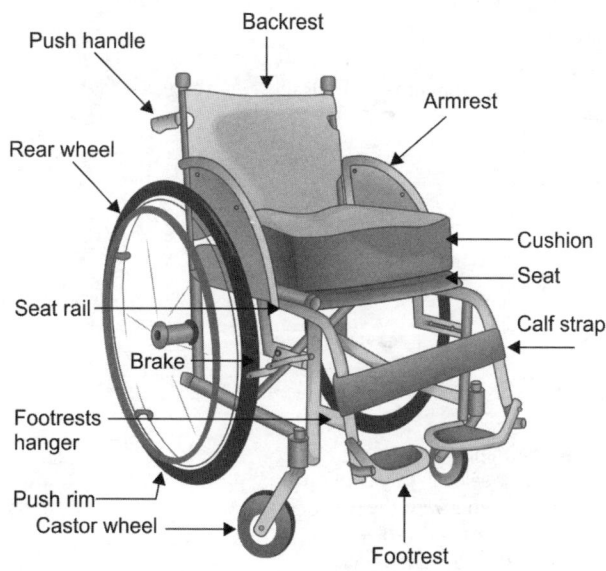

■ WHEELCHAIR SERVICES

Wheelchair services work with wheelchair users to find the most suitable wheelchair among those available for that user. The WHO Wheelchair guidelines outline eight steps that wheelchair service personnel need to carry out to provide a wheelchair. These steps are summarized below:

Steps	Summary
Referral and appointment	The way that wheelchair users are referred will vary. Users may refer themselves or be referred through networks made up of governmental or nongovernmental health and rehabilitation workers or volunteers working at community, district or regional level. Some wheelchair services may need to identify potential users actively if they are not already receiving any social or healthcare services or participating in school, work or community activities.

Steps	Summary	
Assessment	Each user needs an individual assessment, taking into account lifestyle work environment and physical condition.	
Prescription (selection)	Using the information from the assessment, a wheelchair prescription is developed together with the user and family members or caregivers. The prescription (selection) details the selected wheelchair type and size, special features and modifications. It also describes the training the user needs in order to use and maintain the wheelchair properly.	
Funding and ordering	A funding source is identified, and the wheelchair is ordered from stock held by the service or from the supplier.	
Product (wheelchair) preparation	Trained personnel prepare the wheelchair for the initial fitting. Depending on the available product and service facilities, this may include assembly, and possible modification, of products supplied by manufacturers or manufacture of products in the service workshop.	

CHAPTER 19: Wheelchair Management

Steps	Summary	
Fitting	The user tries the wheelchair. Final adjustments are made to ensure the wheelchair is correctly assembled and set up. If modifications or postural support components are required, additional fittings may be necessary.	
User training	The user and caregivers are trained how to use and maintain the wheelchair safely and effectively.	
Maintenance, repairs and follow up	The wheelchair service provides maintenance and repair services for technical problems that cannot be solved in the community. It is appropriate to carry out follow-up activities at the community level as much as possible. Follow-up appointments are an opportunity to check wheelchair fit and provide further training and support. The timing depends on the needs of the user and the other services that are available to them. If the wheelchair is found to be no longer appropriate, a new wheelchair needs to be supplied starting again from step one.	

Source: World Health Organization. Guidelines on the provision of manual wheelchairs in less resourced settings, Table 3.2. Geneva, 2008:76.

SECTION 4: Elderly Individuals and their Services

Wheelchair Mobility Skills

Pushing
- Pushing correctly requires less effort.
- Push from 10 o'clock to 2 o'clock position.
- Use long smooth action to push.

Turning
- Hold one push rim towards the front and the other towards the back.
- Pull the forwards hand backwards and push the backward hand forwards at the same time.

Up slopes
- Lean forward—this helps to stop the wheelchair tipping.
- When practicing, have an assistant stand behind for safety.
- To stop or rest—park the wheelchair sideways on.

CHAPTER 19: Wheelchair Management

Down Slopes	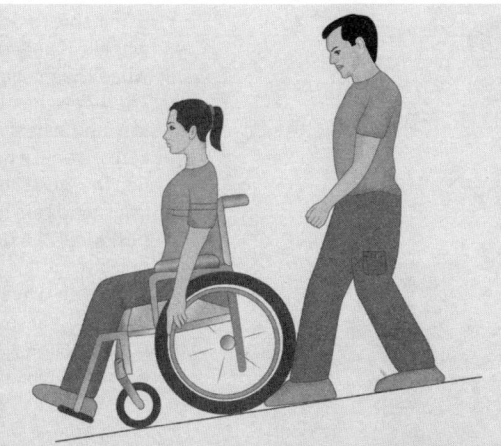	• Lean backwards. • Let the push rim slide slowly through the hands. • Experienced wheelchair users who are able to do a "wheelie" (i.e., balance the wheelchair on the rear wheels only) may roll down a slope on their back wheels. This is very efficient.
Up steps with assistance	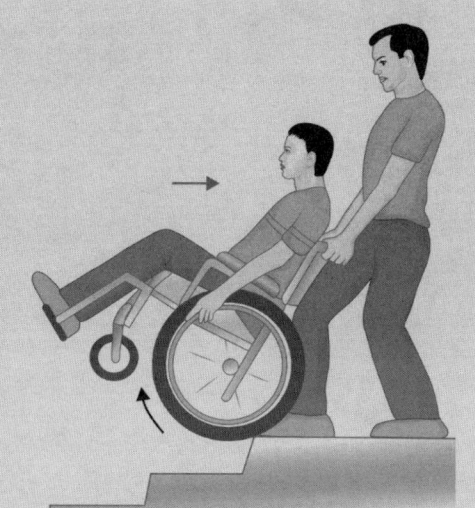	• Go up backwards. • Tilt wheelchair on to back wheels, positioned against the first step. • Assistant pulls backwards and upwards—rolling the wheelchair up. • Wheelchair user can assist by pushing the push rim backwards. • A second assistant can assist by holding on to the wheelchair frame from the front (not footrests).
Down steps with assistance	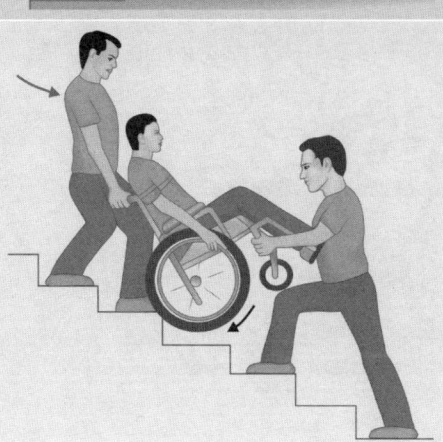	• Go down forwards. • Tilt the wheelchair on to back wheels. • Assistant lets the back wheels roll down slowly, one step at a time. • Wheelchair user can assist by controlling the wheelchair with the push rims. • A second assistant can help by steadying the wheelchair from the front, holding on to the wheelchair frame (not footrests).

Partial wheelie

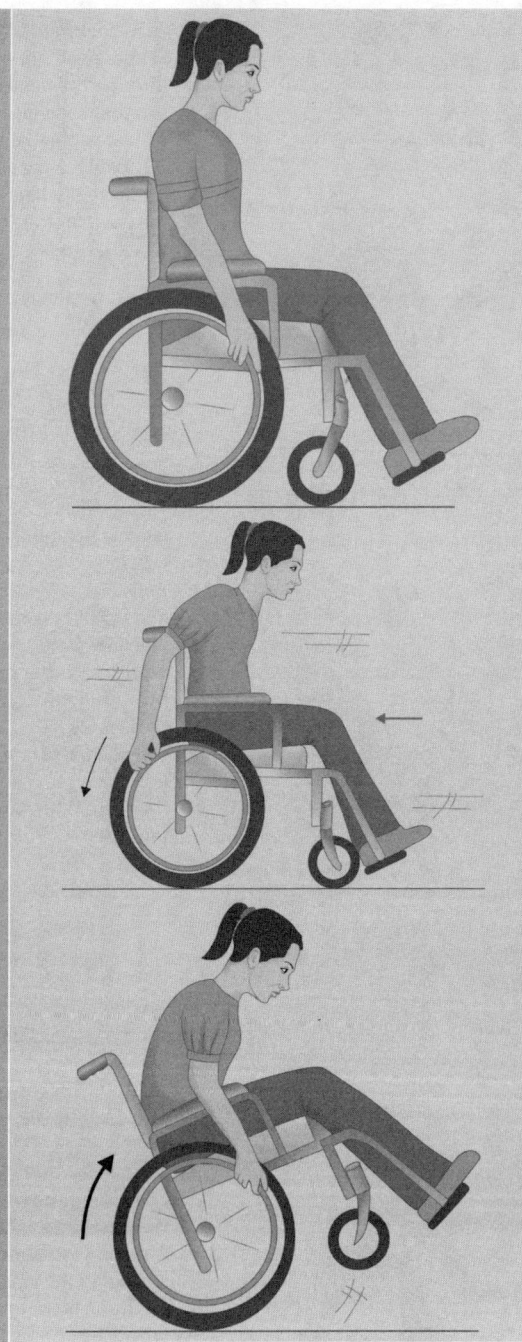

- Being able to do a partial wheelie is very useful for a wheelchair user.
- The wheelchair user can lift the front wheels to clear small kerbs, stones and bumps.
- Roll the wheelchair backwards until hands are in the 10 o'clock position. Then push forwards quickly.
- The castor wheels should come up.
- With practice, it is possible to lift the castor wheels at the right time to clear small obstacles.
- Always make sure that there is an assistant standing behind the wheelchair user when he/she begins to practise this skill.

How to make wheelchair mobility skills training safe

- Do not stand on footrests when getting in and out of the wheelchair.
- Keep fingers clear of the wheel spokes and brakes.
- When learning how to go up hills, or doing a partial wheelie, ALWAYS have an assistant stand behind the person in the wheelchair.
- Do not assist a wheelchair user up and down steps unless you feel very sure that you are able to control the wheelchair safely. If unsure, get help.

■ PRESSURE SORE

A pressure sore is an area of damaged skin and flesh. A pressure sore can develop in a few hours, but the results can last for many months and even cause death.

What Causes Pressure Sores?

The three main causes of pressure sores are the following:
1. **Pressure:** Pressure sores can be caused by pressure on skin from sitting or lying in the same position for too long without moving. Wheelchair users are particularly at risk, because they may spend a long time each day sitting in their wheelchair. Unless the pressure is relieved, a pressure sore can quickly develop.
2. **Friction:** Friction is constant rubbing on the skin. For example, an arm rubbing on a wheel/armrest as a wheelchair is moved can cause a pressure sore.
3. **Shear:** Shear is when the skin stays still and is stretched or pinched as muscles or bones move.

How Can Pressure Sores be Prevented?

- **Use a pressure relief cushion:** A pressure relief cushion will help to reduce pressure. Anyone at risk of developing a pressure sore should be given a pressure relief cushion.
- **Sit upright:** Sitting upright helps to distribute weight evenly. This reduces pressure under bony parts and helps to reduce sores caused by pressure. Sitting upright also helps to avoid pressure sores caused by shear. Wheelchair service personnel can help wheelchair users to sit upright by making sure the wheelchair fits correctly and explaining why it is important to sit upright.
- **Use pressure relief techniques:** Regular pressure relief can be effective in preventing pressure sores.

Pressure relief techniques
- **Bending forward:** A method suitable for most wheelchair users.
- **Side to side leaning:** A method suitable for wheelchair users with limited strength and balance.

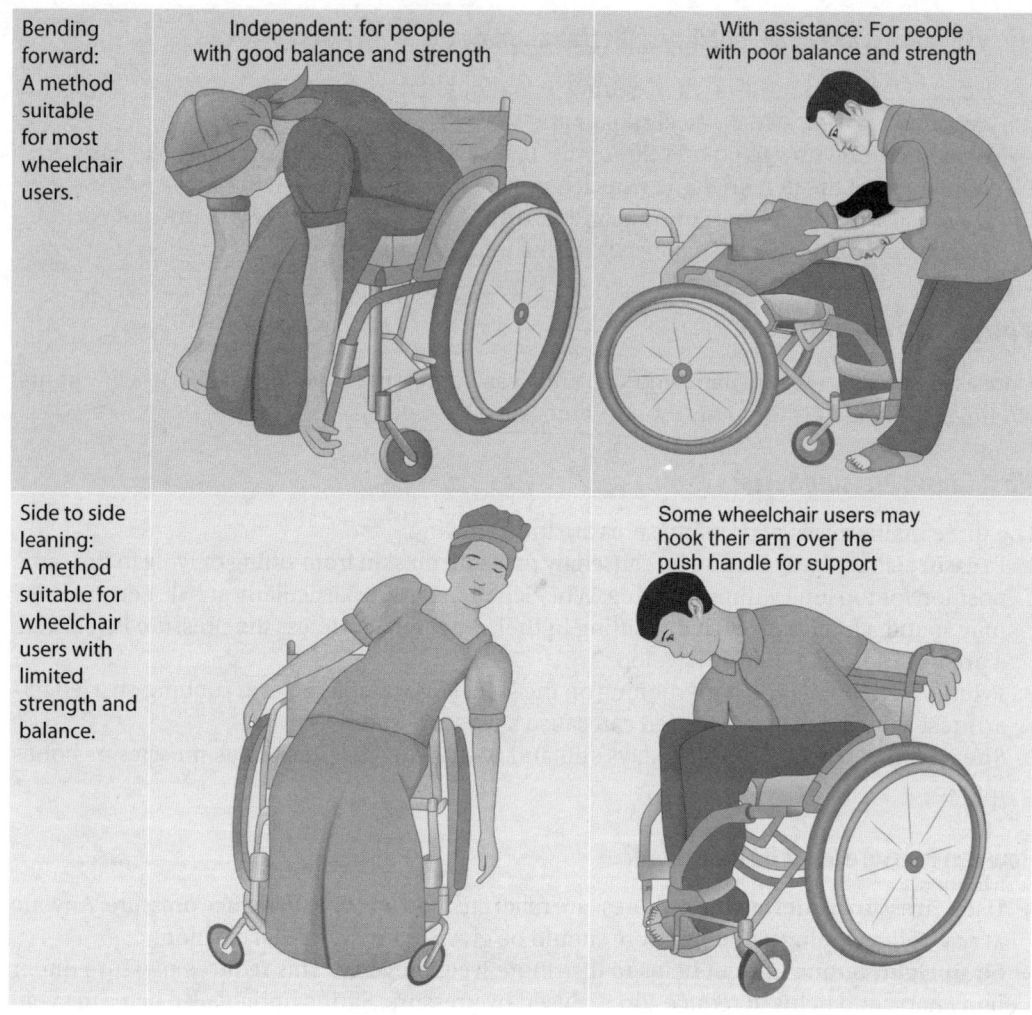

Bending forward: A method suitable for most wheelchair users.

Independent: for people with good balance and strength

With assistance: For people with poor balance and strength

Side to side leaning: A method suitable for wheelchair users with limited strength and balance.

Some wheelchair users may hook their arm over the push handle for support

Eat well and drink lots of water: A well balanced diet with fresh vegetables, fruits and meat can help to prevent pressure sores. Drinking lots of water will help to keep the skin healthy and prevent pressure sores. If you are concerned about a wheelchair user's diet – consider referring him/her to a service that can help.

Avoid friction: Make sure the wheelchair fits correctly and has no rough edges. Teach wheelchair users who cannot feel to check that no parts of their body are being rubbed by the wheelchair. Teach wheelchair users to take care when getting in and out of the wheelchair.

Avoid moisture: Wheelchair users need to be advised to change wet or soiled clothing straight away, and not to use a wet cushion. A bowel and bladder management program can reduce problems with moisture. Refer wheelchair users who have a problem with incontinence to a service that can help them.

Check skin every day: Pressure sores can develop quickly. It is important to identify a pressure sore quickly and take action. Encourage wheelchair users who are at risk to check their skin every day. They can check themselves using a mirror, or ask a family member to check. If they see a red or dark area of the skin (stage 1 pressure sore), they should take all necessary measures to relieve pressure on that spot immediately.

While lying or sitting, change positions regularly: Changing position regularly helps to relieve pressure. For example, change position from sitting to lying. This is particularly important for someone who has a number of pressure sore risk factors, or has a recently healed pressure sore. People who cannot change position by themselves are at risk.

	The four stages of a pressure sore[3]	What to do
1.	A red or dark mark on the person's skin. The redness or change in colour does not fade within 30 minutes after Pressure is removed	• Remove pressure from that area immediately. • Keep pressure off until the skin has fully healed. This may mean bed-rest. • Identify the cause and address this. • Teach the wheelchair user how pressure sores are formed and how to prevent them in future.
2.	A shallow wound. The top layer of skin may start to peel away or blister.	Follow the actions for stage I. Refer for treatment of the pressure sore to an experienced healthcare worker.
3.	A deep wound; the whole layer of skin is lost.	Open pressure sores will need cleaning, dressing and close monitoring to ensure they are healing and do not become infected.
4.	A very deep wound, extending through the muscle and possibly right down to the bone.	Stage 4 wounds may require surgery.

■ APPROPRIATE WHEELCHAIR

An "Appropriate Wheelchair" is a wheelchair that:
❖ Meets the user's needs;
❖ Meets the user's environment;
❖ Is the right match for the user;
❖ Ensures postural support (helps the user to sit upright);
❖ Can be maintained and repaired locally.

Meeting the Wheelchair User's Needs

An appropriate wheelchair should make it easier for wheelchair users to carry out the things they need to do. Wheelchair users need to be able to get in and out of their wheelchair, to push their wheelchair, to fold the wheelchair for transport and storage and carry out their daily activities. The right type of wheelchair can make it easier for the wheelchair user to do all these things. See the examples below.

Transfers

Getting in and Out of the Wheelchair

Wheelchair users get in and out of the wheelchair in different ways, depending on their physical ability. Different wheelchair features can make their transfers easier. Three features that make transfers easier are: armrests, footrests, and brakes.

Removable armrests, or armrests which follow the line of the rear wheels, are easier for people who get in and out of their wheelchair sideways.

People who stand up to get in and out of the wheelchair may need armrests to help them stand up.

Footrests which can be moved out of the way are helpful for people who stand up to get in and out of the wheelchair. People who want to transfer to the floor may prefer a wheelchair with removable footrests.

Brakes are important for all wheelchair users. They are essential for keeping the wheelchair still while the person gets in and out of the wheelchair.

Pushing the Wheelchair

Wheelchair users propel their wheelchair in different ways. Many wheelchair users propel the wheelchair with their arms. Some wheelchair users push the wheelchair with their feet—or with one arm and one foot. Some wheelchair users need someone to push the wheelchair for them some or all of the time. Pushing the wheelchair by hand propelling is easier when the armrests and backrest are the right height.

When the backrest is lower, the wheelchair user has freedom to move the shoulders to push. For a wheelchair user who can sit upright and has good balance, this is a good height for the backrest.

Pushing the wheelchair is easier if the wheelchair user can reach the push rims comfortably.

The rear wheel should be positioned so that when the wheelchair user holds the top of the push rim the elbow is bent at 90 degrees. This is a good pushing position.

If the wheel is further back, it is more tiring for the wheelchair user to push. Some wheelchairs have an adjustable rear wheel position. The position of the rear wheels affects how easy it is to push the wheelchair into a wheelie. Wheelies are useful for going over rough ground, up and down kerbs or down slopes.

If the rear wheels move forwards, the wheelchair is easier to push into a wheelie.

If the rear wheels move backwards, they become more stable but the wheelchair is harder to push and it is harder to perform a wheelie.

Pushing the wheelchair with the feet is easier if the wheelchair user has enough power in one leg and can sit with the pelvis supported by the wheelchair backrest and the feet flat on the floor.

For wheelchair users who push with their feet, the height of the seat from the floor (including the cushion) is very important. Footrests that swing out of the way are also essential. Some users who push with their feet may like a tray or armrests so that they can lean forward while pushing.

A heavy wheelchair takes more energy to push—whether hands, feet or assistant-propelled. However, if the wheelchair is well designed and well balanced, the weight may not be such a problem. The weight of the wheelchair is particularly important in the case of children. If the wheelchair is heavy, this may make the chair hard for the child to control.

Folding the Wheelchair

To transport or store the wheelchair, it needs to fold. Wheelchairs fold in two main ways. Wheelchairs with a cross-folding frame fold so that both sides come together. Sometimes it is possible to remove the wheels as well.

Cross-folding wheelchairs can be helpful for wheelchair users needing to "squeeze" through narrow doorways. For transport, some people prefer a cross-folding wheelchair. For example, it may fit better in the aisle of a bus.

A disadvantage with some cross-folding frames is that the folding mechanism can weaken, making the wheelchair feel unstable. It then becomes harder to push.

Some rigid frame wheelchairs also fold. However, instead of the two sides folding together, the backrest folds down and the rear wheels come off. One advantage of rigid frames is that they can be more durable, as there are fewer moving parts.

Carrying Out Activities

There are several features of a wheelchair which affect how easily a wheelchair user can carry out the activities of daily life. For example, the features that help a wheelchair user to push (described above) will dictate how easily he/she can participate in activities. Here are some other examples.

Wheelchair frame length: The overall length of a wheelchair can affect how easy or difficult it is to use in small spaces. For someone who spends a lot of time indoors, a wheelchair with a short length may be the best choice. The frame length is measured from the furthest back part of the wheelchair to the furthest front part.

Armrests: High armrests may make it difficult for the user to get close to a table or desk.

Meeting the Wheelchair User's Environment

Different types of Wheelchair are suited to different environments. The main features which affect how a wheelchair works in a different environment are:
* Distance between the front and rear wheels (wheelbase);
* The size and width of the wheels.

Distance between the front and rear wheels (wheelbase). The distance between the front and rear wheels is important.

When the wheels are further apart, this is called a "long-wheelbase". When the wheels are closer together, this is a "short-wheelbase".

Long-wheelbase wheelchairs are more stable and less likely to tip forward. They can be a good choice for a person who will spend most of the time outdoors and moving over rough or uneven surfaces.

There are three-wheel and four-wheel long-wheelbase wheelchairs.

Three-wheel long-wheelbase wheelchairs are usually very stable and suitable for outdoors on rough terrain.

The four-wheel long-wheelbase wheelchairs have the front castor wheels under the footrests instead of behind. This gives the wheelchairs a longer wheelbase.

Shorter-wheelbase wheelchairs are more suited to use in places where the ground is flat or the space is confined—indoors, for example. Short-wheelbase wheelchairs are more likely to tip forward if going downhill, or if the front wheels hit a bump.

Wheelchair users with good mobility skills may use a short-wheelbase wheelchair outdoors by balancing on the back wheels to go down hills and over rough ground.

Size and Width of Wheels

The larger the wheel, the easier it is to push over uneven ground. Wide rear wheels and large and wide front castors help prevent the wheelchair from sinking into sandy or muddy ground.

Providing Proper Fit and Postural Support

All wheelchair users are different sizes. The wheelchair must fit the user correctly to provide proper fit and support. Fortunately, many wheelchairs come in a range of different sizes, or have size adjustments. It is easier to make sure these wheelchairs fit the user than if there is only one size available. The following components or features of a wheelchair will affect how well the wheelchair fits and how well it helps the user to sit upright.

Seats

Seats: Wheelchair seats may be either solid or slung. The picture on the left shows a solid seat. Solid seats may be made from wood or plastic. Solid seats should always have a cushion over the top. Slung seats are usually made from canvas. Slung seats are made from fabric attached to each side of the frame. Poor-quality slung seats can sometimes stretch and sag so they fail to provide good support. The man pictured on the left is sitting in a wheelchair with a slung seat which has become loose and saggy. It does not provide him with support. This makes it difficult for him to sit upright.

Backrests: Backrests may be slung or solid. All solid backrests should have some padding/cushioning. Wheelchairs come with different backrest heights. Some wheelchairs have adjustable backrest heights. The correct backrest height needs to be selected for each user.

Armrests: Armrests can also provide support. Some armrests are height-adjustable. If they are not, they can sometimes be modified to give more support for a user who needs it.

Cushions: The cushion provides comfort, helps to relieve pressure, and also provides support and helps to stop the user from sliding.

Footrests: Footrests help to support the user. It is very important that footrests are adjusted correctly. For this reason, the height of the footrests is usually adjustable. Some footrests can also be adjusted by angle, and the distance away from the wheelchair.

■ WHEELCHAIR SPECIFICATIONS

Prepare the wheelchair in the following order:
- ❖ Check that the wheelchair seat width and depth measurements are correct for the prescription (selection).
- ❖ Check that the cushion width and depth match the seat.
- ❖ Adjust (where possible):
  - Backrest height and angle;
  - Armrests height;
  - Rear wheels position;
  - Brakes position;
  - Footrests height;
  - Push handles height;
  - Any other adjustments.
- ❖ Carry out a "wheelchair safe and ready" check.

CHAPTER 19: Wheelchair Management

Wheelchair Safe and Ready Checklist

Use the checklist below to make sure that the wheelchair is safe to use and all parts are working. Always do this before the wheelchair user tries the wheelchair.

Checklist: Is the wheelchair safe and ready to use?

For the whole wheelchair		How to check
There are no sharp edges.	☐	Check all over the wheelchair with eyes and hands.
No parts are damaged or scratched.	☐	
The wheelchair travels in a straight line.	☐	Push the wheelchair away from you, making sure the castor wheels are in the "trail" position.
Front castor wheels		
Spin freely.	☐	Tip the wheelchair on to the back wheels. Spin the castor wheels.
Spin without touching the fork.	☐	
Bolts are tight.	☐	Check. They should feel firm, do not over tighten.
Front castor barrels		
Castor fork spins freely.	☐	Tip the wheelchair on to the back wheels. Spin the castor fork around.
Rear wheels		
Spin freely.	☐	Tip the wheelchair sideways on to one rear wheel. Spin the other wheel. Check the other side.
Axle bolts are tight.	☐	Check. They should feel firm. Do not over tighten.
Tyres (if those are pneumatic) are inflated correctly,	☐	Press on the tyres with your thumb. The wheel should depress a little, but no more than 5 mm.
Push rims are secure.		Check.
Brakes		
Function properly.	☐	Apply brakes. Check the wheelchair cannot be moved.
Footrests		
Footrests are securely attached.	☐	Check.
Frame		
Cross-folding wheelchair folds and unfolds easily.	☐	Fold the wheelchair to check that the folding mechanisms are working correctly.
Fold-down backrest—the backrest folds and unfolds easily.	☐	
Cushion		
The cushion is in the cover correctly.	☐	Usually the cushion cover is done up at the back of the cushion, underneath.
The cushion is sitting on the wheelchair correctly.	☐	If the cushion is contoured, the "well" for the seat bones should be at the back of the seat.
The cushion cover fabric is tight but not too tight.	☐	The cushion cover should not stretch tightly over any contours of the cushion.
The cushion fully covers the seat.	☐	Check that no part of the seat is visible from under the cushion. This is particularly important for solid seats.

■ CUSHION

A cushion is a very important part of every wheelchair. Cushions provide:
- Comfort;
- Posture support (help people to sit more upright);
- Pressure relief.

All wheelchair users should be comfortable in their wheelchair, and a good cushion helps them to sit upright easily and comfortably. That is why every wheelchair user should have a cushion. It is not necessary for every wheelchair user to have a pressure relief cushion.

Different Types of Cushions

Cushions can be described in different ways, including:
- The material they are made from (for example, foam, coir);
- The material they are filled with (for example, air, fluid or gel);
- Their main function (for example, pressure relief, comfort, posture support);
- Their shape (for example, flat or contoured);
- How they are made (for example, foam cushions may be "moulded" from one piece of foam or "layered"—made from a number of layers of foam).

The most commonly available cushion is a foam cushion. Foam cushions are also usually the least expensive. They are easy to make where foam is available and easy to modify to suit individual wheelchair users.

Who needs a Cushion?

Every wheelchair user should have a cushion.

Wheelchair users at risk of developing a pressure sore should use a pressure relief cushion.

Pressure Relief Cushions

There are different types of pressure relief cushions including:
- Foam contoured pressure relief cushions;
- Air/fluid/gel filled cushions.

Foam Pressure Relief Cushions

The key features of a foam pressure relief cushion are the following:

Firm stable base: The base of a pressure relief cushion should be firm. This will make sure the cushion provides good support for the user and does not move when the user moves.

Top layer: Over the base layer there should be a "comfort layer". This is a layer (or more than one layer) of softer foam. The top layer should be soft enough to allow the seat bones to sink into it, but should not be so soft that the seat bones can sink all the way to the bottom and rest on the solid base or seat of the wheelchair.

Advantages
- Can be made locally (where there is high-quality foam).
- Can be modified locally to accommodate different needs.

❖ Not subject to "sudden collapse" (a puncture in the air/fluid/gel cushions can cause the release of the materials from the cushion and stop the cushion from relieving pressure, causing "sudden collapse" of the cushion).
❖ The top layer of a layered foam cushion can be replaced easily and at a low cost (rather than replacing the whole cushion).

Pressure relief cushions help to reduce pressure by:
❖ Distributing a wheelchair user's weight as evenly as possible across the seat surface;
❖ Reducing pressure under high-pressure risk areas (seat bones, hip bones, coccyx/tail bone);
❖ Reducing shear by assisting the wheelchair user to sit upright.

Shaping on a Pressure Relief Cushion

Pressure relief cushions vary. Shaping that you may see on a pressure relief cushion includes:
❖ A "well" under the seat bones to reduce pressure;
❖ Support under the hip bones to help distribute weight;
❖ A shelf in front of the seat bones to keep the pelvis more upright and prevent sliding forward;
❖ Grooves or gutters for the legs.

Air/Fluid/Gel Pressure Relief Cushions

❖ Flotation cushions include those filled with air and those that have a fluid or gel pack.
❖ Gel-pack cushions should have a firm foam base very similar to a foam contoured cushion.
❖ Over the base layer there is a gel/fluid pack.
❖ The gel pack automatically matches the shape of the wheelchair user's body. This helps to distribute the user's weight evenly and reduces pressure under bony areas

Advantages

Pressure is distributed evenly over the seat surface.
   The gel pad automatically adapts to the body when the wheelchair user moves or changes position.

Cushion Covers

A pressure relief cushion should have a cover which can be removed for washing and is water-resistant. The material used for a pressure relief cushion cover should be either stretchy or loose enough to allow the seat bones to sink into the foam. If the cover fabric is not stretchy, a thin fabric is best. Folds in a thin fabric will be less likely to mark the skin and cause a pressure sore. If thin plastic is used under a fabric cover, this also needs to be loose enough to allow the seat bones to sink into the foam.
   Always advise wheelchair users that if their cushion or cushion cover becomes wet it needs to be dried and replaced only when dry. For wheelchair users who are incontinent and at risk of developing a pressure sore, provide two cushions which may be used in turn.

What to do if there is no water-resistant cushion cover?

Wherever possible, wheelchair users who are incontinent need a cushion cover which is water-resistant and will keep fluid away from the user's skin. If there is no water-resistant cover:
❖ Investigate what assistance can be provided to reduce incontinence;
❖ Provide a second cushion—so that one can be drying while the user sits on the other;

- Protect the cushion with a very thin plastic bag inside the cover.

If using a plastic bag:
- Check that the plastic bag does not cause the user to "slide" on the cushion;
- Make sure that there are no creases in the plastic bag that could cause a pressure sore;
- The wheelchair user must ensure that fluid does not "pool" over the plastic, as this increases the risk of a pressure sore;
- The wheelchair user should ensure that the cover is dried out if it becomes wet and the plastic bag cleaned or replaced.

Cushion Fabrication

If foam is available, wheelchair service personnel can make a foam pressure relief cushion with just a few tools. Personnel need to know what foam to use, and a few important dimensions. Discuss with your trainers the foams that you have available in your location, to find out which ones would be suitable for a pressure relief cushion. The instructions below show how to make a basic foam pressure relief cushion, with two key contours. These are a "well" under the seat bones and a shelf in front of the seat bones.

Cushion Features and Dimensions

The main features of the basic foam contoured cushion are the following. A base layer, made with a firm foam (for example, "chip" foam)

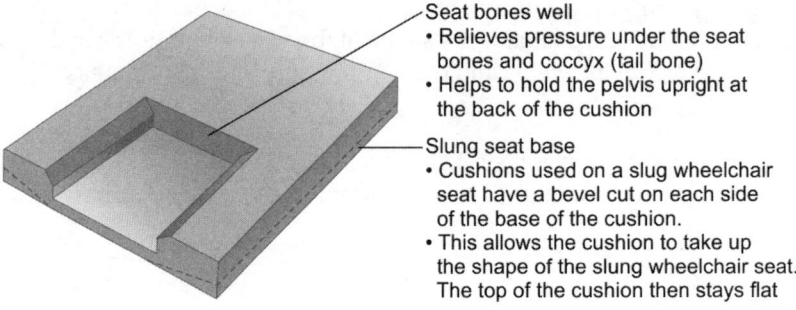

Seat bones well
- Relieves pressure under the seat bones and coccyx (tail bone)
- Helps to hold the pelvis upright at the back of the cushion

Slung seat base
- Cushions used on a slug wheelchair seat have a bevel cut on each side of the base of the cushion.
- This allows the cushion to take up the shape of the slung wheelchair seat. The top of the cushion then stays flat

1. A top layer, made with a soft "comfort" foam

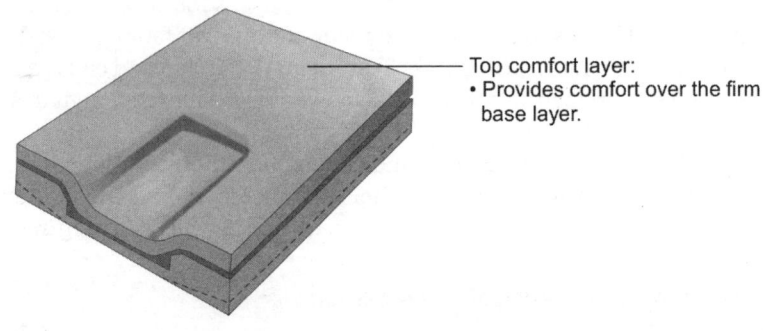

Top comfort layer:
- Provides comfort over the firm base layer.

How to Make a Pressure Relief Cushion Base?

The following instructions provide a cushion of dimensions 400 mm wide × 400 mm deep × 50 mm high. The seat bones well is 200 mm wide × 200 mm deep × 35 mm high. This cushion would be suitable for a wheelchair user with a seat width of 400 mm.

Adapt the dimensions to suit the size of each wheelchair user as described in the box below.

❖ **Mark out the cut lines on the firm foam.**
- Start with a piece of firm foam 400 mm × 400 mm × 50 mm.
- The center of the seat bones well must be on the center line of the cushion.
- For this size cushion, the seat bones well should measure 200 mm × 200 mm × 35 mm.
- Draw the cut lines with a dark colored marker on all six sides of the base foam.

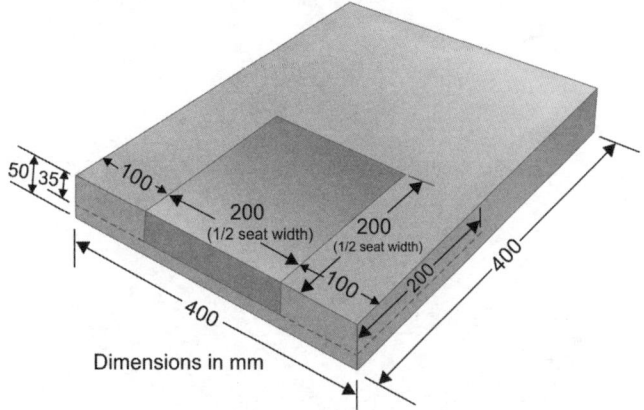

Dimensions in mm

Seat bones well dimensions

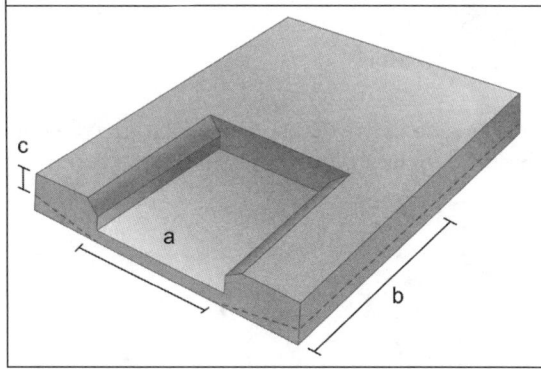

Adjust the dimensions of the cushion and the seat bones well to suit individual wheelchair users as follows:
- seat bones well width = ½ the wheelchair user's seat width or 200 mm (whichever is less) [a];
- seat bones well depth (front to back) = ½ the wheelchair user's seat width or 200 mm (whichever is less) [b];
- seat bones well height = 35 mm for adults and 20–25 mm for children [c].

2. Cut out the seat bones well

Use a sharpened Hacksaw blade or long knife. Use long slow strokes, cutting mostly when pulling to improve control.
❖ First cut through the back of the cushion to the depth of the seat bones well.

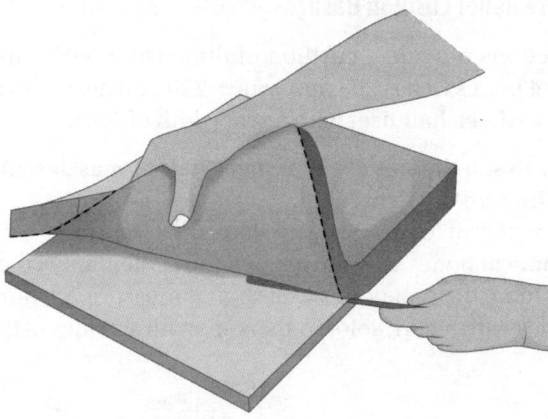

- Then slice out the seat bones well.

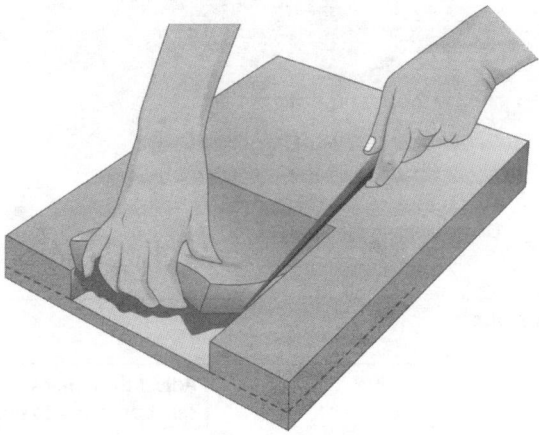

- Glue back into place the two "flaps" left on either side of the seat bones well. Allow the glue to set until not completely dried and slightly sticky to touch. Then press the foam together.

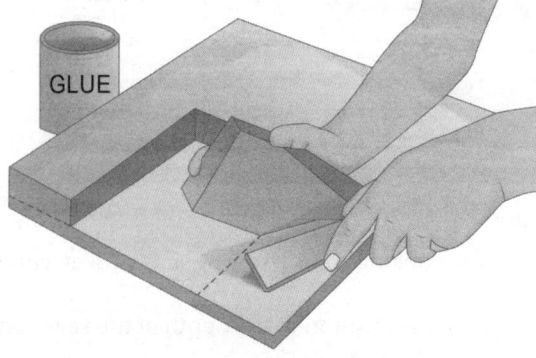

CHAPTER 19: Wheelchair Management

3. Cut off (bevel) the corners inside the seat bones well

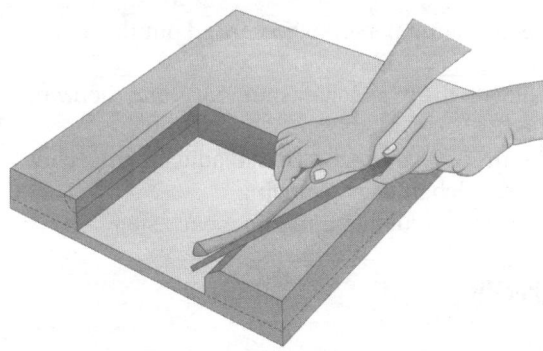

4. For a slung seat cushion: make an angled cut (bevel) on both sides of the base (under-side)
* Mark out as shown and cut.
* This cut helps the base of the cushion to match the shape of a slung wheelchair seat.

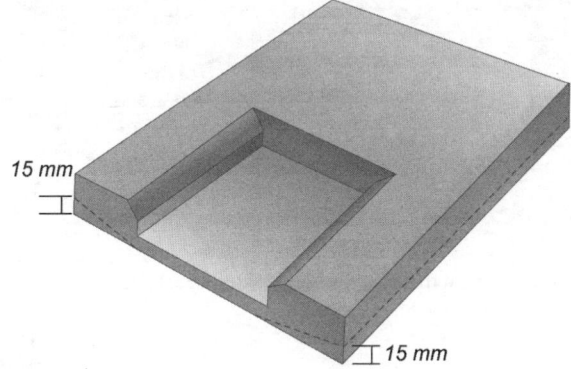

5. Place the top foam layer on top of the cushion
* Both the base and top layer are placed in the cushion cover together.
* The two layers do not need to be glued together.
* If the top layer becomes soiled or worn, it can be washed and dried, or replaced.
* A lift can be added within the cover to increase the depth of the seat bones well.

■ WHEELCHAIR FITTING

During fitting, the wheelchair user and personnel together check that:
* The wheelchair is the correct size and all the necessary modifications and adjustments have been made to ensure an optimum fit;
* The wheelchair and cushion support the wheelchair user in sitting upright;
* If a pressure relief cushion has been prescribed, the cushion really relieves pressure.

SECTION 4: Elderly Individuals and their Services

Good Practice in Fitting

- ❖ Wherever possible, the same person who carried out the assessment should carry out the fitting.
- ❖ Always check the fit with the wheelchair stationary, and then while the wheelchair user self-propels or is pushed.
- ❖ Carry out fitting in this order: check size and adjustments; check posture; check pressure; check fit while the wheelchair user is moving.
- ❖ Use the fitting checklist provided to remember each step.

Wheelchair Fitting Checklist

1. Is the wheelchair ready?

Has the wheelchair been checked to make sure it is safe to use and all parts are working?

2. Check size and adjustments

Seat width
Should fit closely.

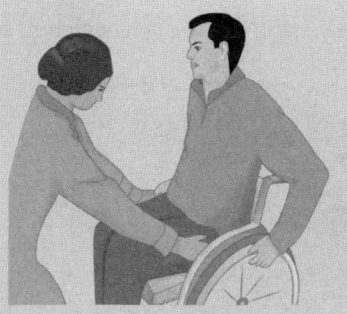

Seat depth
Two fingers' gap between the back of the knee and the seat/cushion.

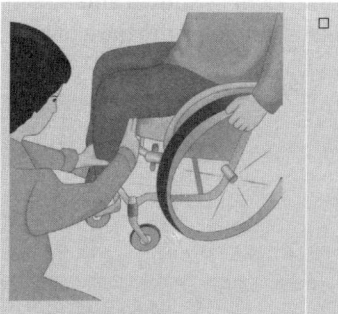

Footrests height:
The thigh is fully supported on the cushion, with no gaps. Each foot is fully supported on the footrest, with no gaps.

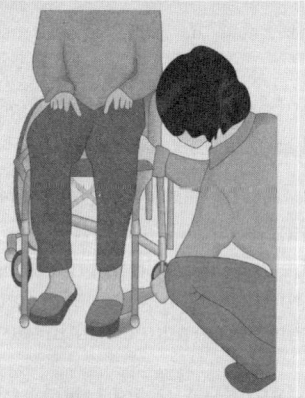

Backrest height:
The wheelchair user has the support they need and freedom to move their shoulders to push (if self-propelling).

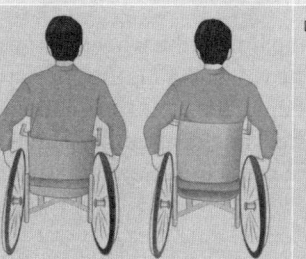

CHAPTER 19: Wheelchair Management

Rear wheels position (for hand propelling): The wheelchair user's arm should be in line with the rear axle when hanging down. When hands are placed on the push rim, the user's elbow should be at a right angle.	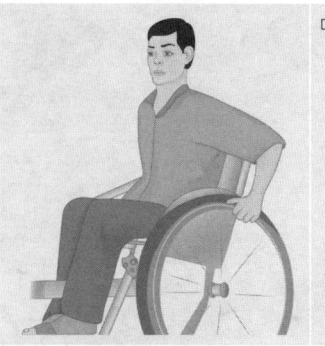 ☐
Brakes: Are the brakes working?	☐
Seat height (for foot propelling): With the wheelchair user sitting upright, the back should be comfortably supported by the backrest, with feet resting flat on the floor.	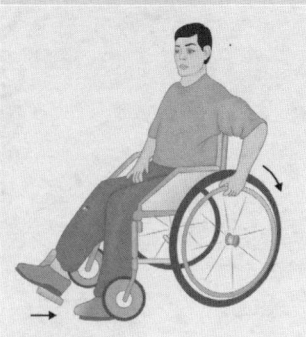

3. Check posture

Is the wheelchair user able to sit upright comfortably?	☐
Check posture from the side.	☐
Check posture from front/back.	☐

4. Check pressure

Check pressure under seat bones for all wheelchair users at risk of developing a pressure sore.	
A 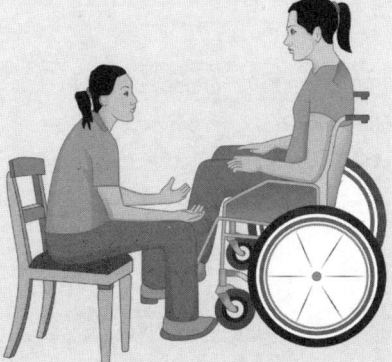	Explain the test to the wheelchair user.

B	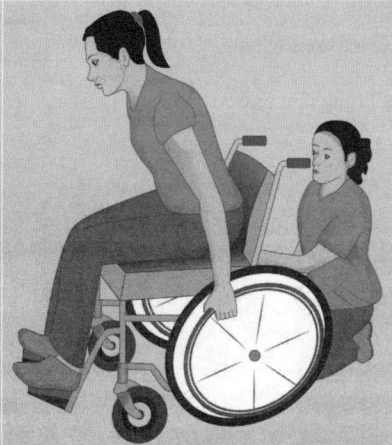	Ask wheelchair user to lean forward or push up. Place fingertips under wheelchair user's seat bone.
C	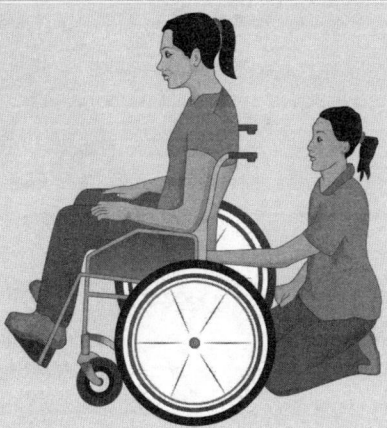	Ask the wheelchair user to sit back down on your fingers. Make sure the user sits upright with hands on thighs.
D	Identify the pressure: **Level 1 = safe:** Fingertips can wriggle up and down 5 mm or more. **Level 2 = warning:** Fingertips cannot wriggle, but can easily slide out. **Level 3 = unsafe:** Fingertips are squeezed firmly. It is difficult to slide fingers out.	
E	Repeat under the second seat bone.	

5. Check fit while the wheelchair is moving

Does the backrest allow the wheelchair user freedom to move the shoulders to push?	☐
Does the backrest give the wheelchair user enough support?	☐
Do the wheelchair user's feet stay on the footrests?	☐
Is the rear wheels position correct for the user?	☐

6. Action?

Is any further action necessary? Write any actions in the wheelchair user's file.	☐

CHAPTER 19: Wheelchair Management

Wheelchair User Training Checklist

	Skills to teach	Skills taught
Wheelchair handling		
Folding the wheelchair	☐	☐
Lifting the wheelchair	☐	☐
Using quick-release wheels	☐	☐
Using the brakes	☐	☐
Using the cushion including positioning correctly	☐	☐
Transfers		
Independent transfer	☐	☐
Assisted transfer	☐	☐
Other	☐	☐
Wheelchair mobility		
Pushing correctly	☐	☐
Up and down a slope	☐	☐
Up and down a step	☐	☐
On rough ground	☐	☐
Partial wheelie	☐	☐
Preventing pressure sores		
Checking for pressure sores	☐	☐
Pressure relief lifts	☐	☐
Eat well and drink lots of water	☐	☐
What to do if a pressure sore develops	☐	☐
Looking after the wheelchair at home		
Clean the wheelchair; wash and dry the cushion and cushion cover	☐	☐
Oil moving parts	☐	☐
Pump the tyres if they are pneumatic	☐	☐
Tighten nuts and bolts	☐	☐
Tighten spokes	☐	☐
Check upholstery	☐	☐
Check for rust	☐	☐
Check the cushion	☐	☐
What to do if there is a problem		
Wheelchair needs repairs	☐	☐
The wheelchair does not fit or is not comfortable	☐	☐

■ TRANSFERS

Getting in and out of the Wheelchair

The ability to get in and out of the wheelchair easily and safely, with or without assistance, will help a wheelchair user in daily life. Getting in and out of the wheelchair can be called "transferring".

Why do Wheelchair Users Need to Learn how to Transfer?

Wheelchair users may need to get in and out of their wheelchair several times a day. They need a method which is safe, quick and does not use much energy. Wheelchair users practice different methods, depending on their abilities. Some wheelchair users can get in and out of the chair by themselves, and others need help. Some users can stand up to transfer, while for others this is not possible.

Three Ways to Get in and Out of the Wheelchair

Before recommending or practising a transfer with a wheelchair user you need to know whether he/she can transfer independently or needs help.
- ❖ For transferring independently through sitting, check that the wheelchair user can lift his/her weight upwards by pushing with the arms. If the user cannot do this, he/she needs help to transfer.
- ❖ For transferring independently through standing, check that the wheelchair user can stand up and take his/her own weight through the legs. If he/she cannot do this, he/she needs help to transfer. Some different ways to transfer are shown below.

Independent Transfer Through Sitting (Wheelchair to Bed)

Position the wheelchair close to the bed, apply brakes.
- ❖ Take feet off and swing away or remove (where applicable) the footrests.
- ❖ Remove armrest closest to the bed.
- ❖ Push up on hands and move to the front of the wheelchair.
- ❖ With one hand on the bed and the other on the wheelchair, push up and lift on to the bed.
- ❖ If the user has poor balance or cannot lift high enough or move sideways far enough, he/she may use a transfer board.

If transferring to a bed, some wheelchair users prefer to place their legs on to the bed before transferring.

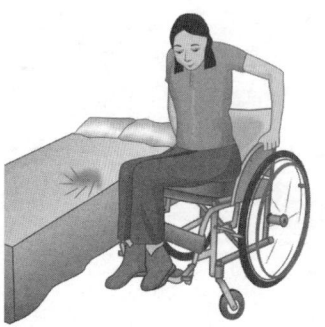
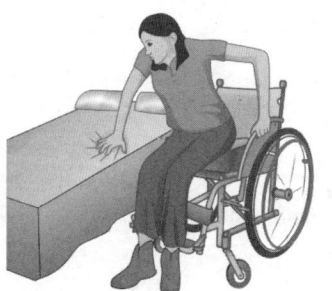
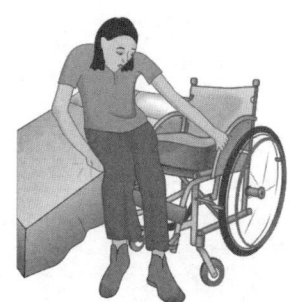

CHAPTER 19: Wheelchair Management

■ WHEELCHAIR TO BED

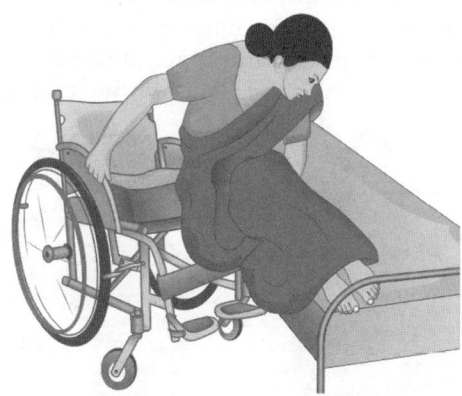

■ WHEELCHAIR TO BED BY PLACING LEGS ON THE BED

Assisted transfer through sitting with a transfer board (wheelchair to bed)
* Position the wheelchair close to bed, apply brakes.
* Take feet off and swing away or remove (where applicable) the footrests.
* Remove armrest closest to the bed.
* Assist user to move forward.
* Put a transfer board under buttocks across the wheelchair and bed.
* User to assist as much as possible by pushing up on wheelchair and bed to take own weight.
* Assistant stands behind user, and moves user's buttocks over to the bed.

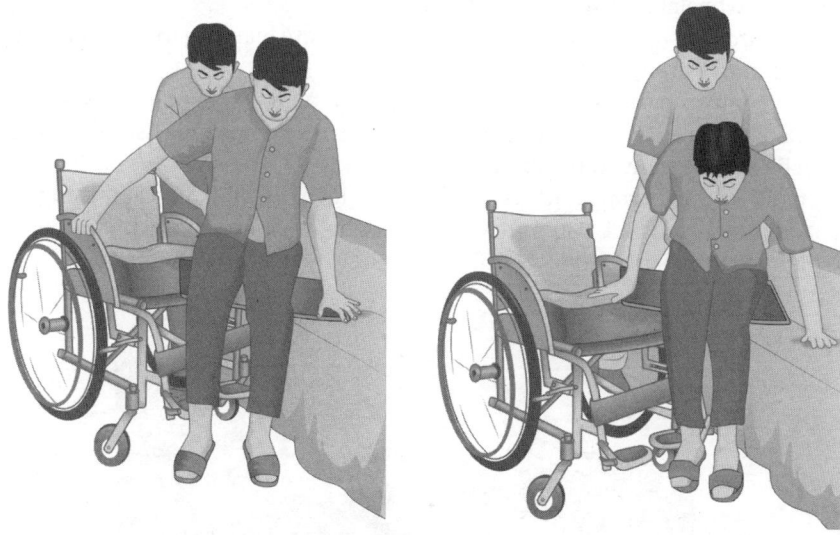

Assisted Standing Transfer (Bed to Wheelchair)

* Position the wheelchair, apply brakes.
* Take feet off and swing away or remove (where applicable) the footrests.

- Remove armrest closest to the bed.
- Assist the user to move forward on the bed and place feet on the floor.
- Support the user's knees from the side (do not push against knees from the front).
- Bring user's body forwards and upwards by supporting around the shoulder blades.
- Twist the user towards the wheelchair and allow him/her to sit down gently.

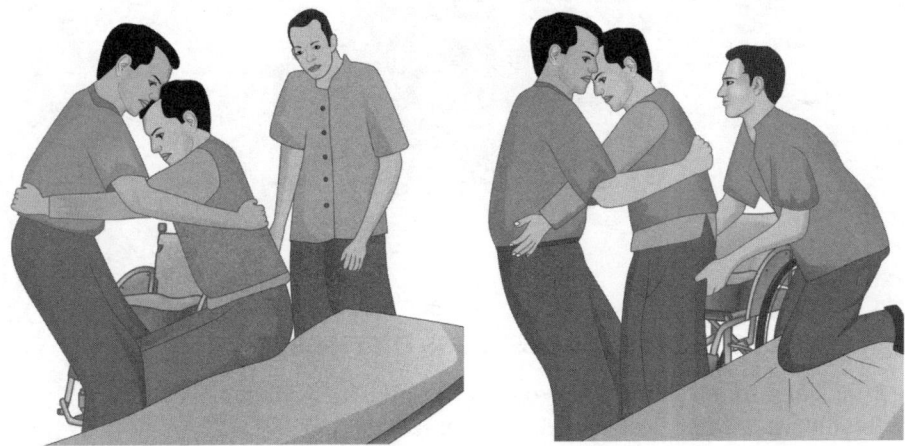

■ ASSISTED STANDING TRANSFER

What is a Transfer Board?

A transfer board is a strong, thin board which can help to bridge the gap between the wheelchair and surface the wheelchair user is transferring to.

Transfer boards are useful for wheelchair users who are learning to transfer independently, or who have limited strength in their arms.

The wheelchair user can carry out the transfer in a series of small lifts, rather than one big lift. A transfer board can also reduce the assistance a wheelchair user may need. Transfer boards can be made locally from wood or plywood.

They should be thin, strong and very smooth. Reduce the thickness at the edges.

Suggested dimensions are 300 mm × 600 mm. The thickness of the board depends on the strength of the material, but a typical thickness is between 20 and 25 mm.

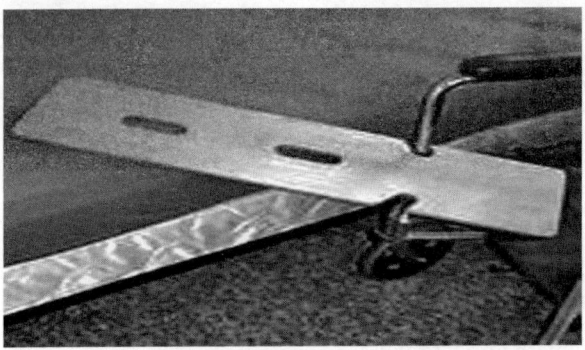

Transfer Board

■ TRANSFER BOARD

SCALES

SF-36 QUESTIONNAIRE

Name: Ref. Dr:................................. Date:...................

ID#:...............   Age: ....Gender: M / F.............

Please answer the 36 questions of the Health Survey completely, honestly, and without interruptions.

GENERAL HEALTH:
In general, would you say your health is:
☐ Excellent   ☐ Very Good   ☐ Good   ☐ Fair   ☐ Poor

Compared to one year ago, how would you rate your health in general now?
☐ Much better now than one year ago
☐ Somewhat better now than one year ago
☐ About the same
☐ Somewhat worse now than one year ago
☐ Much worse than one year ago

LIMITATIONS OF ACTIVITIES:
The following items are about activities you might do during a typical day. Does your health now limit you in these activities? If so, how much?

Vigorous activities, such as running, lifting heavy objects, participating in strenuous sports.
☐ Yes, Limited a lot   ☐ Yes, Limited a Little   ☐ No, Not Limited at all

Moderate activities, such as moving a table, pushing a vacuum cleaner, bowling, or playing golf
☐ Yes, Limited a lot   ☐ Yes, Limited a Little   ☐ No, Not Limited at all

Lifting or carrying groceries
☐ Yes, Limited a Lot   ☐ Yes, Limited a Little   ☐ No, Not Limited at all

Climbing several flights of stairs
☐ Yes, Limited a Lot   ☐ Yes, Limited a Little   ☐ No, Not Limited at all

Climbing one flight of stairs
☐ Yes, Limited a Lot   ☐ Yes, Limited a Little   ☐ No, Not Limited at all

Bending, kneeling, or stooping
☐ Yes, Limited a Lot   ☐ Yes, Limited a Little   ☐ No, Not Limited at all

Walking more than a mile
☐ Yes, Limited a Lot   ☐ Yes, Limited a Little   ☐ No, Not Limited at all

Walking several blocks
☐ Yes, Limited a Lot   ☐ Yes, Limited a Little   ☐ No, Not Limited at all

Walking one block
☐ Yes, Limited a Lot   ☐ Yes, Limited a Little   ☐ No, Not Limited at all

Bathing or dressing yourself
☐ Yes, Limited a lot   ☐ Yes, Limited a Little   ☐ No, Not Limited at all

PHYSICAL HEALTH PROBLEMS

During the past 4 weeks, have you had any of the following problems with your work or other regular daily activities as a result of your physical health?

Cut down the amount of time you spent on work or other activities

☐ Yes ☐ No

Accomplished less than you would like

☐ Yes ☐ No

Were limited in the kind of work or other activities

☐ Yes ☐ No

Had difficulty performing the work or other activities (for example, it took extra effort)

☐ Yes ☐ No

■ EMOTIONAL HEALTH PROBLEMS

During the past 4 weeks, have you had any of the following problems with your work or other regular daily activities as a result of any emotional problems (such as feeling depressed or anxious)?

Cut down the amount of time you spent on work or other activities

☐ Yes ☐ No

Accomplished less than you would like

☐ Yes ☐ No

Didn't do work or other activities as carefully as usual

☐ Yes ☐ No

SOCIAL ACTIVITIES

Emotional problems interfered with your normal social activities with family, friends, neighbors, or groups?

☐ Not at all ☐ Slightly ☐ Moderately ☐ Severe ☐ Very severe

PAIN:

How much bodily pain have you had during the past 4 weeks?

☐ Not at all ☐ Slightly ☐ Moderately ☐ Severe ☐ Very severe

During the past 4 weeks, how much did pain interfere with your normal work (including both work outside the home and housework)?

☐ Not at all ☐ A little bit ☐ Moderately ☐ Quite a bit ☐ Extremely

■ ENERGY AND EMOTIONS

These questions are about how you feel and how things have been with you during the last 4 weeks. For each question, please give the answer that comes closest to the way you have been feeling.

Did you feel full of pep?

☐ All of the time
☐ Most of the time
☐ A good bit of the time
☐ Some of the time

☐ A little bit of the time
☐ None of the time

Have you been a very nervous person?

☐ All of the time
☐ Most of the time
☐ A good Bit of the time
☐ Some of the time
☐ A little bit of the time
☐ None of the time

Have you felt so down in the dumps that nothing could cheer you up?

☐ All of the time
☐ Most of the time
☐ A good bit of the time
☐ Some of the time
☐ A little bit of the time
☐ None of the time

Have you felt calm and peaceful?

☐ All of the time
☐ Most of the time
☐ A good bit of the time
☐ Some of the time
☐ A little bit of the time
☐ None of the time

Did you have a lot of energy?

☐ All of the time
☐ Most of the time
☐ A good bit of the time
☐ Some of the time
☐ A little bit of the time
☐ None of the time

Have you felt downhearted and blue?

☐ All of the time
☐ Most of the time
☐ A good bit of the time
☐ Some of the time
☐ A little bit of the time
☐ None of the time

Did you feel worn out?

☐ All of the time
☐ Most of the time
☐ A good bit of the time
☐ Some of the time
☐ A little bit of the time
☐ None of the time

Have you been a happy person?

☐ All of the time
☐ Most of the time
☐ A good bit of the time
☐ Some of the time
☐ A little bit of the time
☐ None of the time

Did you feel tired?

☐ All of the time
☐ Most of the time
☐ A good bit of the time
☐ Some of the time
☐ A little bit of the time
☐ None of the time

SOCIAL ACTIVITIES

During the past 4 weeks, how much of the time has your physical health or emotional problems interfered with your social activities (like visiting with friends, relatives, etc.)?

☐ All of the time
☐ Most of the time
☐ Some of the time
☐ A little bit of the time
☐ None of the Time

■ GENERAL HEALTH

How true or false is each of the following statements for you?

I seem to get sick a little easier than other people

☐ Definitely true ☐ Mostly true ☐ Don't know ☐ Mostly false ☐ Definitely false

I am as healthy as anybody I know

☐ Definitely true ☐ Mostly true ☐ Don't know ☐ Mostly false ☐ Definitely false

I expect my health to get worse

☐ Definitely true ☐ Mostly true ☐ Don't know ☐ Mostly false ☐ Definitely false

My health is excellent

☐ Definitely true ☐ Mostly true ☐ Don't know ☐ Mostly false ☐ Definitely false

CHAPTER 19: Wheelchair Management

FIM™ Instrument

LEVELS		No helper / Helper
	7 Complete independence (Timely, safely) 6 Modified independence (Device)	No helper

	Modified dependence
	  5 Supervision (subject = 100%+)
	  4 Minimal assist (subject = 75%+)
	  3 Moderate assist (subject = 50%+)
	
	Complete dependence
	  2 Maximal assist (subject = 25%+)
	  1 Minimal assist (subject = 75%+)
		Helper

	Admission	Discharge	Follow-up
Self-care A. Eating B. Grooming C. Bathing D. Dressing - upper body E. Dressing - lower body F. Toileting			
Sphincter control G. Bladder management H. Bowel management			
Transfers I. Bed, chair, wheelchair J. Toilet K. Tub, shower			
Locomotion L. walk/wheelchair M. Stairs	W Walk C Wheelchair B Both	W Walk C Wheelchair B Both	W Walk C Wheelchair B Both
Motor subtotal score			
Communication N. Comprehension O. Expression	A Auditory V Visual B Both V Vocal N Nonvocal B Both	A Auditory V Visual B Both V Vocal N Nonvocal B Both	A Auditory V Visual B Both V Vocal N Nonvocal B Both
Social cognition P. Social interaction Q. Problem solving R. Memory			
Cognitive subtotal score			
Total Fim score			

Note: Leave no blanks. Enter 1 if patient not testable due to risk

■ BIBLIOGRAPHY

1. Frost S, Mines K, Noon J, Scheffler E, Stoeckle RJ. Wheelchair service training package: basic level. World Health Organization; 2012.
2. https://apps.who.int/iris/bitstream/handle/10665/78236/9789241503471_reference_manual_eng.pdf?sequence=1
3. https://apps.who.int/iris/bitstream/handle/10665/246227/9789241549080-workbook-eng.pdf

CHAPTER 20

Environment Modifications for People with Disabilities and Elderly Individuals

Deepti Nandlal Wadhwa

LEARNING OBJECTIVES

Through this chapter, the reader will be able to:
- Environment modifications with reference to access to building
- Internal corridors and accessible routes, floors, doors, ramps, gradient, stairs, handrails, grab bars, furniture, kitchen, bathroom, bedroom area, clear floor space, electrical points, controls
- Outlets, faucets/taps, windows, heating units: drinking water, signage, lifts, accessible toilets, water closet, washroom accessories, emergency evacuation and plans, refuge area, parking

■ ACCESS TO BUILDING

- It should connect all major entrances and exits of the building from the alighting and boarding point of vehicles/car park
- If there is more than one entry to the dwelling, the most accessible should be selected
- The accessible entrance should be clearly signed and easy to locate
- Symbol should be displayed at all other non-accessible entrances
- A clear, firm and level landing of at least 1,800 mm × 1,800 mm
- The clear width of the accessible entrance door should not be less than 900 mm, preferable 1 m and the width of the corridors or passageways leading to and from such access door should not be less than 1,200 mm
- Internal floor surfaces should be anti-skid/non-slip
- Steps should not be greater than 7 in (180 mm) high with a minimum depth of 11 in (280 mm)
- Nosings are the 0.5 in (13 mm) curved overhangs on the front edge of stairs
- Texture difference in the floor can be provided
- Beepers may be put at all main entrances
- A tactile layout plan of the building along with Braille and audio-systems should be provided
- Glazed entrance doors must have manifestations on the glass preferably at two levels, i.e., one between 800 to 1,000 mm and another between 1,400 to 1,600 mm above the floor

Internal Corridors and Accessible Routes

- Width—the minimum clear with of an accessible route should be 1,500 mm
- Resting areas should be provided at frequent intervals not exceeding 30 meters

CHAPTER 20: Environment Modifications for People with Disabilities and Elderly Individuals

- Obstacles or other protrusions should be avoided in pedestrian areas such as corridor
- Floor surface should be stable, firm, level and slip-resistant and preferably matt finish
- If carpet is used, it should be fixed firmly with a pile not higher than 12 mm
- Lighting—minimum illumination level in the corridor should be 150 lux
- Where a door opens into an infrequently used corridor such as emergency exit, the corridor width should allow a clear space of 900 mm
- Atactile floor guidance path should be provided

Floors

- Floors should be nonslip and level
- When carpeting is used, a dense, low pile 0.635 to 1.27 cm, low-level loop generally provides for easiest movement
- Avoid carpeting with bold patterns of mixed colours which may be visually confusing

Doors

- Doorways should be levelled with minimum clear openings of doorways should be not less than 900 mm
- Door handle to be between 850 mm and 1,100 mm from finished floor level—not to require fine finger control
- Vision panel for two-way swing doors with visibility between 800 mm and 1,500 mm height
- Glass doors to have permanent manifestations contrasting visually with background
- Bathroom (toilets/washroom) doors should swing out/should be two-way opening type
- Automatic doors should have a push button system to open them
- All external doors should have warning blocks installed 300 mm before entrances
- The presence of a glass door should be within 800–1,000 mm from the floor and within 1,400–1,600 mm from the floor
- Double-leaf doors: In case the door has two independently operated door leaves, at least one active leaf should have minimum width of 900 mm
- Where a forward approach is used, a clear knee space of at least 900 mm wide, 480 mm deep and 650 mm high should be provided

Door Hardware

- Be mounted at a height of 850–1,100 mm from the floor
- All door furniture should contrast visually with the surface of the door
- Operable devices such as handles, pulls, latches and locks should be operable by one hand

Door Handles

- Use D-shaped handles as they reduce the risk of catching on clothing, or injuring from the exposed lever end
- Lever handles to be preferred on latched doors
- Doorknob is not recommended

Kerb Ramps

- A short ramp cutting through a curb or built up to it or a Kerb is a drop
- Be provided where the vertical rise is less than 150 mm
- Do not require handrails
- Have a slip-resistant surface
- Be free from any obstruction such as signposts, traffic lights, etc.

Ramps

- Ramps and landing surfaces should be slip resistant
- The minimum clear width of a ramp should be 1,200 mm
- Landings should be provided at regular intervals of not more than 9,000 mm of every horizontal run and should have a level platform of not less than 1,500 mm
- Ramps should have a level landing at the top and bottom of each run and also where the run changes direction
- Large ramps are typically constructed of wood or concrete; smaller ramps can be made from aluminum or fiber glass
- Small, commercially available ramps can be used for traversing curbs and small step heights.

Gradient

Level difference	Minimum gradient	Ramp width
≥150 mm to ≤300 mm	1:12	1,200 mm
≥300 mm to ≤750 mm	1:12	1,500 mm
≥750 mm to ≤3,000 mm	1:15	1,800 mm
≥3,000 mm	1:20	1,800 mm

Stairs

- They should be supplemented by lifts and/or ramps
- There should be no more than 12 risers in one flight run
- Treads should be 300 mm deep and risers not higher than 150 mm
- The stairs landing should be minimally 1,200 mm deep
- Width—minimum 1,500 mm
- Projecting nosing and open stairs should not be provided to minimize the risk of stumbling.
- Warning blocks should be installed 300 mm before the beginning and 300 mm after the end of each flight of steps
- Step edges must contrast in color to the risers and the treads
- Contrast color bands 50 mm wide should be provided on the edge of the treads

Handrails

- A rail used in circulation areas such as corridors, passageways, ramps and stairways to assist in continuous movement.
- Be slip-resistant with round ends and should be on both sides
- Have a circular section of 38–45 mm in diameter

CHAPTER 20: Environment Modifications for People with Disabilities and Elderly Individuals

- Be free of any sharp or abrasive elements
- Have continuous gripping surfaces, without interruptions or obstructions that can break a hand hold
- minimum of 34 in (865 mm) and a maximum of 38 in (965 mm) high for stairs, ramps, and level walking surfaces
- At least one handrail should extend a minimum of 12 in (305 mm) beyond the foot and top of the stairs
- Placed at a height of between 760 mm and 900 mm above the floor level
- Extended horizontally for a distance of not less than 300 mm beyond the top and bottom of the ramp

Grab Bars

- A bar used to give a steadying or stabilizing assistance to a person engaged in a particular function
- Be slip-resistant with round ends
- Have a circular section of 38–45 mm in diameter
- Be able to bear a weight of 250 kg
- Be free of any sharp or abrasive elements
- It should be manufactured from a material which contrasts with the wall finish (or use dark tiles behind light-colored rails), be not too warm/cold to the touch and provide good grip
- It should be properly fixed, since considerable pressure will be placed on the rail during maneuvering.
- One L-shape grab bar: 600 mm long horizontal and 700 mm long vertical should be mounted on the side wall closest to the water closet
- A hinged type horizontal grab bar should be installed adjacent to the water closet between heights of 200–250 mm from the top of the water closet seat and extending 100–150 mm beyond the front of the water closet
- An emergency alarm-cum-call switch should be provided within easy reach on the wall near water closet at two levels: at 300–900 mm from the floor level

Furniture

- An initial step is to move as much furniture as possible against the walls to increase clearance and stability (i.e., prevent sliding of furniture during movement transitions).
- One can modify the current furniture by placing a fitted wooden board under the seat cushion and behind the seat back (if removable).
- Clear passage must be allowed from one room to the next
- The chair should be the height of the seat should allow the knees to flex approximately 90° with the feet flat on the floor, a firm cushioned seat, a firm cushioned back that provides adequate upright support, and double arm rests

Kitchen

- The ideal height of counter surfaces should be no greater than 31 in (794 mm) from the floor with a knee clearance of 27.5–30 in (705–769 mm).
- Counter space should provide a depth of at least 24 in (615 mm)
- Stools (preferably with back and footrests) may be placed strategically at the main work area(s).

- Placing colored tape along the border of the countertop that contrasts sharply with the color of the counter surface will help identify boundaries of the workspace
- A spray-hose fixture allows filling heavy pots without needing to lift them from a sink.
- Motorized adjustable sinks can be mounted against a wall between two stationary cabinets with free space beneath.
- A small cart with casters may be helpful to improve ease of moving articles from refrigerator to counter or table
- Adjustable shelves are preferable and should be placed 16 in (410 mm) above the countertop
- Large-print label-making devices and large-print stencil overlays can be used to enlarge
- Electric stoves are generally preferable to open-flame gas burners
- Wall-mounted ovens (separate from the stove) should be placed 30–34 inch (76–102 cm) from the floor with a side-opening door.
- Dishwashers should be elevated 9 in (228.6 mm) and be front-loading, with pull-out shelves and front-mounted controls
- Access to the refrigerator will be enhanced by use of a side-by-side (refrigerator-freezer) model.
- A standard or remote-control smoke and carbon monoxide detector should be available

Bathroom

- An elevated toilet seat can be used to facilitate transfers
- Power-lift toilet seats with grab bars are designed to assist the patient to standing (elevation initiated from the posterior aspect of the seat)
- Grab bars securely fastened to a reinforced wall will assist in both toilet and tub transfers
- Grab bars should have a circular cross-section diameter of 1.25 in (32 mm) minimum and 2 inch (51 mm) maximum and be knurled
- Two grab bars are secured horizontally to the back wall for use in tub transfers. One is placed 33–36 inch (840–915 mm) from tub floor and the second 9 in (230 mm) above top rim of the bathtub
- A tub transfer bench (tub seat) may be recommended for bathing.
- A space-saving design combines a toilet and shower seat into one assembled seat
- In shower stall areas, a collapsible seat may be permanently attached to the wall
- Nonskid adhesive strips may be placed on the floor of the tub or shower area
- Additional bathroom considerations may include a hand-spray attachment to the bathtub or shower faucet, antiscald valves to prevent water temperature from rising above a present limit (also called scald-guard valves or high temperature stops), water volume-control mechanisms (to prevent a sudden surge of water with resultant change in temperature)
- Sinks should provide clear knee space below and any exposed hot water pipes should be insulated to prevent burns

Bedroom Area

- The bed should be stationary and positioned to provide ample space for transfers
- The height of the sleeping surface must be optimal for transfers. Furniture risers can be used to raise bed height
- The mattress should provide a firm, comfortable surface.
- A bedside nightstand (or small table) should be available; it can be used to hold a lamp, telephone necessary medications, and call bell if assistance is needed from a caregiver

CHAPTER 20: Environment Modifications for People with Disabilities and Elderly Individuals

- The closet clothes bar should be lowered to 52 inch (132 cm) from the floor
- Wall hooks also may be a useful addition to the closet area and should be placed between 40 inch (101.6 cm) and 56 inch (142.2 cm) from the floor.
- Wardrobe lifts can increase closet storage capacity while maintaining accessibility
- Shelves also can be installed and should not exceed 115 cm

■ CONTROLS AND OPERATING MECHANISMS

Clear Floor Space

- It should be at least 900 mm × 1,200 mm
- A clear knee space of at least 900 mm wide, 480 mm deep and 650 mm high should be provided, which may overlap the clear floor space by a maximum of 480 mm

Electrical Points, Controls and Outlets

- Touch pad dimmer switches can be used to activate lamps with small control knobs. The dimmer module is plugged into a wall outlet and the lamp attached to the module.
- Located adjacent to the clear floor space
- Located at a height of between 600 mm and 1,100 mm from the floor with the exception of vending machines where the upper limit is maximum of 100 mm
- Operable with a force less than 22 N
- Rocker switches are available with lighted surfaces and with occupancy (motion) sensor devices that automatically turn on or off
- Power strips (surge protectors) can be used to increase the number of outlets, as well as improve access
- A ground fault circuit interrupter (GFCI) should be installed in wet locations such as bathrooms to prevent against electrical shock
- Inexpensive, programmable electrical timers can be used to regularly turn lights on and off throughout the day and night.

Faucets/taps

- It should be hand-operated or electronically controlled
- Require no tight grasping, pinching or twisting of the wrist
- Require a force less than 22 N to activate
- Have handles of lever type (not self-closing) operable with a closed fist.

Windows

- To reduce glare, window films can be installed; frosted films are effective at diffusing light without appreciably reducing ambient light
- Remote control systems for closing or opening window

Heating Units

- The heating source should be clear of combustible material and clutter.
- Smoke alarms and carbon monoxide detectors should be in the home and checked regularly by pressing the test button
- They should be appropriately screened off or insulated with pipe covers to prevent burns

Drinking Water

- Clear floor space of 900 mm × 1,200 mm
- Provision of 2 drinking water facilities at different heights preferable
- Lever type tap and comply with requirements

Signages

- Any room number, name tag, building directory, or similar object containing a printed message and/or symbol. Signage and signs are used synonymously in this document.
- Information may take the form of visual information (e.g., signs, notice boards)
- Audible information (e.g., public address and security systems, induction loops, telephones, and infrared devices)
- Tactile information (e.g., signs with embossed lettering or Braille)
- Use of tactile letters/symbols: Visual contrast and lighting, finished surfaces of materials used for signs and symbols should be non-reflective, simultaneous use of audible cues

The Location, Accessibility, Layout and Height of Signs

Viewing distance	Size of signage
Up to 7 meters	60 mm × 60 mm
7–8 meters	100 mm × 100 mm
Exceeding 8 meters	200 mm × 200 mm to 450 mm × 450 mm

Lifts

- The lift brings the wheelchair user from the ground level to the landing level to access the entrance to the home (these lifts can be used indoors as well)
- Dimensions—1,500 mm wide × 1,500 mm deep
- Lift door should have a clear opening of minimum 900 mm
- Door closing time for an automatic door should be more than 5 seconds
- Call buttons should be installed at a height between 800 mm and 1,000 mm and be supplemented in Braille/raised letters and in sharp contrast from the background to aid people with visual impairments.
- Grab bars/handrails to be fixed on both sides and the rear at 900 mm height from floor level
- Voice announcement system along with a visual display
- Where it is impracticable to provide a lift or a ramp, a wheelchair stair-lift or platform lift should be considered as a reasonable alternative for vertical circulation within the building
- For maximum level changes of 2,500 mm, vertical movement platform lifts may be installed
- Platform lifts are often installed adjacent to stairs with an upper landing and are available in a variety of dimensions with lengths ranging from 54 to 60 inch (137.16–152.4 cm) and widths ranging from 34 to 42 inch (86.36–106.68 cm).

Accessible Toilets

- One unisex accessible toilet should be provided in each toilet block on each floor.
- It should have the international symbol of accessibility displayed outside for wheelchair access.

- Minimum internal dimensions of 2,200 mm × 2,000 mm
- All fixtures and utilities should provide a clear space of 900 mm × 1,200 mm for wheelchair users to access them

Toilet Doors

- Be provided with a horizontal pull-bar, at least 600 mm long, on the inside of the door, located so that it is 130 mm from the hinged side of the door and at a height of 1,000 mm
- Should be outward opening or two-way opening or a sliding type door and should have a clear opening width of at least 900 mm
- Be capable of being locked from the inside by a device that is operable by one hand, activated by a force not more than 22 N

Water Closets

- Be located between 460 mm and 480 mm from the centreline of the water closet to the adjacent wall
- It should have a clear dimension of 750 mm from the front edge of the water closet to the rear wall to facilitate side transfer
- The top of the water closet seat should be 450–480 mm from the floor
- There should be an adequate clear floor space of at least 1,350 mm depth and 900 mm width, both in front and on the transfer side, adjacent to the water closet
- The flush control should either be lever type or automatic, and located on the transfer side of the water closet and not be located more than 1,000 mm from the floor

Washroom Accessories

- A mirror—the bottom edge at a height of not more than 1,000 mm from the floor and mirror should be tilted at an angle of 30° for better visibility of wheelchair user
- Have the toilet roll dispenser and hand water faucet
- Towel, soap dispensers, hand dryer and waste bin should be positioned such that the operable parts and controls are between 800 mm and 1,000 mm from the floor
- Cloth hook mounted on a side wall not more than 1,200 mm from the floor and projecting not more than 40 mm from the wall

Emergency Evacuation and Plans

- Alarm panels—fire alarm boxes, emergency call buttons and lighted panels should be installed between heights of 800–1,000 mm from the finished floor surface
- It should be adequately contrasted in color and tone from the background wall
- It should be labeled with raised letters and also in Braille.
- It should indicate the designated emergency evacuation routes as well as location of refuge areas should be displayed at all public areas of the building
- It should incorporate raised letters, tactile routes and Braille for benefit of persons with visual impairments
- Orientation and direction signs should be installed frequently along the evacuation route and these should preferably be internally illuminated
- Designating evacuation routes shall be at least 1,500 mm wide and it should be free of any steps or sudden changes in level and should be kept free from obstacles such as bins

Alerting Systems

- Audible alarms with "voice instructions" should be installed
- These alarms may be connected to central control room for on-the-spot broadcasts
- Non-auditory alarms (visual or sensory) to alert persons
- Non-auditory alarms include flashing beacons

Refuge Area

- A place of relative safety where persons who may not be able to negotiate inaccessible egress routes may await rescue assistance
- Every required area of refuge is to be accessible from the space it serves by an accessible egress route
- Every area of refuge shall have direct access to an exit stairway
- Each area of refuge must be separated from the remainder of the story by a smoke barrier having minimally 1 hour fire resistance rating
- The size of the refuge—not less 750 mm by 1,200 mm.
- It shall be not less than one for every 200 persons of calculated occupant load served by the area of rescue assistance
- A method of two-way communication, with both visible and audible signals, shall be provided between each area of rescue assistance and the primary entry.

Parking

- **Dimensions:** 5,000 mm × 3,600 mm
- **Location:** Nearest to the accessible entrance and/or lift lobby within 30 meters
- Two accessible parking lots should be provided for every 25 car parking spaces

■ BIBLIOGRAPHY

1. Guidelines and Space Standards for Barrier Free Built Environment for Disabled and Elderly Persons. https://cdn.nic.in/SJ/PDFFiles/GuidelinesIndia.PDF
2. Harmonized Guidelines and Space Standards for barrier Free Built Environment for Persons with Disability and Elderly Persons. 2016 http://tcpo.gov.in/Harmonized-Guidelines.
3. Manual on guidelines and space standard Barrier Free Environment for Disabled and elderly, Ministry of Urban Affairs. 1998 https://cpwd.gov.in/Publication/agedanddisabled.pdf
4. Planning a Barrier Free Environment. Office of the Chief Commissioner for Persons with Disabilities https://cdn.nic.in/SJ/PDFFiles/PlanningForBarrierFreeEnvironment
5. Shishu Sarothi, Overview of the Harmonized Guidelines and Space Standards for Barrier Free Built Environment for Persons with Disability and Elderly Persons, 2020. https://gmda.assam.gov.in/sites/default/files/swf_utility_folder/departments/gmda_webcomindia_org_oid_4/do_u_want_2_know/overview_of_the_harmonized_guidelines

CHAPTER 21

Integrated Treatment Approach for Neuromuscular Dysfunction in Elderly

Sanjivani Kamble

LEARNING OBJECTIVES

Through this chapter, the reader will be able to:
- Introduction of ageing
- Common health issues that come with ageing
- The brain's aging
- Key elements of the assessment of neurologic examination in geriatric
- Integrated treatment approach
- Advantages of integrated treatment approach
- Long-term care setting for integrated therapy

■ AGEING

Ageing is caused by the accumulation of a wide range of molecular and cellular damage over time. This results in a steady decline in physical and mental function, an increased risk of disease, and, eventually, death. These changes are not linear nor consistent, and they are only tangentially related to a person's chronological age. The diversity exhibited in old age is not coincidental. Aside from biological changes, ageing is frequently connected with other life transitions such as retirement, move to more suitable housing, and the death of friends and companions.

■ COMMON HEALTH ISSUES THAT COME WITH AGEING

Hearing loss, cataracts and refractive errors, back and neck pain and osteoarthritis, chronic obstructive pulmonary disease, diabetes, depression, and dementia are all common illnesses in the elderly. People are more likely to encounter multiple ailments concurrently as they age. Older age is also marked by the appearance of various complex health conditions known as geriatric syndromes. Frailty, urine incontinence, falls, confusion, and pressure ulcers are all common outcomes of several underlying causes.

■ THE BRAIN'S AGING

The size, vasculature, and cognition of the brain change with age. With advancing years, the brain shrinks and undergoes changes at all levels, from chemicals to morphology. Along with memory loss, dementia, white matter lesions, and stroke, there are changes in neurotransmitter and hormone levels as people age. Increased cognitive effort in the form of schooling or occupational attainment, as well as protective variables that lower cardiovascular risk, such as regular exercise, a balanced diet, and low to moderate alcohol use, seem to benefit the ageing brain. The strongest defence against the changes brought on by an ageing brain may be living a physically and intellectually healthy life. It may also be crucial to take additional precautions against cardiovascular disease.[2,5]

■ KEY ELEMENTS OF THE ASSESSMENT OF NEUROLOGIC EXAMINATION IN GERIATRIC POPULATION

Mental status	Attention, executive function, language, memory
Cranial nerves	Vision and hearing, eye movements, visual fields, facial symmetry
Motor/symmetry	Coordination and speed of limb use; muscle tone, test for pronator drift, involuntary movements
Sensation	Joint position, double simultaneous stimulation
Reflexes	Pathologic or asymmetric reflexes
Gait	Arising from chair, casual, and tandem gait

■ INTEGRATED TREATMENT APPROACH FOR NEUROMUSCULAR DYSFUNCTION IN ELDERLY

- To maintain muscle strength and prevent contracture
- To develop postural control
- To increase respiratory capacity
- Biofeedback in patients
- Task specific training
- To prevent falls in elderly

To Maintain Muscle Strength and Prevent Contracture

Exercise has numerous psychological and physical advantages, including the:[6]
- Preservation of muscle strength
- The prevention of contractures
- Increase flexibility
- To decrease energy expenditure
- Relief from fatigue
- The reduction of pain
- The reduction of depression
- The reduction of social isolation
- The maintenance of mobility
- An improvement in quality of life

However, there are not many studies that provide strong information about the kind, degree, frequency, and speed of exercise. The etiology, onset, severity, and course of the condition, the patient's age and sex, as well as the recommended exercise's intensity and frequency, should all be taken into account when choosing a potential exercise programme.[3]

- ❖ **Stretching and regular range-of-motion exercise**
  - In order to do the static stretching, which is typically employed to treat NMDs, the joint must be properly aligned, and the muscle must be stretched to its maximum length along the joint while the unmoving joints are stabilised.
  - The position is held for at least 10 seconds after the movement comes to a finish, then it is repeated.
  - The suggested frequency of stretching for healthy people is one to two repetitions per day or three to seven repetitions per week, however, there is no set recommendation for neuromuscular dysfunction.
- ❖ **Resistance training**
  - One of the best ways to increase the neuromuscular system's functional capability is through resistance exercise training. However, there is ongoing debate in the literature regarding the advantages and disadvantages of strength training in neuromuscular illnesses.[1]
  - Exercises that gradually build muscle strength are frequently used to treat neuromuscular problems. Lean body mass, muscle protein mass, contractile strength, strength, and bodily function are all improved by progressive strengthening workouts.[1]
  - This improvement varies depending on how quickly the sickness is developing. The benefits of mild to moderate intensity strength training (25–40% of maximal weight) on muscle strength without apparent negative effects, notably for slow-progressing neuromuscular illnesses, have gained widespread acceptance in recent years.[3]
  - It is not advised to utilise high-intensity eccentric or concentric training programs on dystrophic types with rapid progression and membrane instability since they would put mechanical stress on muscle fibres and worsen muscular weakness (such as Duchenne muscular dystrophy).[3]
- ❖ **Electrical stimulation**
  - Neuromuscular diseases should be treated with prudence while using electrical stimulation, which is frequently utilized in clinics for strengthening. Since all muscle fibers contract at the same time with electrical stimulation, it can increase degeneration in patients with low muscle fiber counts. For this reason, patients with muscle strength below three should use current types that will not cause fatigue.
- ❖ **Aquatic therapy:** The best form of exercise for this population of patients is in the water. The water lift allows for functional movement, supports weak muscles, and in some circumstances can also be utilized as a resistance workout. All muscle groups are worked on during pool exercises, which also increase the patient's aerobic capacity. Patients with low energy levels respond well to it very well. The literature suggests exercising for 45 minutes twice a week. Pool therapy has accessibility issues and financial restrictions.
- ❖ **Aerobic endurance Training**
  - Strength training does not produce the same physiological effects as aerobic endurance training. For aerobic exercise involving the utilization of large muscle groups and lasting 30 minutes, an intensity of 50–85% of VO_{2max} is sufficient.[3]
  - The heart, the peripheral circulation, and the musculoskeletal system are all stimulated by aerobic exercise.[3,7]
  - More oxygen is thereby circulated throughout the body, increasing cardiac output, capillary density, and vascular transmission. Exercises that are less taxing on the musculoskeletal system, such swimming, walking, and cycling, can be done for this advantage.[3]

- Aerobic exercise stimulates the heart, the peripheral circulation, and the musculoskeletal system. As a result, the body receives more oxygen, which raises cardiac output, capillary density, and vascular transmission. For this benefit, you can engage in activities like swimming, walking, and cycling that are easier on your musculoskeletal system.[4]

To develop Postural Control

- One of the initial steps of mobility is the movement from the supine position to the sitting posture. This is an important action of the body against gravity.[3]
- The trunk flexors muscles contract concentrically whereas the trunk extensor muscles contract eccentrically during this activity, which is crucial for muscle sufferers as well. Due to the patient's difficulties getting into a sitting posture, it is important to consider the risk of mobility issues and take measures with the trunk during therapy.[3]

To Increase Respiratory Capacity

- Airway cleaning methods such air stacking (glossopharyngeal breathing), mechanical coughing, and manual coughing should be used as soon as feasible if there is a coughing weakness in the patient.[3]
- Breathing exercises, diaphragm breathing exercises, and thoracic expansion exercises should all be given to patients in order to increase pulmonary capacity and maximise lung expansion.[3]
- The forced inspiratory vital capacity is increased through pulmonary expansion therapy and maximal insufflation therapy (mask or mechanically assisted hyperinsufflation and prevents atelectasis.[8]
- To this patient population, traditional chest physiotherapy treatments for clearing the airways should be introduced. This entails moving the patient into various positions before clapping, vibrating, and coughing on the chest wall.[8]
- Strength and endurance can be increased by exercising the respiratory muscles strength training is typically carried out by performing a maximal static maneuver against a closed glottis or a nearly closed glottis in studies of respiratory muscle training closed resistance valve.[10]
- Inspiratory and expiratory muscles can also be strengthened by nonrespiratory exercises like sit-ups and bicep curls.[10]

Biofeedback in Patients

- A biofeedback system recommends both external (i.e., augmented information, which is a learning technique that is provided on demand from an external source) and intrinsic feedback, which is response-produced training that is (a) interactive, (b) safe, and (c) allows the individual motivation to discover and relearn motor skills and thereby to regain cognitive capacities.[8]
- Knowledge of performance (KP), also known as kinematic feedback, and knowledge of results (KR), enhanced information, are two common categories for external feedback.[8]

Task specific Training

- An method to rehabilitation known as task-specific or task-oriented therapy focuses on the performance of functional tasks that are important to the individual.[9]

- The biomechanics of movement can be utilized to ensure that the most effective technique is trained in a variety of neurological diseases, particularly Parkinson's disease.[9]
- The context of functional tasks, such as walking (with variations in movement speed, direction, and distance), climbing stairs, sitting down, turning around, navigating obstacles, picking up items from a shelf and placing them in a cart, hanging clothes on a line, putting items in and taking things out of the refrigerator, picking up items off the floor, etc., is equally important for physical therapy.[8,9]

To Prevent Falls in Elderly

- It includes 5 strengthening exercises—knee extensor, knee flexor, hip abductor, ankle plantar flexors, and ankle dorsi flexors.[11]
- It also includes 11 balance retraining exercises—knee bends, backward walking, walking and turning around, sideways walking, tandem stands, tandem walking, 1-leg stand, heel walking, toe walking, heel-toe walking backward, and stand. The physical therapy aim was to progress participants to a greater level of difficulty over time.[11]

■ HEALTH ADVANTAGES OF INTEGRATED TREATMENT APPROACH

Integrated therapy is crucial because it can help you function and feel your best. As a result of your effort, you may discover that you move better and have healthier relationships. Therapy enhances your overall quality of life.

Some of the other advantages you may gain from therapy are as follows:
- Greater independence
- Enhanced motor function
- Pain alleviation
- Improved circulation
- Increased strength and stamina
- Avoid aggravation
- Disease progression is slowed.

■ WHAT TO LOOK FOR IN A LONG-TERM CARE SETTING FOR INTEGRATED THERAPY

The first thing you might worry about if you or a loved one needs neuromuscular treatment in a long-term care facility is likely to be the expense and insurance coverage. Its crucial to talk about the financial commitment with your family and your provider.

Following aspects you might want to think about include:
- Convenience of the area and the lodging options
- Whether or not the providers are specialists
- The clinic's commitment to using treatments that have been scientifically demonstrated
- One-stop access holistic treatments
  In order to be sure your family member is in good hands.

■ REFERENCES

1. Seraji-Bzorgzad N, Paulson H, Heidebrink J. Neurologic examination in the elderly. Handbook of Clinical Neurology. 2019;167:73-88.

2. Pasnoor M, Dimachkie MM. Approach to muscle and neuromuscular junction disorders. CONTINUUM: Lifelong Learning in Neurology. 2019;25(6):1536-63.
3. Suzuki T (Ed). Neurological Physical Therapy. BoD–Books on Demand; 2017.
4. Embon-Magal S, Krasovsky T, Doron I, Asraf K, Haimov I, Gil E, Agmon M. The effect of co-dependent (thinking in motion [TIM]) versus single-modality (CogniFit) interventions on cognition and gait among community-dwelling older adults with cognitive impairment: a randomized controlled study. BMC geriatrics. 2022 Aug 31;22(1):720.
5. Zgaljardic DJ, Temple RO. Neuropsychological Assessment Battery (NAB): Performance in a sample of patients with moderate-to-severe traumatic brain injury. Applied Neuropsychology. 2010;17(4):283-8.
6. Gleeson E, Wolfson L. Neuromuscular Diseases in Geriatric Patients: Part II.
7. Hou N, Sun X. Effect of aerobic exercise on neuromuscular quality in the elderly. Revista Brasileira de Medicina do Esporte. 2022;28:509-12.
8. Carmeli E. Physical therapy for neurological conditions in geriatric populations. Frontiers in Public Health. 2017;5:333.
9. Volery S, Singh N, de Bruin ED, List R, Jaeggi MM, Mattli Baur B, Lorenzetti S. Traditional balance and slackline training are associated with task-specific adaptations as assessed with sensorimotor tests. European Journal of Sport Science. 2017;17(7):838-46.
10. Haas CF, Loik PS, Gay SE. Airway clearance applications in the elderly and in patients with neurologic or neuromuscular compromise. Respiratory Care. 2007;52(10):1362-81.
11. Liu-Ambrose T, Davis JC, Best JR, Dian L, Madden K, Cook W, Hsu CL, et al. Effect of a home-based exercise program on subsequent falls among community-dwelling high-risk older adults after a fall: a randomized clinical trial. JAMA. 2019;321(21):2092-100.

Appendices

Appendix 1:
Geriatric Assessment

■ SUBJECTIVE ASSESMENT

- ❖ Name:
- ❖ Age:
- ❖ Occupation:
- ❖ Address:
- ❖ Dominance:
- ❖ Chief/complaints:
- ❖ HOPI:
- ❖ Past history:
- ❖ Family history:
- ❖ Drug history:
- ❖ Medical history:
- ❖ Surgical history:
- ❖ Personal history: (a) sleep; (b) diet; (c) appetite; (d) bowel/bladder; (e) addictions
- ❖ Socio/economic status:
- ❖ General physical examination: (a) temperature; (b) BP; (c) PR; (d) RR
- ❖ Pallor:
- ❖ Icterus:
- ❖ Clubbing:
- ❖ Cyanosis:
- ❖ Lymphadenopathy:
- ❖ Edema:

MUSCULOSKELETAL EXAMINATION
0/0

Attitude and posture:	
GAIT: (Use Rancho Los Amigos scale) stance, step length, step width, cadence	
Deformity	
Wasting Edema	
Skin changes	
Inspection: Bony prominence: Scar: Skin changes:	
Palpation: Swelling: Tenderness: Spasm: Crepitus: Joint range of motion: RIC: Joint play: Capsular pattern:	

Fall history:	
1. Onset: sudden/gradual/frequency	
2. Circumstances of fall: Environment: location, floor surface, lighting, quality of chair Direction: forward/backward Activity at the time of fall: recent meals Symptoms Comorbid conditions Previous fall history Recent/past medications	
3. Physical evaluation: Vision: acuity, peripheral fields, depth perception Vestibular: head thrust test, dix halpike, Romberg test Somatosensory: proprioception, vibration	
4. Balance: sitting: static/dynamic Standing: static/standing	
5. Coordination test: non-equilibrium test/equilibrium tests	

Screening for gait instability/risk of falls: "Timed get up and go" test Just before the test, open the examination room door and place a marker on the floor ten feet from the patient's chair. To test the patient, give the following instructions: (a) Rise from the chair; (b) Walk to the line on the floor (10 feet); (c) Turn; (d) Return to the chair; (e) sit down again	

Fitness for Activity—Performance-based Measures

Seated step test (SST): The SST is a performance based measure of exercise tolerance, fitness for activity, and endurance. (30) The SST was designed to provide a graded exercise test that is less intense than submaximal and maximal treadmill and bicycle ergometer tests of exercise tolerance. To describe the fitness for ADL of frail older people (e.g., having difficulty in performance of more than one ADL task)

■ HOME ENVIRONMENT EVALUATION

Environmental, Home, and Work (Job/School/Play) Barriers

("Environmental, home, and work barriers" in subsequent tabs)

Environment, home, and work recommendations		
Category	*Areas to be assessed*	*Recommendations*
Entry route	Driveway surfaces	Make smooth, level and well-lit
	Stairs	Adjust height to <7 inch; adjust depth to >11 inch
	Handrail height	Adjust height to 34–38 inch
	Handrail location	Install handrails on both sides
	Ramp grade	1 inch in height is required for every 12 iinch in length If ramp is >30 ft, a platform is required for rest
Entrance	Door clearance	Adjust space beyond swing-out door to 5 × 5 ft and swing-in door to 3 × 5 ft
	Door handles	Adapt door handles depending on patient's hand function
	Door thresholds	Remove, if any
	Door width	Adjust to 32–34 inch
Furniture	Sofas and chairs	Use furniture with height that is even with WC; seating should be firm
Lighting	Room lighting	Make well-lit
	Night lights	Install in hallways and rooms
Halls	Hallway width	Adjust to 36 inch
Smoke and carbon monoxide detectors, fire extinguishers	Smoke detector	Install on each level; one in each sleeping area
	Carbon monoxide detectors	Install on each level; one in each sleeping area; one by any major gas burning appliances
	Fire extinguishers	Install in the kitchen, garage, basement, and sleeping areas
Floors	Floor surfaces	Use nonskid surface
	Small area rugs	Remove, if any
	Large area rug	Secure with carpet tape
Electrical controls	Switches and outlets	Make accessible

Contd...

Contd...

Category	Areas to be assessed	Recommendations
	Types of switch	Adapt switches for patient with limited control
Interior doors	Door handles	Adapt door handles depending on patient's hand function
	Door thresholds	Remove, if any
	Door width	Make at least 32 inch
Driving	Opening and closing door, including locks	Modify for patient with limited hand function
	Driver's seat	Adjust height to ensure easy transfer from WC or scooter
	WC or scooter storage	Ensure sufficient storage space
	Driving ability	Adapt steering, brake, and acceleration systems for patient with limited hand function

School function assessment—measures the performance of students in grades K through 6 in the classroom, bathroom, and playground/recess, as well as during transitions, mealtime, and transportation. It includes the supports and assistance needed.

Source: Available at http://www.proedinc.corn/Scripts/prodList.asp

■ HAND FUNCTION

Strength with dynamometer: Mass grasp: Release:	
Grasp: Spherical Cylindrical Hook	
Grip: Pulp to pulp Tip to tip Three jaw chuck	

■ CARDIORESPIRATORY EVALUATION

- ❖ Breathlessness
- ❖ Chest pain
- ❖ Cough dry/wet
- ❖ Palpitations

Past History

- ❖ Hypertension
- ❖ DM
- ❖ CHD
- ❖ CAD

Past Surgical History

History of Hospitalization
- No. of times
- Duration of each admission
- Investigations
- Diagnosis
- Drugs if any

Family History

Personal History
Environmental history: work and home (pollutants)

O/O:
- Position of trachea
- Dilated veins
- Trails sign
- Use of accessory muscles of breathing

O/P
- Apex beat
- Tracheal position
- Parasternal heave
- Thrills

Investigations: radiographs, ABG reports, RA factor any other relevant

AROUSAL, ATTENTION AND COGNITION

Sl. No.	Test	Result
	Glasgow coma scale	
1.	Galveston orientation and amnesia test	
2.	RLA levels of cognitive function	
3.	MMSE	

Assistive and Adaptive Devices
- Determine the need for an assistive or adaptive devices and equipment for functional activities
- Asses components alignment for and adaptability to care for assistive devices and equipment
- Asses wheel chair mobility tasks: propulsion on level surfaces and ramps, opening doors, completing a wheelie

Neurological Examination

❖ Cranial nerve integrity: check for all 12 nerves
❖ Sensory examination: superficial and deep
❖ Balance static and dynamic: sitting/standing

Depression Scales

The PHQ-9 has increasingly been used to detect and monitor depression symptoms among elder adults. The PHQ-9 provides a reliable and valid measure of depression severity.

Functional status: Functional status of the patient is the ability to perform activities necessary or desirable in daily life. Functional status is directly influenced by health conditions, particularly in the context of an elder's environment and social support network. Changes in functional status (e.g., not being able to bathe independently) should prompt further diagnostic evaluation and intervention. Measurement of functional status can be valuable in monitoring response to treatment and can provide prognostic information that assists in long-term care planning.

Functional Status Questionnaire

The FSQ is a self-report measure of physical, psychological, and social role functions in patients who are ambulatory. The FSQ has been widely used to screen and monitor functional status

■ BIBLIOGRAPHY

1. Jette AM, Davies AR, Cleary PD, et al. The Functional Status Questionnaire: reliability and validity when used in primary care. J Gen Intern Med. 1986;1:143-9.
2. Kroenke K, Spitzer RL, Williams JB. The PHQ-9: validity of a brief depression severity measure. J Gen Intern Med. 2001;16:606.
3. Mehta PJ.
4. Physical rehabilitation, 6th edition, Chapter 4.
5. Smith EL, Gilligan C. Physical activity prescription for the older adult. The Physician and Sports Medicine. 1983;11:91-101.

Appendix 2:
Orthosis Prescription Assessment

■ SUBJECTIVE ASSESSMENT

Demographic Data

Name:　　　　　　　　　　　　　　　Date:
Age:　　　　　　　　　　　　　　　　Sex:
Occupation:　　　　　　　　　　　　Address:
Referring doctor:
Primary diagnosis:

Case History

Chief complaints:

Past Medical History

Date of onset:
Medical history:
Previous medications:
　　　　　Medicine　　　　　　Dosage　　　　　　Frequency
Previous surgeries
　　　　　Surgery name　　　　Date　　　　　　　Complication

■ PREVIOUS DIAGNOSTIC TEST REPORTS

General Medical History

Personal history
Family background:
Hereditary complaint:

Occupational history
Related to present illness:
Occupational hazards for illness:

Social History

❖ Do you live alone and what type of work do you do in and outside of the home?
❖ How has this problem affected your ability to perform your job?
❖ Do you have to climb stairs to get into your house? Reach the bedroom?

Economic History

1. Onset of pain:
   Sudden: Yes/No
   Gradual: Yes/No
   Congenital onset: Yes/No
2. Location of pain:
   Has the pain change in location: Yes/No if yes, where?
   Spread to other areas: Yes/No if yes, where?
   Become more focused: Yes/No if yes, where?
3. Intensity of pain (ask the patient to rate his or her pain on visual analog scale):

■ OBJECTIVE ASSESSMENT

Mental Status

- ❖ Level of consciousness:
- ❖ Orientation to person, place and time:
- ❖ Vital signs: Blood pressure:
   Respiratory rate:
   Pulse rate:
   Temperature:

Observation

- ❖ General posture:
- ❖ Ability to perform status:
- ❖ Changing the position:
- ❖ Ambulate to the examining room:
- ❖ Built of the patient: Ectomorphic/mesomorphic/endomorphic

Inspection

- ❖ **Postural alignment:**
  - Anterior view:
  - Posterior view:
  - Lateral view:
- ❖ **Contour and alignment of bone and joints:**
  - Impression
- ❖ **Size and contour of soft tissue structure:**
  - Soft tissue edema:
  - Joint effusion:
  - Muscle atrophy:
  - Cysts, rheumatoid nodules:
  - Ganglion:
  - Impression:
  - Muscle rupture:
  - Muscle hypertrophy:

❖ **Colour and texture of skin:**
- Cyanosis:
- Pallor:
- Scars:
- Thickening, thinning and hair loss:
- Highly pigmented hairy areas:
- Erythema:
- Yellow skin:
- Open wounds:
- Old scar:

▌PALPATION

❖ **Bony Prominence:**
- Anterior surface:
- Posterior surface:
- Lateral surface:

❖ **Soft tissue structures:**
- Pain:
- Spasm:
- Swelling:
- Nodules:
- Fascia tightness:

- Density and extensibility of soft tissues:
- Impression:
- Tenderness:
- Trigger points:
- Mobility of soft tissue:

❖ **Skin:**
- Warmth:
- Edema:
- Peripheral pulses:

- Extensibility of skin:
- Density:
- Grade:

Anthropometric Measurements

❖ Limb length:
- True length: (Rt)   (Lt)
- Apparent length: (Rt)   (Lt)

❖ Circumference measurement:
Upper arm: (Rt)   (Lt)
- Upper:
- Middle:
- Lower:

Forearm: (Rt)   (Lt)
Midthigh: (Rt)   (Lt)
- Upper:
- Middle:
- Lower:

Calf: (Rt)   (Lt)
Chest:
- Upper:
- Middle:
- Lower:

Examination

- ❖ **Assessment of range of motion:**
- ❖ **Assessment of muscle strength:**
- ❖ **Assessment of muscle length:**
- ❖ **Assessment of Sensation:**
  - Superficial
  - Deep
- ❖ **Assessment of posture:**
- ❖ **Assessment of gait:**
- ❖ **Assessment of functional activity:**
- ❖ **Assessment of environment:**
- ❖ **External devices used:**
- ❖ **Other systems examination:**
  - Nervous system:
  - CVS:
  - Bladder/bowel: retention/constipation/autonomous/autonomic bladder:
  - Respiratory system:
  - Sexual function:
  - Physical diagnosis:
  - Functional diagnosis:
  - **Professional diagnosis:**
  - **Problem list:**
  - **Management:**

Appendix 3: Prosthesis Prescription Assessment

■ SUBJECTIVE ASSESSMENT

Demographic Data

Name:
Age:
Occupation:
Referring doctor:
Primary diagnosis:

Date:
Sex:
Address:

Case History

Chief complaints:

Past Medical History

Date of onset:
Medical history:
Previous medications:

| Medicine | Dosage | Frequency |

Previous surgeries

| Surgery name | Date | Complication |

■ PREVIOUS DIAGNOSTIC TEST REPORTS

General Medical History

Personal history
- Family background:
- Hereditary complaint:

Occupational history
- Related to present illness:
- Occupational hazards for illness:

Social History
- Do you live alone and what type of work do you do in and outside of the home?
- How has this problem affected your ability to perform your job?
- Do you have to climb stairs to get into your house? Reach the bedroom?

Economic History

1. Onset of pain:
   Sudden: Yes/No
   Gradual: Yes/No
   Congenital onset: Yes/No
2. Location of pain:
   Has the pain change in location: Yes/No if yes, where?
   Spread to other areas: Yes/No if yes, where?
   Become more focused: Yes/No if yes, where?
3. Intensity of pain (ask the patient to rate his or her pain on visual analog scale):

■ OBJECTIVE ASSESSMENT

Mental Status

- ❖ Level of consciousness:
- ❖ Orientation to person, place and time:
- ❖ Vital signs: Blood pressure:
  Respiratory rate:
  Pulse rate:
  Temperature:

Observation

- ❖ General posture:
- ❖ Ability to perform status:
- ❖ Changing the position:
- ❖ Ambulate to the examining room:
- ❖ Built of the patient: Ectomorphic/mesomorphic/endomorphic

Inspection

- ❖ **Postural alignment:**
  - Anterior view:
  - Posterior view:
  - Lateral view:
- ❖ **Contour and alignment of bone and joints:**
  - Impression
- ❖ **Size and contour of soft tissue structure:**
  - Soft tissue edema:
  - Joint effusion:
  - Muscle atrophy:
  - Cysts, rheumatoid nodules:
  - Ganglion:
  - Impression:
  - Muscle rupture:
  - Muscle hypertrophy:

❖ Colour and texture of skin:
- Cyanosis:
- Pallor:
- Scars:
- Thickening, thinning and hair loss:
- Highly pigmented hairy areas:
- Erythema:
- Yellow skin:
- Open wounds:
- Old scar:

■ PALPATION

❖ Bony prominence:
- Anterior surface:
- Posterior surface:
- Lateral surface:

❖ Soft tissue structures:
- Pain:
- Spasm:
- Swelling:
- Nodules:
- Fascia tightness:

- Density and extensibility of soft tissues:
- Impression:
- Tenderness:
- Trigger points:
- Mobility of soft tissue:

❖ Skin:
- Warmth:
- Edema:
- Peripheral pulses:

- Extensibility of skin:
- Density:
- Grade:

Anthropometric Measurements

- ❖ Limb length:
  - True length: (Rt)   (Lt)
  - Apparent length: (Rt)   (Lt)
- ❖ Circumference Measurement:
  Upper arm: (Rt)   (Lt)
  - Upper:
  - Middle:
  - Lower:

  Forearm: (Rt)   (Lt)
  Midthigh: (Rt)   (Lt)
  - Upper:
  - Middle:
  - Lower:

  Calf: (Rt)   (Lt)
  Chest:
  - Upper:
  - Middle:
  - Lower:

Examination

- ❖ **Assessment of range of motion:**
- ❖ **Assessment of muscle strength:**
- ❖ **Assessment of muscle length:**
- ❖ **Assessment of Sensation:**
  - Superficial
  - Deep
- ❖ **Assessment of posture:**
- ❖ **Assessment of gait:**
- ❖ **Assessment of functional activity:**
- ❖ **Assessment of environment:**
- ❖ **External devices used:**
- ❖ **Other systems examination:**
  - Nervous system:
  - CVS:
  - Bladder/bowel: retention/constipation/autonomous/autonomic bladder:
  - Respiratory system:
  - Sexual function:
  - Physical diagnosis:
  - Functional diagnosis:
  - **Professional diagnosis:**
  - **Problem list:**
  - **Management:**

■ GERIATRIC DEPRESSION SCALE (LONG FORM)

Patient's name: Date:

Instructions: Choose the best answer for how you felt over the past week.

No.	Question	Answer	Score
1.	Are you basically satisfied with your life?	Yes/No	
2.	Have you dropped many of your activities and interests?	Yes/No	
3.	Do you feel that your life is empty?	Yes/No	
4.	Do you often get bored?	Yes/No	
5.	Are you hopeful about the future?	Yes/No	
6.	Are you bothered by thoughts you cannot get out of your head?	Yes/No	
7.	Are you in good spirits most of the time?	Yes/No	
8.	Are you afraid that something bad is going to happen to you?	Yes/No	
9.	Do you feet happy most of the time?	Yes/No	

Contd...

Appendix 3: Prosthesis Prescription Assessment

Contd...

No.	Question	Answer	Score
10.	Do you often feel helpless?	Yes/No	
11.	Do you often get restless and fidgety?	Yes/No	
12.	Do you prefer to stay at home, rather than going out and doing new things?	Yes/No	
13.	Do you frequently worry about the future?	Yes/No	
14.	Do you feel you have more problems with memory than most?	Yes/No	
15.	Do you think it is wonderful to be alive now?	Yes/No	
16.	Do you often feel downhearted and blue?	Yes/No	
17.	Do you feel pretty worthless the way you are now?	Yes/No	
18.	Do you worry a lot about the past?	Yes/No	
19.	Do you find life very exciting?	Yes/No	
20..	Is it hard for you to get started on new projects?	Yes/No	
21.	Do you feel full of energy?	Yes/No	
22.	Do you feel that your situation is hopeless?	Yes/No	
23.	Do you think that most people are better off than you are?	Yes/No	
24	Do you frequently get upset over little things?	Yes/No	
25.	Do you frequently feel like crying?	Yes/No	
26.	Do you have trouble concentrating?	Yes/No	
27.	Do you enjoy getting up in the morning?	Yes/No	
28.	Do you prefer to avoid social gatherings?	Yes/No	
29.	Is it easy for you to make decisions?	Yes/No	
30.	Is your mind as clear as it used to be?	Yes/No	
Total		**Total**	

This is the original scoring for the scale: One point for each of these answers.
Cutoff: normal—0–9; mild depressives—10–19; severe depressives—20–30.

1. No	6. Yes	11. Yes	16. Yes	21. No	26. Yes
2. Yes	7. No	12. Yes	17. Yes	22. Yes	27. No
3. Yes	8. Yes	13. Yes	18. Yes	23. Yes	28. Yes
4. Yes	9. No	14. Yes	19. No	24. Yes	29. No
5. No	10. Yes	15. No	20. Yes	25. Yes	30. No

Courtesy: Yesavage JA, Brink TL. Rose TL, et al. Development and validation of a geriatric depression screening scale: a preliminary report. J Psychiatr Res. 1983;17:37-49.
CME Outfitters, LLC Available for download at www.neuroscienceCME.com

■ FUNCTIONAL REACH TEST

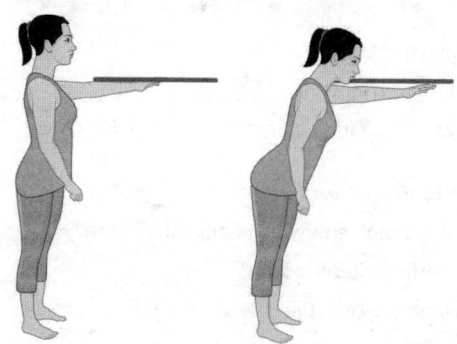

The functional reach test is a single item test developed as a quick screen tor balance problems in older adults.

■ INTERPRETATION

A score of 6 or less indicates a significant increased risk tor talis. A score between 6 and 10 inches indicates a moderate risk for falls.

Age related norms for the functional reach test:

Age	Men (In inches)	Women (in inches)
20–40 years	16.7 ± 1.9	14.6 ± 2.2
41–69 years	14.9 ± 2.2	13.8 ± 2.2
70–87	13.2 ± 1.6	10.5 ± 3.5

Requirements

The patient must be able to stand independently for at least 30 seconds without support and be able to flex the shoulder to at least 90 degrees.

Equipment and Setup

A yard stick is attached to a wall at about shoulder height. The patient is positioned in front of this so that upon flexing the shoulder to 90 degrees, an initial reading on the yard stick can be taken. The practitioner takes a position 5-10 feet away from the patient, viewing the patient from the side.

Instructions

Position the patient close to the wall so that he/she may reach forward along the length of the yardstick. The patient is instructed to stand with feet shoulder distance apart then make a list and raise the arm up so that its parallel to the floor. At this time, the practitioner takes an initial reading on the yard stick, usually spotting the knuckle of the third metacarpal. The patient is instructed to reach forward along the yardstick without moving the feet. Any reaching strategy is allowed, but the hand should remain in a fist. The practitioner takes a reading on the yardstick of the farthest reach attained by the patient without taking a step. The initial reading is subtracted from the final to obtain the functional reach score.

■BILIOGRAPHY

1. Duncan, PW, Weiner DK, Chadler J, Studenske S. Functional reach: A new clinical measure of balance. J Gerontol. 1990;45:M192.
2. Mann GC, et al. Functional reach and single leg stance in patients with peripheral vestibular disorders. J Vestib Res. 1996;6:343.
3. Ouncan PW, et al. Functional reach: Predictive validity in a sample of elderly male veterans. J Gerontol. 1992;47:M93.
4. Weiner DK, et al. Does functional reach improve with rehabilitation. Arch Phys Med Rehab. 1993;74:796.

Appendix 4:
Short Falls Efficacy Scale—International

Below are some questions about how concerned you are about the possibility of falling. Please reply thinking about how you usually do the activity. If you currently do not do the activity (for example, if someone does your shopping for you), please answer to show whether you think you would be concerned about falling if you did the activity. For each of the following activities, please check the box which is closest to your own opinion to show how concerned you are that you might fall if you did this activity.

		None	A little	Medium	A lot
		No concern	Somewhat concerned	Fairly concerned	Very concerned
1.	Getting dressed or undressed	1	2	3	4
2.	Taking a shower or bath	1	2	3	4
3.	Getting in or out of a chair	1	2	3	4
4.	Going up or down stairs	1	2	3	4
5.	Reaching for something above your head or on the ground	1	2	3	4
6.	Walking up or down a slope	1	2	3	4
7.	Going out to a social event (religious service, family gathering, club meeting)	1	2	3	4
	Total				

Courtesy: Kempen GIJM, Yardley L, Haastregt JCM van, Zijlstra GAR. Beyer N, Hauer K, Todd C. Prevention of Falls Network Europe, Falls Efficacy Scale International.

Scoring: Low Concern: 7-8; Moderate Concern: 9-13; High Concern: 14-28.

■ THE MODIFIED FALLS EFFICACY SCALE

	Not confident at all		Fairly confident								Completely confident	
	(0)	(1)	(2)	(3)	(4)	(5)	(6)	(7)	(8)	(9)	(10)	
Items from Tinetti et al[1]												
1. Get dressed and undressed												
2. Prepare a simple meal												
3. Take a bath or shower												
4. Get in/out of a chair												
5. Get in/out of bed												
6. Answer the door or telephone												
7. Walk around the inside of your house												
8. Reach into cabinets or closets												
9. Light house keeping												
10. Simple shopping												
Additional items												
11. Using public transportation												
12. Crossing roads												
13. Light gardening or hanging out the wash*												
14. Using front or rear steps at home												

The items on the scale are scored from 0 to 10, with 0 meaning "not confident/not sure at all," 5 being "fairly confident/fairly sure," and 10 being "completely confident/completely sure. Subjects are asked, "How confident/sure are you that you do each of the activities without falling?"

* Rate most commonly performed of these activities

[1]Tinetti M, Richman D, Powell I. Falls efficacy as a measure of fear of falling. J Gerontol. 1990; 45:P239-43.

Courtesy: Hill K, Schwarz J, Kalogeropoulos A, Gibson S. The Modified Falls Efficacy Scale Arch Phys Med Rehabil. Aol 77, October 1996.

Index

Page numbers followed by *f* refer to figure and *t* refer to table.

A

Academic program 81
Accessibility 141, 172, 181, 237
Accessible format 157
Accessible multimedia 137
Accessible toilets 276
Accredited Social Health Activist 103, 173, 175, 196
    workers, roles and responsibilities of 175
Acid attack victims 26, 109
Acknowledging seniors 234
Activity
    documentation of 47
    limitation 158, 265
    theory 225
Adaptive devices 289
Adaptive technology 96, 97
ADIP scheme 113
Administrative setup 226
Adolescent pregnancy 18
Adolescents groups 51
Advanced balance exercises 30
Aerobic endurance training 281
Aerobic exercise 30, 34, 35, 194
    stimulates 282
Aerobic fitness 189
Affective disorders 62
Affirmative action 108
Affordability 172
Aganwadi, grassroots level of 94
Agarbatti maker hand rolling 92
Agencies 180
Aging, theories of 225
Aids and assisted devices 112
Air/fluid/gel pressure relief cushions 253
Alerting systems 278
Ali Yavar Jung National Institute of Speech and Hearing Disabilities 92, 116
All human rights, equal enjoyment of 137
Alma ata declaration 83, 188
Amendments 156
Amputation
    home exercise program for 30
    upper limb levels percentage of 163
Anganwadi worker 173, 174, 196
Ankle toe movements 219*f*
Annual regional conferences 233
Anoxia 165
Anthropometric measurements 293
Anxiety 62
Appoint Maintenance Officers under Section 18 (1) 233
Appropriate technology 96
    assistive devices used for disabled 96
Aquatic exercise 194
Aquatic therapy 281
Architectural barriers, removal of 108
Arm component 159
    combining values for 159
Arm ergometer 34
Arm raise 220*f*
Armrests 249, 250
Arousal, attention and cognition 289
Arthritis 86
Article 41 of constitution 232
Artificial Limbs Manufacturing Corporation 90, 118, 228
Assisted standing transfer 263, 264
Assistive devices 91, 97, 103, 289
Assistive technology 96, 97
Atelectasis, prevents 282
Audible information 276
Audio and visual indicators 136
Authentic texts 157
Autism 115
    spectrum disorder 26
Autoimmune theory 225
Automatic door 276
Autonomous body 89
Auxiliary nurse midwife 173, 175, 178, 196
    functions of 178
Awareness-raising 140

B

Back pain 279
    management of 178
Backrest 250
    fold-down 251
    height 258
    and angle 250
Badhte kadam (awareness and community interaction) 112

Balance exercises 36, 218
Banks and Funding Agencies 21
Barrier free environment 91, 105
Basic balance and coordination exercises 30
Basic infrastructure 88
Basic Minimum Services Program 176
Bathroom 274
    doors 271
Bedroom area 274
Behavior therapy 94
Behavioural disorders 62
Bending forward 245, 246
Bill of Rights 121
Biofeedback in patients 282
Biological theories 225
Birth trauma 165
Blindness 26, 109, 158
Blood disorder 110
Body 158
    composition 190
    measurements 238
Borg's perceived exertion 35
Braille 137, 145
    facilitating learning of 147
Brain
    aging 279
    lesion 29
Breastfeeding 185
Breathing exercises 282
Building, access to 270
Burns, prevent 275

C

Call button 135
Calm and peaceful 267
Cardiorespiratory evaluation 288
Cardiorespiratory fitness exercises 218
Cardiovascular conditioning 34
Cardiovascular disease 280
Cardiovascular exercise 30
Cardiovascular fitness 29, 30
Caregiver stress 221
Caregiver Training Scheme 111
Carrying out activities 249
Cataracts 279
Celebrate successes 46
Cellular theory 225
Central braille press 92
Central Government Health Scheme 180
Central Government Schemes for Disabled Persons 113
Central nervous system 34
Central Public Sector Enterprises Schemes 117
Central Sector Scheme of Integrated Program for Older Persons 227
Cerebral palsy 12, 14, 26, 27, 109, 110, 115, 186
    home exercise program for 27
Certain medications, avoidance of 18

Certificate, contents of 7
Certification, guidelines for 7
Cervical
    intervertebral disc lesions 162
    spine injuries 161
Chair sitting and standing 218
Chest wall 282
Child Labour (Prohibition and Regulation) Act 185
Child Marriage Restriction Act 16
Child-rearing responsibilities 146
Children with special needs 114
Christian Marriage Act 16
Chronic neurological condition, home exercise program for 29
Chronic obstructive pulmonary disease 279
Circulation dimensions 125
Civil society 152
Clear floor space 275
Clinician skills 79
Clock drawing test 221
Cognitive behavior therapy 94
Cognitive impairment 221
    screening for 221
Collect and analyze information 45
Comfort layer 252
Committee dies 153
Committee with other bodies, relationship of 154
Committee's responsibilities 153
Common health issues 279
Communication
    alternative 145
    augmentative 145
    method of two-way 278
    process, develop effective 45
    technologies 139
Community 72
    based rehabilitation 65
    bonding 234
    capacity building 55
    developer 50
        role of 50
    engagement 55
    leaders 51
    members 42, 49
    participation 173
    stakeholders, identify 45
    types of 48
Community development 41, 42, 46, 49, 50
    activities and programs, implementation of 47
    aims 43
    asset-based 49
    characteristics of 43
    components of 44
    concept of 41
    effective approaches to 49
    emphasizes 49
    initiatives 49

literature 50
objectives of 43
possesses 43
practitioners 45
principles of 42
process of 44, 45
programme 42, 44
    types of 48
values of 43
worker, role of 50
Community health centre 178
    role of 179
Community in rehabilitation
    principles and role of 58
    role of 71
Community physiotherapy 75*f*, 76, 79
    evidence-based in 74
    in social context 75*f*
Community-based approach 65
Community-based organization 54
Community-based rehabilitation 13, 22, 41, 53, 64, 65, 83
    advantages of 67*t*
    basic principles of 23
    components of 66
    disadvantages of 67*t*
    multisectoral support of 67
    objectives of 66
    principles of 66
    programme 23
Community-dwelling adults 221
Comorbid physical illness 222
Consistency, seed producers of 92
Constitute Appellate Tribunals under Section 15 (1) 233
Constitute Maintenance Tribunals under Section 7 (1) 233
Constitution of India 101
Consumer Law Applicable to Health Services 183
Continuity theory 225
Contraindications and safety 194, 195
Contributions to society 233
Control panel 135
Controls and operating mechanisms 275
Convention 139
    pursuant to law 139
Convergence 66
Coordinated activities, principles of evaluation of 159
Coordination exercises 36
Counseling and medical rehabilitation 102
Couple therapy 94
Cranial nerves 280
Criminal law and health 182
Criminal procedure, code of 233
Critically appraise evidence 78
Cruising 27
Crutch 123
    user
        space allowance for 130
        space requirement for 130*f*

Cultural rights 181
Cushions, types of 252
Cut out seat bones well 255
Cylindrical grasp 160

D

Daily living
    activities of 36, 221
    instrumental activities of 221
    skills, activities of 23
Deaf 109, 147
    community 147
Deafblind 147
Deendayal Disabled Rehabilitation Scheme 88, 113
Defence medical services 180
Delirium 221
Dementia 221, 234, 279
    old person with 227
Dentist Act 184
Department for Divyangjan 88
Department of Social Justice and Empowerment 229
Dependence 62
Depositary 155
Depression 37, 62, 221, 222, 279
    scales 290
Designating evacuation routes 277
Desktop video magnifier 98
Detection of disability, early identification and intervention for 158
Develop postural control 282
Development, timing stages of 164
Developmental Activities of Society 61
Developmental screening 166
De-worming 86
Diabetes 279
Diabetic foot
    assistive technology in 99
    types of 99
Diagnosis-related group 221
Diary, maintaining 56
Diet and nutrition 190
Diet and physical activity 190*f*
Dietician 63
Disabilities 2, 4, 5, 100
    Act 115
    affects entire family 71
    and health 1, 36
    and law 186
    and physiotherapy rehabilitation 25
    awareness generation, early detection and intervention 88
    basis of 137
    cause of 66
    certificates, issue of 105
    certification 7
    children with 105, 140
    classification of 25

Index

developmental 66
evaluation of 159
extent of 7
families of people with 71
grades of 6
impairment and handicap 4
in social environment, secondary prevention of 18
laws 15
legislation, role of 119
live in poverty
    moderate 101
    severe 101
management and treatment of 19
medical model of 10
models and acts 9
moral models of 9
pensions 68
people with 55, 71, 83
permanence of 7
prevention 13, 17, 19, 60, 66
    and early detection of 12, 108
    and rehabilitation 85
    management and rehabilitation 17
related problems 10
severe 5
social model of 10
types of 5-7, 26, 158
Disabled at secondary stage 115
Disabled people
    movement 100
    organisations 68
    rehabilitation of 19
Disabled person 102
Disengagement theory 225
DISHA scheme 111
Disposable paper, delivery of items for 92
District Disability Rehabilitation Centres 87, 88, 90, 103, 116
District Management Team 88, 116
District rehabilitation center, role of 83
Divyangjan Adhikaar Kanoon 26
Divyangjan Swavalamban Yojna 117
Door 129, 134
    double-leaf 271
    handles 271
    hardware 271
Down steps with assistance 243
Down syndrome 27
Drinking water 276
Drugs and Cosmetics Act 183
Drugs and magic remedies 183
Dwarfism 26, 109
Dyslexic students 11

■ E

Early detection
    and intervention 102
    program 164

Early intervention 165
    service approach 167
    strategy 166
Early intervention program 165
    activities of 168
Eat well and drink lots of water 246
Economic conditions 68
Economy 237
Education 60
    and training opportunities, provision of 66
    law 16
    phase 51
Educational loan 118
Educational opportunities, denial of 119
Educational program 81
Educational rehabilitation 64
Educational sector, support from 69
Educational support 112
Effective evidence-based practice, strategies for 79
Effective Home Exercise Program 37
Electrical points, controls and outlets 275
Electrical stimulation 281
Embossed lettering, signs with 276
Embracing health technologies 37
Emergency evacuation 277
    and plans 277
Emergency room visits 221
Emergency services 141
Emotional and psychological care 18
Emotional health problems 266
Emotional problems 268
Emphasising ability 70
Emphysema 6
Employee State Insurance 180
    Act 184
Employment 12
    agencies 21
    and labor sector, support from 69
    in government establishments 104
Empowerment 67
    phase 51
Endurance 189
Energy
    and emotions 266
    lot of 267
Enhanced motor function 283
Environment and health 183
Environment Protection Laws 183
Environmental barriers 37
Environmental issues 43
Epidemic Diseases Act 184
Equal opportunities 5, 7, 186
    and protection of rights 114
Equal protection and equal benefit of law 139
Equal recognition before law 142
Equality and non-discrimination 139
Equality of opportunity 138

Equipment 90
    and setup 300
Equitable distribution 173
Essential drugs, provision of 173
Evaluation of permanent physical impairment in lower extremity, guidelines for 159, 160
Evidence-based community physiotherapy, steps in 76
Evidence-based health care 74
Evidence-based physiotherapy 74
    in community physiotherapy, methodology for 81
Evidence-based practice 74, 76
    in community, methodology for 81f
    seven steps of 78f
    steps of 76f
Evil behaviour, punishment for 9
Exercise 192
    duration 191
    frequency 191
    intensity 191
    prescription and program 191
    simple 28f
Exposure and response prevention therapy 94
Extremity, combining values for 160

F

Factories Act 184
Falls Prevention Programs 86
Family 63, 94
    and kinship 234
    law 16
Feasibility 172
Feeding bottles 185
Feel tired 268
Feel worn out 267
Female health worker 175
Feminiaation of aging 225
Firm stable base 252
First referral units 179
Fitness 189, 196
    applications, thousands of 38
    components of 189
    encouraging cardiovascular fitness 29
    exercises for geriatrics, types of 194
    for activity 287
    training, principles of 189
Flexibility 34, 189
Floor 271
    comfortably 238
Floor to wheelchair transfers using
    backward approach 39f
    frontward approach 39f
    sideways approach 40f
Flotation cushions 253
Foam pressure relief cushions 252
Food laws and health measures 186
Food Safety and Standards Act 186
Foot propelling 259

Footrests 250
    height 250, 258
Frame Rules under Section 32 233
Free radical theory 225
Freedom from
    exploitation 143
    expression and opinion 145
    torture or cruel 143
Friction 245
    avoid 246
Front castor
    barrels 251
    wheels 251
Functional independence 60
Functional reach test 300
Functional skills 237
Functional status 290
    questionnaire 290
Fundamental freedoms 137, 140, 146
Funding and ordering 240
Furniture 273

G

Gait 280
Gait instability 223
    evaluating patients with 222
    screening for 223
Gait training 27
    exercises 30
Gel-pack cushions 253
Gene mutation theory 225
General health 268
General tertiary education 147
Genetic counselling 18
Genuine participation 43
Geriatric assessment 285
Geriatric depression scale 298
Geriatric functional assessment 221
Geriatric health 86
Geriatric homed-based rehabilitation 35
Geriatric population, neurologic examination in 280
Geriatric syndromes 279
Gharaunda 111
Glass doors 271
Glossopharyngeal breathing 282
Glottis 282
Good practice in fitting 258
Government Concessions for Disabled 119
Grab bar 131, 131f, 133, 273, 276
Grievance redressal 109
Ground fault circuit interrupter 275
Grower with mushrooms 92
Growth chart monitoring 174
Guide 50
    problem-solving 45
Guilt, feelings of 9

H

Habilitation and rehabilitation 148
Hamstrings 29
   and iliotibial band 28
Hand component 159
   combining values of 160
Hand function 288
Hand stretch by dumbbells 30
Handicap 4
Handles 129
Handrail 131, 133*f*, 272, 276
   for extension 131*f*
   for ramps 132*f*
   for steps 131*f*
   standards 132
Hand-written notes 56
Happy person 268
Head injury 165
Health 147
   and disability, framework for 1
   and quality of life 236
   biomedical model of 9
   education 174
   guides, duties assigned to 174
   insurance 180, 231
   law 15
   personnel, role of 187
   professionals 147
   promotion, and disease prevention 190*f*
   sector, support from 68
   services 147
   workers 85
Health care 172
   and fitness 171
   characteristics of 172
   levels of 173
   secondary 178
Health fitness for
   geriatric, strategies of 194
   women and geriatric, strategies of 192
   women, strategies of 192
Health system 172, 178
   components of 172
Healthy weight, maintain 192
Hearing
   deaf and hard of 6
   hard of 109
   impairment 6, 26, 109, 115, 158
   loss 279
Heart pumping 30
Heating units 275
Heel raise 218*f*
Heights and widths 129
Hemophilia 26, 110

Hindu Marriage Act 16
Hip
   abduction 30
   adduction 30
   bones 253
   flexor 29
   raise, standing 218
   thrust 30
Home and family, respect for 145
Home automation 98
Home environment evaluation 287
Home Exercise Program 23, 25, 26, 36, 56
   adherence to 36
   barriers for 37
Home-based physical activity for individuals with disability, benefits of 36
Home-based Rehabilitation Program 23
Homeopathy Central Council Act 184
Hook grasp 160
Hormone 280
Hospitals 180
Human diversity 146
Humanitarian emergency, situations of risk and 141
Hydrotherapy 29
Hypothyroidism 19
   effects of 19

I

Ideal Home Exercise Program 26
Iliotibial band muscles 29
Immunization 85, 174
Impairment 4, 158
Implement plan 45
Implementation phase 51
Implementing agency, identification of 88
Income tax relief for handicapped 119
Independent transfer through sitting 262
India's Rehabilitation Council Act 186
Indian Constitution Limits Discrimination 15
Indian Medical Council Act 184
Indian Medicine Central Council Act 184
Indian Nursing Council Act 184
Indian Penal Code 183
   and Code of Criminal Procedure 182
Indian Sign Language in Audiovisual and Social Media 94
Indian Sign Language Research and Training Center 94, 116
Indian Society 226
Indira Gandhi National Disability Pension Scheme 114
Indira Gandhi National Old Age Pension Scheme 228
Individual level barrier 37
Infant foods (regulation of production) 185
Infant milk substitutes 185
   distribution of 185
Infant, safety measures for 18
Infectious diseases, complication of 165

Informal apprenticeships 69
Information, access to 145
Infrared devices 276
Initiating community development, steps for 46
Injury, level and completeness of 237
Inquiry, cultivate spirit of 77
Insecurity, feeling of 62
Inspection 286, 292
Institutional rehabilitation 64
    programs 54
    strategies 53
Institution-based rehabilitation
    advantages of 65*t*
    disadvantages of 65*t*
Insurance Schemes Launched by National Trust 88
Integrated Education for Disabled Children 12
    Scheme 103
Integrated Program for Older Persons 227
Integrated therapy 283
    long-term care setting for 283
Integrated treatment, health advantages of 283
Intellectual disability 6, 26, 66, 109
Intellectual impairment 100
Intellectual retardation 7
Interdisciplinary approach 167
Internal physiological deterioration 225
International Classification of Functioning 1
    disability and health 1
International Day for Older Persons 229
International Human Rights Instruments 120
International Human Rights Law 141
International Humanitarian Law 141
International instruments 120
International Law 139, 150
    role of 120
International Legal Framework 120
International Legislations for People with Disability 119
International Plan on Aging 232
Interpreting international standards 120
Intervertebral disc lesion 162

J

Job identification 13
Justice, access to 142
Juvenile Justice (Care and Protection) Act 186

K

Keep calm and hydrate 192
Kerb ramps 272
Kitchen 273
Knee
    clearance 125*f*
    raise, standing 30
    rotations 30
Kothari commission 12

L

Labour and Industrial Law Legislations 184
Labour law 16
Labour sectors promote vocational training 69
Language interpretation 94
Lap height 124
Late-life suicide 222
Law for Universal Health Coverage 182
Learning disabilities 6
Learning technique 282
Legal backings 232
Legal duties 110
Legal rights and benefits related to health 180
Legislations 233
    for Conduct of Medical Profession 184
Leprosy 7
    cured 115
        person 26, 109, 114
Lesions, and stroke 279
Liberty and security of person 142
Life and property, protection of 231
Life insurance company 119
Lift 134, 276
    accessories, placement of 134*f*
    control panel, controls layout of 136*f*
    size of 134, 135*f*
    specifications of 136*f*
Living alone 222
Living and social protection, adequate standard of 149
Living facilities, assisted 234
Local dais 174
Locomotor
    disability 6, 12, 26, 109, 115, 158-160
    evaluation of 7
Logical considerations 79
Loneliness 62
Low energy expenditure deconditioning syndrome,
    disabilities with 36
Low vision 26, 109, 115, 158
Lower extremity stretches 34
Lower limb
    amputation of 59
        level of 164
    functional exercises 30
    levels percentage of amputations 164
    muscular strengthening exercises 30
    stretching exercises 30
Lumbar and lumbosacral spine fracture 162

M

Madrid international plan 232
Maintenance and Welfare of Parents and Senior Citizens
    Act 233
Male gender 222
Male health worker 175

Mass media, encouraging 145
Maternity Benefit Act 184
Mechanical coughing 282
Media, support from 70
Medical care, provision of 176
Medical complications 237
Medical doctors, type of 63
Medical ethics, principles of 187
Medical laws 183
Medical model 100
Medical rehabilitation 60, 61
Medical technology, advancement of 99
Medical Termination of Pregnancy Act 185
Medicinal plants, cultivator of 92
Medicine, indigenous system of 180
Meeting wheelchair user's needs 247
Mental abilities 83
Mental behavior 109
Mental health 84, 87
    Act 14, 186
    and Illness 66, 94
Mental illness 6, 26, 109, 115, 158
Mental retardation 110, 115, 158, 186
Mental Retardation and Multiple Disabilties Act 14
Mental status 280
Metabolic equivalent threshold 218
Micronutrient management 85
Millennium development goals 236
Mind 158
Mines Act 184
Minimum Needs Program 176
Min-mental state examination score 221
Misuse, regulation and prevention of 185
Mobile camps 117
Mobile devices, use of 37
Mobility 59, 60, 160
Mobility component 160
    combining values for 161
Mobilize community 175
Modified falls efficacy scale 303
Moisture, avoid 246
Mortality and morbidity statistics 3
Mother and child, postnatal care of 108
Motivational enhancement therapy 94
Motorized tricycles 113
Movement and nationality, liberty of 144
Multidisciplinary approach 167
Multiple disabilities 6, 26, 110, 186
    Act 110
Multiple sclerosis 6, 26, 110
Multi-rehabilitation workers 84
Multi-sectoral coordination 83
Muscle
    endurance 34
    expiratory 282
    inspiratory 282
    principles of evaluation of strength of 159, 160

strength
    maintain 280
    principle of evaluation of 160
strengthening 29, 34
sufferers 282
tightening of 29
Muscular dystrophy 26, 109
    home exercise program for 28
Musculoskeletal examination 286
Musculoskeletal patients 37
Musculoskeletal system 281
Museums 150

N

Narcotic Drugs and Psychotropic Substances Act 184
National Awards 229
National Awards for Empowerment of Persons with Disabilities 118
    scheme of 118
National Awards for Senior Citizens, scheme of 229
National Cancer Institute 59
National Council for Senior Citizens 229
National Handicapped Finance and Development Corporation 104, 117, 118
National Healthcare Delivery System 171
National Implementation and Monitoring 151
National Institute for Empowerment of Persons with Intellectual Disabilities 93, 116
National Institute for Locomotor Disabilities 94, 116
National Institute of Mental Health and Rehabilitation 94
National Institutes and Composite Regional Centre 115
National Institutes for Capacity Building 90
National Institutes for Rehabilitation 84
National institutes, role of 83
National Institutions for Protection 152
National Iodine Deficiency Disorder Control Programme 102
National Legislation 120
National Leprosy Eradication Programme 85, 102
National Mental Health Programme 85
National Policy for Older Persons 229
National Policy for Persons with Disabilities 102
National Policy on Older Persons 230
National Policy on Senior Citizen 234
National Program for Health Care for Elderly 85, 230
National Programme for Control of Blindness 85, 102
National Programme for Prevention and Control of
    Cancer, Diabetes, CVD and Stroke 85
    Deafness 85, 102
    Fluorosis 102
National Programme on Orientation of Medical Officers Working in Primary Health Centers for Disability Management 85
National Rural Health Mission 103, 175
National Skill Development Corporation 104
National Social Assistance Programme 228
National Trust 186

Index

National Trust for Welfare of Persons with Autism 14, 110
Nationality Arbitrarily 144
Neck exercise 27
Neck pain 279
Neck rotation 219f
Neighborhood bonding 234
Nervous person 267
Nervous system 159
Neurological conditions, chronic 26
Neurological examination 290
Neuromotor exercise 189
Neuromuscular dysfunction 279, 280
Neuromuscular systems functional 281
Neuroplasticity 34
Neurosurgeon 20
Newborn 165
Non-communicable diseases 86
Non-formal pre-school education 174
Non-governmental organizations 21, 72, 227
   and local community, support from 68
   promotion of 106
   variety of 68
Non-governmental sector 68
Nonviolent direct action 55
Notice boards 276
Nursery workers 92
Nursing mothers 174
Nutrition 18, 192

O

Obesity 36
Object detection by visually impaired 130f
Objectionable advertisements 183
Occupational Health Laws 184
Occupational therapist 63
Occupational therapy 93, 102
Offices and factories, modifications of 13
Old age
   homes, maintenance of 227
   problems with 226
Older people, general exercises for 218
Older persons, volunteers bureau for 228
Organic producers 92
Organs, encouraging all 140
Orthopedic surgeon 20
Orthosis 34
   prescription assessment 291
Orthotics 93
Orthotist 63
Osteoarthritis 279
Osteoporosis Education and Management Programs 178
Overhead shoulder stretch 34

P

Pain 37
   management 178
      assessment of 178

Palliative care 178
Palpation 286, 293
Pamphlet 56
Panchayati Raj Institutions 227
Paraplegia 34
Parking 278
Parkinson's disease 26, 35, 110, 283
   home exercise program for 35
   society 35
Participation in cultural life, recreation, leisure and sport 150
Participation restrictions 158
Passive circulatory techniques, utilization of 80
Pension scheme 230
People with disabilities
   and elderly individuals, environment modifications for 270
   rehabilitation of 84
Permanent physical impairment
   and disability certification 5
   guidelines for 6
Person, protecting integrity of 143
Personal mobility 144
Personality
   disorders 62
   premorbid 61
Persons with disabilities (Divyangjan) 100, 123, 144, 186, 236
   accessibility for 123
   economic rehabilitation of 104
   education for 103
   empowerment of 115
   in rural areas 88
   provisions for 101
   rehabilitation and empowerment of 94
Persons with Disabilities Act 11, 85, 103, 107
   scheme for implementation of 88, 113
Persons, category of 119
Pharmacy Act 184
Phenylketonuria 19
Physical activity 36
   guidelines 194
Physical attributes 237
Physical disability 109
Physical health 268
Physical medicine and rehabilitation 93
Physical rehabilitation
   measures 102
   strategies 102
Physiotherapist 63
   in community development, role of 51
   in primary health care, role of 177
   role of 21, 57f, 170
Physiotherapy 93, 102
   at subcentres, role of 176
   in primary health care, role of 86
   role of 86t
   services 177

Picot format, clinical questions in 77
Pillow, kneeling on 32f
Placing disability issues 66
Plan and prepare activity 47
Plantation Labour Act 185
Plastic surgeon 20
Play and drama therapist 21
Plus clock draw test 221
Plyometrics 195
Policy and Programs for Welfare 226
Policy formulation and implementation 106
Political and public life, participation in 149
Political empowerment 65
Polygamy, case of 16
Population requiring early intervention, nature of 166
Postmenopausal women's health 87
Postnatal exercises 194
Post-stroke recovery 30
Posture, check 259
Poverty reduction strategies 236
Power conflict approach 49
Practicing community physiotherapist 76
Pradhan Mantri Vaya Vandana Yojana 228
Pregnant and lactating mother, care of 17
Pregnant and postnatal women, fitness exercise for 193
Pregnant mother and newborn, immunization for 18
Pregnant women 174
Prepare time and cost estimates 47
Prerna 112
Pressure 245
    check 259
Pressure relief cushion 245, 252
    base 255
    shaping on 253
Pressure relief techniques 245
    use 245
Pressure sore 245
    causes 245
    prevention 245, 261
    stages of 247
Prevention of Food Adulteration Act 186
Primary health care 68, 173
    elements of 173
    principles of 65, 173
Primary health centre 108, 173, 176, 196
    functions of 84
    manpower 177
    role of 83, 84, 176
    types of 176
Primary level health care
    centres 84, 175
    schemes 174
Prioritize issues and problems 46
Prisoners, treatment of 187
Privacy, respect for 145
Private entities, urging 145
Private sector (business and industry) 72
    wage employment in 104
Product preparation 240

Professional associations, highly visible role for 80
Program planning and task completion 45
Program, managers of 68
Prohibit discrimination 139, 147
Promote Voluntary Action for Persons with Disabilities, scheme to 88, 113
Promoting Awareness-training Programmes 140
Promoting self-care 59
Proper fit and postural support 250
Prosthesis 98
    prescription assessment 295
Prosthetic rehabilitation program exercises 33f
Protection and Security for Children with Disabilities 105
Proximal joint of stump 32
Psychiatrist 20
Psychological symptoms 37
Psychosocial rehabilitation 61
Psychosocial theories 225
Psychotherapy treatment 94
Pt. Deendayal Upadhyaya National Institute for Person with Physical Disabilities 93, 116
Public health 171
    sector 180
Pulse-Polio Programme 102
Pyramid for quality of evidence 77f

R

Railway employees, health care of 180
Ramps 272
    large 272
Range of motion
    exercise 281
        active and passive 28f
    of joints, principles of evaluation of 159
Range of movement, principles of evaluation of 160
Rashtriya Madhyamik Shiksha Abhiyan 115
Rashtriya Vayoshri Yojana 228
Rational emotive therapy 94
Rear wheels 251
    position 259
Re-conception and pre-natal diagnostic techniques 185
Recycle planning and implementation processes 48
Red Cross Society 89
Referral beneficiaries 174
Reflexes 280
Refuge area 278
Regional geriatrics centres 230
Regional integration organization 155
Regular information on persons with disabilities, collection of 106
Regular stretches 28
Rehabilitation 19, 59
    approaches to 64
    assistance, shortage of 65
    common goals of 60t
    cycle 59f
    goals of 59
    institution-based 22, 53, 64, 83

methods, types of 83
model 10
nurse 63
objectives of 60
outreach program for 70
outreach-based 83
principles of 70
process of 61
professionals, development of 103
programs 19
services, provision of 66
team 20, 21, 62, 62*f*
types of 60, 62, 62*t*
worker 167
Rehabilitation Council 89
    Act 14, 112
Report of committee 154
Research 107
    and manpower development 13, 109
    methods 79
Reservations 156
Resistance exercises 35
Resistance training 281
Resource Management and Administration of Environment Laws 183
Resource mapping 47
Respiratory capacity, increase 282
Respiratory endurance and strengthening 35
Respite care 111
Retardation and Multiple Disability Act 110
Right to Education 16
Right to Health 182
    core components of 181
Rights and full participation, protection of 5, 186
Rights for person with disability 137
    Act 13, 109
Rights of child, convention on 187
Rights of disabled persons, declaration on 188
Rights of mentally retarded persons, declaration on 187
Rights of Persons with Disabilities, committee on 152
Rights to wheelchairs 235
Rise from chair 223
Robotic wheelchair, low-cost 97
Rural communities 48, 100
Rural Rehabilitation Extension Centers 117

■ S

Safe 182
    water supply and basic sanitation 173
Sarva Shiksha Abhiyan 103, 114
Schemes and Legislations for Person with Disabilities 100
Scholarship schemes of department 89
Screening test 221
Search best evidence 77
Seat 250
    bones 253
        well dimensions 255
    height 124, 259

Sector Skill Council for Persons with Disabilities 104
Self care 60
Self-advocacy 67
Self-determination 43
Self-employment 104
Self-help 42
Self-neck stretching 219*f*
Self-responsibility 42
Semi-autonomous body 89
Semi-urban and urban 235
Sensation 280
    principles of evaluation of 160
Sensory impairment 100
Service provision 169
Sharpened hacksaw blade 255
Shifting services 23
Short-wheelbase 249
Shoulder
    openers 30
    stretching exercises, assisted 34
Sickle cell disease 26, 110
Side to side leaning 245, 246
Sign language
    facilitating learning of 147
    use of 145
Signages 276
Signs with braille 276
Single leg stand 218
Sit to stand 220*f*
Sit upright 245
Sitting balance 27
Skill development
    and employment 108
    composite regional centre for 94, 115
Skill training workshops 117
Skin every day, check 246
Sleep
    and stress management 190
    in prone lying 32
    influence of 190
    solves everything 193
Slice out seat bones 256
Slip-resistant 271
Slung seat cushion 257
Small Industries Development Bank 104
Social activities 266, 268
Social and cultural rights 187
Social barriers 37
Social capital formation 55
Social justice 15
Social life, aspects of 10
Social model 100
Social participation 60
Social rehabilitation 61
Social sector, support from 68
Social security 13, 106, 109
Social worker 21
Soft tissue structures 293

Software applications 37
Solid seat 250
Special education and rehabilitation psychology 92
Special Recreational Centers 13
Specific leaning disabilities 26
Speech and language
    disability 6, 26, 109
    pathologist 63, 105
Speech impairment 7
Spherical grasp 160
Spinal cord injury disability, home exercise program for 34
Spine, disabilities evaluation of 161
Sports, recreation and cultural life 107
Stability component 160, 161
Standard armchair 223
Standards and guidelines, development of 139
Standing balance 27
    exercises 32f
State government, role of 90
States parties 147, 151, 153, 155, 156
    and committee, cooperation between 154
    conference of 155, 156
    obligations 151
    reaffirm 141
    recognize 140, 146
Statistics and data collection 151
Strengthening exercise 195
Strengthening muscles, resistance exercises for 30
Stress
    getting relaxed from 193
    influence of 190
Stretches, regular passive 29
Stretching 27, 34
    exercises 36, 195
    frequency of 281
Stroke 29
    home exercise program for 29
    survivors 30
Sub-centre, role of 175
Sudden collapse 253
Sugamya Bharat Abhiyan 115
Suicidal tendencies 62
Supplementary nutrition 174
Support circle, strengthening of 192
Surgical scars, taking care of 17
Sustainable development goals 84
Swami Vivekanand National Institute of Rehabilitation Training and Research 93, 116
Swimming 29

T

Tactile communication 137
Tai chi 195
Tandem standing 218
Tandem walking 218
Task-oriented therapy 282

Task-specific
    therapy 282
    training 282
Tax benefits 231
Team members role 63
Technical assistant 50
Tendo-Achilles 28, 29
Territorial constituency 102
Tertiary health care 179
Tetraplegia 34
Thalassemia 26, 110
Therapeutic recreational therapist 63
Thoracic and thoracolumbar spine injuries 162
Threat and beliefs 37
Toe
    loss of 164
    raise 218f
Toilet doors 277
Torture and other cruel, convention against 187
Torture convention 187
Traditional birth attendants 85
Traffic in persons, convention for suppression of 187
Training disabled in community 20
Transdisciplinary approach 167
Transfemoral residual limb bandaging 31f
Transfer 247, 262
    Board 264, 265
    devices 98
    of property, revocation of 233
Transplantation of Human Organs Act 184
Transportation 237
Transtibial exercises 32f
Transtibial residual limb bandaging 31f
Treatment maneuvers ranging, strategy of 25
Trunk bends 30
Trunk extensor muscles 282
Turning radius and clear floor space 125f
Typical handrail extensions 132f

U

Unfamiliar terminology 11
Unique disability identity
    card 88
    project 105
United Nations Organs 154
Universal design 138
Universal health care system, part of 58
Universal health coverage 84, 180
Universal Immunisation Programme 102
Upper body stretches 34
Upper limb
    amputation, level of 163
    bilateral 32
    functional exercises 30
    muscular strengthening exercises 30
    strengthening of 32
    stretching exercises 30

Urban communities 48
Urine incontinence 279
User training 241

V

Validity period 7
Varishtha Pension Bima Yojana 228
Vayoshreshtha Samman 229
Vikaas (day care) 111
Village health guide 85, 173, 196
    scheme 174
Village level workers 42
Violence and abuse 143
Vishesh Microfinance Yojana 118
Vision
    field of 129f
    zone 128, 129f
Visual contrast 276
Visual disability 92
Visual impairment 6, 109
Vital role 23
Vitamin
    A 85
    lack of 165
Vocational counselor 21
Vocational rehabilitation 61, 64
    centers 64, 116
    specialist 63
    system 10
Vocational training 89
    centres 70
    facilities 12
Voice announcement system 276
Voice instructions 278
Voluntary health agencies 180

W

Walkers 98, 123
Warm-up
    exercises 35
    period 191
Washroom accessories 277
Water-resistant cushion cover 253
Wear and tear theory 225
Wearable technology 98
Wearing orthoses 29
Welfare approach 49
Welfare of persons with
    autism 186
    disabilities 12
Welfare of senior citizens 230
Wheelchair 97, 113, 123, 236, 276
    accessibility of 124
    affect selection of 237
    appropriate 247

    benefit of 236
    castor width 124
    fitting 257
    fold 124
        cross-folding 251
    folding 248
    footrest 124
    foundation components of prescriptive 38f
    frame length 249
    getting in and out of 247, 262
    handling 261
    long-wheelbase 249
    management 235
    manual 124
    measurements 237
    need for 235
    parts of 239
    pushing 248
    ready 258
    safe 251
    services 239
    specifications 250
    standard dimensions 124f
    transfer techniques 38
    whole 251
Wheelchair mobility 261
    skills 242
        training safe 245
Wheelchair to bed 263
    by placing legs on bed 263
Wheelchair user 124, 235, 262
    area 125
    range of reach of 126f
    training checklist 261
    weight 253
White cane user 130
Windows 129
Women and Health Laws 185
Women self-help group 55
Women with disabilities 105, 140
Women's health 87
Work 60
    and employment 148
Workmen's Compensation Act 185
World Confederation for Physical Therapy 74, 75
World Health Organization, constitution of 180, 188
World Programme of Action Concerning Disabled Persons 120
Wrist curls by weight 30

Y

Young working-age persons, migration of 226

Z

Zero rejection policy for education 114